SHORT-TERM PSYCHIATRIC
HOSPITALIZATION OF ADOLESCENTS

Short-Term Psychiatric Hospitalization of Adolescents

Aman U. Khan, M.D.
Department of Psychiatry
Southern Illinois University School
of Medicine
Springfield, Illinois

YEAR BOOK MEDICAL PUBLISHERS, INC.
Chicago • London • Boca Raton • Littleton, Mass.

1 2 3 4 5 6 7 8 9 0 YR 94 93 92 91 90

Library of Congress Cataloging-in-Publication Data
Khan, Aman U.
  Short-term psychiatric hospitalization of adolescents / Aman U. Khan
  p. cm.
    Includes bibliographical references.
    ISBN 0-8151-5126-8
    1. Psychiatric hospital care. 2. Adolescent psychiatry.
  I. Title.
  [DNLM: 1. Hospitalization. 2. Mental Disorders—in adolescence.   WS 463 K45s]
  RJ504.5.K43 1990   89-22622
  362.2'1'0835—dc20   CIP
  DNLM/DLC
  for Library of Congress

Sponsoring Editor: Richard Wallace
Associate Managing Editor, Manuscript Services: Deborah Thorp
Production Project Coordinator: Carol A. Reynolds
Proofroom Supervisor: Barbara M. Kelly

PREFACE

Delivery of psychiatric care to adolescents has changed drastically during the 1980s. The escalating cost, resistance on the part of third-party payers to reimburse these costs, development of prepaid health maintenance organizations (HMOs), and impending threats of intrusion of DRGs in psychiatry have forced adolescent psychiatry to utilize different models to provide short-term psychiatric care. Long-term care models to bring about conflict resolution and characterological changes have largely been replaced by short-term care models focusing on crisis resolution and treatment of acute symptoms, leaving subacute and chronic care of emotional problems to community agencies.

The number of acute adolescent psychiatric units has mushroomed in the late 1970s and 1980s to fill the gap left by closing and shrinking of a large number of residential treatment facilities. Most patients hospitalized in acute care units are discharged after a few weeks of treatment. However, pressure on psychiatry continues unabated by third-party payers and HMOs to further reduce the duration of in-hospital treatment. This attitude is deeply ingrained in misconceptions about the psychopathology of mental illness. It may be possible to discharge a chronic schizophrenic after two weeks if he was hospitalized in a state of acute exacerbation because he had stopped taking his medication. However, most mental disorders do not respond in a predictable fashion. A patient with major depression may not respond to antidepressants and continue to be a suicidal risk for several weeks. The situation is further complicated with children and adolescents. The younger the child, the more dependent he is on his immediate environment, and his psychopathology is influenced more by the factors in his family, school, and community, and in relationships with peers. Most of these factors relating to the child's environment are not specific to any type of psychopathology, as they may have different psychological meanings and exert different amounts of influence in creating a problem. Diagnostic evaluation would thus include not only the determination of multiple etiological factors, but the weight of each factor contributing to a specific psychopathology. Discharge of an adolescent from the hospital may be delayed because his family continues to interpret his behavior as manipulative. Similarly, a runaway adolescent may stay in the hospital longer for her own protection because she refused to compromise with her family on house rules and finds an easier escape in running away.

Psychiatric diagnoses rarely specify treatment. The choice of a treatment modality depends upon the outcome of treatment desired. For example, the therapeutic goal of a conflict resolution and characterological change would certainly require long-term treatment, whereas a therapeutic objective of crisis resolution may indicate short-term intervention. Chapter 8 describes several working models for short-term hospital care. According to these models, the sole criteria for psychiatric hospitalization of an adolescent is the inability of the available community mental health resources to sustain the adolescent in the community. These models also emphasize the need for determination of a clear focus for hospital treatment in order to return the patient back to his community.

Actual therapeutic work with the hospitalized adolescent and his environment (family, community, school) is focused on helping them understand the factors that contributed to the hospitalization and helping to initiate the steps to modify those factors to avoid recurrence of admissions. Of course, a great deal of initial time is spent in working with the resistance of the patient and his family before they are able to understand and accept the rationality of the therapeutic approach. It may be emphasized that the short-term treatment models view hospitalization as the last resort in the treatment of acute crisis. The hospitalization may also be used for diagnostic evaluation and initiation of therapy. Most of the therapeutic work, however, should be carried out in the patient's natural environment. A strict adherence to short-term models would necessitate the development of appropriate community resources to provide multiple modalities of therapeutic services. This book focuses on the application of short-term models in therapeutic work with hospitalized adolescents.

Aman U. Khan, M.D.

CONTENTS

1 | Hospital Treatment for Emotionally Disturbed Adolescents

Hospital treatment of emotionally disturbed adolescents may be conceptualized in terms of the following phases:

1. Crisis phase.
2. Evaluation phase.
3. Treatment phase.
4. Discharge planning.

CRISIS PHASE

Crisis intervention starts with a telephone call from a family, a physician, or a community agency. Many admissions to the hospital may be avoided if the receiver of the call is experienced in dealing with an acute crisis and knowledgeable about community mental health resources. The crisis frequently reflects a recent intensification of an ongoing problem between the adolescent and his family. It also indicates that the family's tolerance limit for their disturbed adolescent has been reached and that the family can endure him no more. Other factors that may precipitate and/or exacerbate the crisis include sickness in the family, loss of a job, and strained spouse relationships. There is a great deal of anxiety and confusion in the family at this time. These families may have never worked together in dealing with a difficult problem. Different members of the family may have different opinions about the nature of the problem and the best methods to deal with it. It is not uncommon for some parents to take extreme measures such as asking the adolescent to leave home or requesting the local police to intervene. Similarly, psychiatric hospitalization is frequently presented as a threat rather than as a helpful and appropriate form of treatment. The crisis is generally experienced and expressed more by the parents than the adolescent. The highly developed capacity of adolescents to deny and project may be partly responsible for their apparently calm demeanor. There are, however, some adolescents who protest loudly and aggressively. They may threaten their familes with violence and promise to take revenge. Most hospitalized adolescents tend to blame their families for their difficulties and rarely acknowledge their contribution to the creation of the crisis. Consequently, any help initially offered to them is rejected. It is a rare occasion when an adolescent requests his own hospitalization. Even after serious suicidal attempts or aggressive acts, most adolescents refuse help.

Thus, the decision to hospitalize the disturbed adolescent must usually be made by the parents. Most parents, however, are very ambivalent about making such a decision and change their minds several times before deciding to hospitalize their adolescent. It is not uncommon for parents to bring an adolescent to the emergency room of the hospital for admission but then to change their minds and return home. Some parents may use a hospital visit as a threat to the adolescent, without actually intending to hospitalize him. Even after the hospitalization, doubts and indecision continue to prey upon the minds of some parents. The adolescents of such parents are at a high risk for early discharge against medical advice. This can be prevented, however, if the parents' ambivalence and their need for extra support is recognized. Several counseling sessions with the parents during the first week of their adolescent's hospitalization and daily brief telephone contacts with them will usually produce an atmosphere of cooperation.

Admitting an adolescent to the hospital is generally very stressful for all parties involved. It is not uncommon to hear an adolescent begging his parents not to hospitalize him and making all kinds of false promises: "I will never drink again"; "I will stop hitting you"; "I will go back to school." Some parents who are determined to hospitalize their adolescent when they first arrive may not remain as strongly determined after a period of begging and pleas from their adolescent. The apologies and promises of better conduct (which they may not have heard for a long time) sound like music to their ears, and the parents cave in and cancel admission, hoping that the threat of admission was sufficient to turn the adolescent around.

Other adolescents terrorize their parents. The parents feel that they are no longer in control and are afraid of mentioning hospital treatment for fear of violence or threats of running away from home. They frequently seek the help of relatives, friends, or the local police to bring the adolescent to a psychiatric facility. Unfortunately, such help is scarce and many times inappropriate. The local police in many towns and cities do not want to get involved in aiding the family to hospitalize their child. Many adolescents are thus brought to a hospital under false pretext, such as for a physical examination or a blood test. Such adolescents are likely to become violent when first hearing about their admission from the admitting psychiatrist. The presence of hospital security officers may be necessary to curtail their outbursts of violence.

Since most admissions of adolescents are carried out against their will, one can expect some form of resistance to be manifested during the admission process. Passive resistance is quite common. Adolescents refuse to give any information about themselves or acknowledge any problems. Some blame their parents for all their problems. Some adolescents withdraw into themselves, whereas others fight back in a desperate attempt to find some escape. Some may even bring false accusations of physical and sexual abuse against their parents. It should be emphasized that the decision to admit frequently creates in the adolescent a feeling of entrapment, helplessness, and a sense of the loss of newly found freedom. All of what is said in the admission room should be interpreted in the light of this intense emotional turmoil in the adolescent, a turmoil compounded by feelings of guilt, shame, and doubt of the parents. All accusations made by the adolescent should be noted down in the admission record, but no hasty legal action should be taken before further confirmation is obtained.

Frequently, admission procedures are often carried out in a hasty manner. Little or no time is spent in calming and dispersing the intense emotional climate surrounding the admission. (Ideally, an experienced mental health professonal should be available in the admission room to do this.) The goal of this therapeutic intervention is to minimize the adolescent's feeling of helplessness and the parents' guilt feelings over "abandoning their adolescent." The adolescent needs to feel that he has full control over his treatment. It should be emphasized to the adolescent that the current conflict between him and his family has been a source of severe hardship and stress for both him and his family. He and his family have tried to resolve the conflict in their own way, but they have not been successful. In fact, the family situation has become worse, putting more emotional strain on him as well as on other members of his family. It is clear that neither he nor his family can turn things around by themselves. They have to work together with the professional staff to regain family peace and tranquility. He and his family need outside help in order to resolve their differences and restore family happiness. His admission to the hospital is only the first step along the path to restore family harmony. The nature and the purpose of the hospital treatment should be explained in enough detail to help the adolescent understand the treatment program and allay some of his fears. The emphasis on family conflict as the primary source of the problem induces some adolescents to demand that their parents be hospitalized too since they are also part of the problem. The therapist should assure the adolescent that his family will also be participating in the treatment program. His hospitalization provides him with the opportunity to learn more about himself and his contribution to the family problems.

The parents' attitude toward hospitalizing their adolescent varies greatly. At one extreme are parents who are angry at their adolescent for having caused so many problems and for forcing them to employ an expensive and time-consuming remedy. They want the psychiatrist to "fix" their kid so they can be spared from similar ordeals in the future. They usually have no insight into the causes of the problem and are unaware of their contribution to the conflict. They are generally very resistant to getting involved in the therapeutic process. They strongly believe that all the problems of the adolescent are caused entirely by events outside the family. "If he would straighten out, everything would be just fine."

At the other extreme are parents who feel very guilty about bringing their adolescent to the hospital. They are overly attached and make all kinds of false promises to the adolescent, including telling him that they will take him out of the hospital in a few days. They are willing to acknowledge the existence of problems in the family but tend to minimize them. They believe that a few days' stay in the hospital will somehow magically cure all the adolescent's problems.

Parents have mixed emotions about court-ordered or social agency–ordered psychiatric evaluation of their adolescent. Some parents feel angry at the legal system and do not want to cooperate with the psychiatric evaluation. Others feel that psychiatric evaluation is useless since the primary problem is the adolescent's misbehavior and misconduct, which, in their opinion, can only be corrected by punishments meted out by a juvenile court.

The crisis phase does not end with the hospitalization of the adolescent. It may continue for several days afterward. As parents return home, they begin to focus upon themselves. They observe and experience other problems in the family that were overshadowed by the constant turmoil caused by the problem adolescent. They may blame each other for mishandling the adolescent's problems. They may experience grave doubts about the wisdom of hospitalizing their adolescent and may ask friends and other mental health professionals for advice. Unfortunately, these people lack knowledge of and have no experience with the hospital treatment of adolescents and thus give the parents contradictory advice. This adds to the parents' confusion about the right type of treatment for their adolescent. The hospitalized adolescent often senses his parents' ambivalence and confusion and does everything possible to exacerbate their guilt and doubt. The adolescent may, for example, tell his parents stories about the insensitivity and uncaring attitude of the hospital staff. He may compare the hospital with a jail with strict and "stupid rules." He may brand other adolescent patients in the program as "crazy and drug addicts," persons obviously having nothing in common with him. He may cry on the telephone and complain of being miserable, lonely, and missing everybody at home. Few parents can listen to this type of verbalization several times a day without beginning to doubt the wisdom of their decision to hospitalize their adolescent. If these parents do not receive strong support from the staff during this critical phase, they are likely to withdraw their adolescent from the treatment program.

Hospitalization of a disturbed adolescent provides temporary relief for most families. It may also halt the adolescent's movement along a self-destructive path. It helps many families to face up to a long-standing problem that has become progressively worse. By summoning up their strength and mobilizing their resources to face the crisis situation, many families come out stronger and better equipped to deal with day-to-day stresses. In fact, the family should be persuaded to view the crisis as a challenge requiring both purposeful problem-solving activities and the discarding of habitual responses and old strategies in favor of new and more effective conflict-resolving responses.

The outcome of the crisis depends upon several factors including personal strength, familial support, sociocultural conditions, and community resources. The personal strength factors include the coping skills of the adolescent and his family and their past experiences dealing with crises. If the present crisis is symbolically linked to or is explicitly similar to past crises, it is helpful to determine how well the family dealt with the previous crisis. Past experience with a problem reduces the probability of a similar problem becoming a new crisis. On the other hand, unsuccessfully resolved past crises are likely to result in repetition of previously unsuccessful solutions before new and more effective solutions are discovered.

There are many drawbacks to hospitalizing adolescents. Some community mental health workers fear that the hospital treatment may focus unduly on the disturbed adolescent, thereby conveying the message to the family that the problem was primarily with the adolescent. They are sometimes afraid that such families receiving treatment in the community agencies may withdraw and become less willing to invest in treatment directed toward a substantial change in the family system. Some families may abandon a disturbed adolescent in the hospital and refuse to take him back. A similar reluctance may be expressed by schools and other community agencies who may perceive the hospitalized adolescent as too disturbed to return to the school and the community and want him to be "sent away" for a long time. The hospitalized adolescent himself may feel safer in the structured environment of the hospital and may express fear and reluctance about returning home. All these issues are important and frequently arise as a consequence of hospitalization. However, most of these problems can be remedied if family therapy is considered an integral part of the hospital treatment and the community agencies and the schools are kept abreast of the adolescent's progress and the discharge plan.

The preceding discussion does not imply that intrafamilial conflict and a breakdown of communication in the family are the only precipitating causes for the hospitalization of adolescents. They are, however, major precipitating factors and are found in most adolescent disorders such as conduct disorders, oppositional disorders, running away, substance abuse, and depression. Biological factors contribute heavily to the etiology of serious psychopathology such as acute psychosis, manic-depressive disorder, and separation anxiety.

EVALUATION PHASE

Hospitalization provides an opportunity to collect data that are not usually available in the outpatient treatment setting. The structure of the hospital milieu helps the staff to collect information on the new patient's adaptive and maladaptive behaviors and on his psychopathology. The observations that are made include the following: eating, sleeping, personal care and hygiene, peer interaction, adult interaction, general attitude, mood changes, obsessions, and compulsions. It is important that the data be gathered in an organized and systematic manner so as to provide information about the adolescent's strengths and weaknesses, the nature of the psychopathology, and its effects on his overall functioning.

A comprehensive hospital evaluation should include the following:

1. Extensive history obtained from different members of the family.
2. Mental status and physical examination of the adolescent.
3. Collateral information from the school and community agencies.
4. Ward observation by the nursing staff.
5. Educational evaluation by the teachers involved in ward education.
6. A use of leisure time evaluation by the recreational therapist.
7. Assessment of participation in group therapy sessions.
8. Assessment of participation in individual therapy sessions.
9. Laboratory tests.
10. Extent of substance abuse.
11. Psychiatric diagnosis.

Since multiple factors usually contribute to the etiology of psychiatric problems, it is essential to gather information on a wide range of possible contributing factors. The above outline of the comprehensive evaluation includes most of the relevant areas. There are several lengthy questionnaires and inventories designed to collect information on newly hospitalized patients. However, most of these were developed by residential treatment centers for planning long-term treatment and are thus not suitable for short-term hospitalization. We have developed several smaller inventories (listed in the Appendix), each designed for collecting information in a specific area. These inventories are used by the members of the multidisciplinary team. The information gathered by each staff member is specific to their area of expertise, relates to a particular aspect of the patient's life, and is not duplicated by other staff. For example, an evaluation by a recreational therapist focuses primarily on the patient's use of leisure time. Similarly, an evaluation by a nursing staff member will include information about the patient's daily habits of eating, sleeping, personal care, peer and adult interactions, general attitude, and dominant mood. These inventories allow each member of the multidisciplinary team to contribute specific information to the overall evaluation and help them to set specific treatment goals in their areas of expertise. For example, a recreational therapist may set a goal of helping an adolescent to discover an area of recreational interest or help him find resources to fulfill his long-standing desire to get involved in a specific recreational activity. Similarly, the nursing staff may set up specific treatment goals based on their own evaluation to improve personal hygiene, peer interaction, and general attitude. If findings of specific learning difficulties are found by the educational evaluation, this leads to planning a specific curriculum and to specific recommendations about the patient to the public school system.

It is often quite difficult to distinguish the immediate precipitating factors from the ongoing chronic factors in the etiology of a psychiatric problem. This distinction, however, is extremely important for planning effective and successful short-term hospital treatment. The primary goals of short-term hospitalization such as crisis resolution and stabilization of acute psychopathology are best achieved by focusing treatment efforts on the precipitating factors. A knowledge of the chronic problems is essential to understand how the current problems relate to the chronic problems in the context of developmental and past history. More durable changes in the psychopathology are brought about by working through these past conflicts. This type of therapy, however, requires long periods of time and is carried out primarily in outpatient settings.

Historical Information

It is usually helpful to divide all the historical information about the patient into two broad categories:

1. Precipitating factors and psychiatric symptoms leading to hospitalization.
2. Long-standing problems including developmental problems, family issues, and psychiatric symptomatology.

This information is obtained from the parents, guardians, and extended members of the family. The first interview is usually quite difficult, both for the family and the interviewer. The interviewer may be unduly preoccupied with obtaining the facts of the history and may not note the presence of anxiety in the family. It is, however, more important to spend a sufficient amount of time to develop a working relationship with the parents before venturing into the facts of the history. It is not uncommon to find most parents to be very anxious during the first interview. Many feel guilty and responsible for their child's problems. The parents may appear very defensive and guarded. They may hide important facts for fear of being incriminated by the psychiatrist. Mothers and fathers frequently perceive the nature and the seriousness of the problem quite differently. The clinician should insist on seeing both parents in intact families during the first interview.

The interviewer must help the anxious parents to feel relaxed and less defensive. The interviewer can do this by maintaining a respectful attitude toward the parents and by talking about a neutral subject for a few minutes (e.g., difficulties in taking time off to come for the interview). The interviewer need not worry about starting the interview because most parents have a lot on their mind and will begin talking about their problems without prompting. It is extremely important to allow the parents to follow their own associations in describing the problem, at least during the first half of the interview. The rest of the interview can be structured to obtain pertinent historical information. Exploration of sensitive issues such as marital relations and child abuse is usually done last when the parents are less defensive and more open.

Some professionals view their role as that of child advocate and develop an adversary relationship with the parents. Such preconceived notions and attitudes are detrimental to overall treatment. Even in cases of suspected child abuse, parental cooperation is necessary to help the child. It is important to develop a fairly good working relationship with the parents. The parents should regard the diagnostic and treatment process as a collaborative effort on the part of the interviewer and themselves. They should be encouraged to explore all factors contributing to the child's problem. However, this type of cooperation is not always achieved, especially with parents who are unwilling participants or who are hostile to helping professionals. Creating an atmosphere of openness and honesty and clearly stating the goals of the interview will promote the development of a good working relationship. Because there are many facets to the diagnostic work-up that may appear irrelevant to the parents, it is helpful to state and clarify the purpose of every aspect of the work-up in order to obtain their full cooperation.

A diagnostic family interview offers an excellent opportunity for the psychiatrist to observe the patterns of interaction among various members of the family and to understand the family dynamics that influence the adolescent. It is important to have all or most members of the family at this interview. Most parents find it difficult to comprehend the need for a family session. Since the parents provide most of the diagnostic information about the child's development and his interaction with other members of the family, they may interpret the psychiatrist's desire to interview the whole family as an expression of his lack of trust in them or in their ability to provide reliable information. Some parents are reluctant to bring their families to the interview because they have not told the siblings about the intended or already accomplished hospitalization. In one case, the parents explained that they did not want to tell the siblings because they were likely to share the information with their friends who would then tease the patient about being "crazy." Some parents fear that the family session may have a traumatic impact on the younger siblings. Talking about an 8-year-old sibling, one parent remarked, "She would not understand. She is just a little, innocent child. She wouldn't know what this is all about." The reluctance of parents to accept the need for family sessions frequently arises from a lack of open communication within the family. Different members of such families keep secrets from one another. Getting together in a family session may imply that everybody will be exposed and that their secrets will no longer remain secrets. The other children in such families offer as much resistance to coming for a family session as do the parents. All kinds of excuses are made to avoid attending the family session. In fact, one may find that the members of such a family rarely ever get together for anything.

The psychiatrist should explain to the parents that the family session is part of the routine diagnostic process and is designed to help the psychiatrist understand the relationships among various members of the family. He should explore the concerns and the feelings of the parents about the family session. He should emphasize strongly that during the family session he will not divulge any information about any family member that was derived from a prior individual interview with that member. The psychiatrist may, however, tell the parents that in his experience children already know about most of the family secrets and that a lack of complete information and family secrecy force children to fill in the gaps with their own imaginings. Moreover, efforts to hide certain family matters from children places a great burden on the parents to maintain that secrecy. This may be interpreted by the children as evidence of parental objection.

Some preparation of the siblings at home before the family session is helpful in ensuring a successful interview. The psychiatrist should suggest that the parents call a family meeting at home and explain to all the siblings the nature of the hospitalization of the adolescent and the importance of the family session with the psychiatrist. They should indicate that the psychiatrist wants to meet the whole family to find out how they all get along and how they can help the hospitalized adolescent. They should be told to act naturally in the psychiatrist's office and to talk about whatever they like without censoring their remarks for fear of parental reprisal.

Families in a psychiatrist's office show different patterns of conflict and anxiety. Typically, the family arrives in a state of tension and apprehension. The children are quiet, reserved, and on their best behavior. The parents or the psychiatrist may reduce the anxiety by talking about the problems. Each child may be asked to express his perception of the problem.

Family therapists frequently regard the family as a functioning unit and consider the problem(s) of an individual member as being the result of some basic underlying problem(s) in the family system. Although different family members, by virtue of differing ages and mental capacities, may express the problem differently, they are regarded as reacting to the same basic problem. Thus, after anxiety is reduced and communication improves, the psychiatrist may try to find the nature of the basic problem(s) in the family system. Various types of family systems and family interactions have been recognized. For example, some families put up a good front as if nothing is wrong, and no one in the family is allowed to criticize or talk negatively about other family members. At the other end of the spectrum, there are families in which nobody agrees on anything, and there is a constant bickering and arguing over every matter. Recognition of the various patterns of family functioning is helpful in both diagnosis and planning treatment.

The hospitalization of one sibling may precipitate severe problems in other siblings. Another sibling may become the focus of abnormal attention and/or the recipient of expressions of pathology. Occasionally a younger sibling may become very upset over the absence of the hospitalized sibling and develop symptoms of severe anxiety, a school phobia, and nightmares. The parents' preoccupation with the hospitalized adolescent may result in less time spent with the other siblings and may be perceived by the other siblings as neglect.

Mental Status Examination of the Adolescent

An interview with an adolescent requires special sensitivity. The adolescent aspires to being treated like an adult and resents any reference to or suggestion of being a child. Many adolescents are suspicious and have negative feelings toward the psychiatrist because they view all adults (including the parents and the psychiatrist) as plotting against them. It is quite common for the adolescent to be belligerent and uncommunicative in the initial sessions. The psychiatrist should respect the adolescent's right to behave in that manner. The psychiatrist may have to make intense efforts to win the confidence of the adolescent. The effort, however, should be genuine. Trickery and deception have no place in dealing with children or adolescents. Since the primary goals of short-term hospitalization are to solve the immediate crisis and to return the patient to the community for further treatment, this can be openly stated to the adolescent. Most hospitalized adolescents like to hear any mention of leaving the hospital. It should be emphasized, however, that the hospitalization has resulted from problems that need to be resolved before the discharge can occur and that the sooner they get down to the business of working on their problems, the earlier they will leave. The adolescent should have impressed upon him the fact that most of his behavior problems are the result of an interaction between him and his environment, such as the family, the school, and the community. The adolescent needs to work on his part of the problem, while his family has to work on its. This point should particularly be emphasized with adolescents who have conduct problems and who have little or no insight into the causes of their problems. They tend to blame their environment for their problems. They also minimize substance abuse and view their habits as recreational.

Most depressed adolescents are not aware of their depressed mood. They are more aware of their anger and dysphoria or irritability. The physical symptoms of depression such as a poor appetite or excessive eating, sleeping problems, a low energy level, and diminished interests are frequently denied by adolescents in spite of the fact that these symptoms can easily be observed by the members of the family and the hospital staff. Similarly, adolescents have very little insight into the problems of anorexia, bulimia, and anxiety disorders.

Physical Examination

This is an important part of the evaluation. However, most adolescents, especially females, are reluctant to be examined. A great deal of support from the nursing staff may be necessary to carry out a physical examination on an uncooperative adolescent. The majority of the adolescents are in good physical health and rarely show an abnormal physical finding. The medical history and presenting complaints guide the physician to focus on certain areas during the examination. It is important to check for needle marks, bruises, burns, and cuts on every patient and to carefully record these findings.

Pelvic examination is not included in a routine physical examination. Parental permission should be obtained if a pelvic examination appears necessary. A recent history of rape and suspicion of venereal disease warrants a pelvic examination. Most hospitals have a standardized protocol for the examination of rape victims. Such an examination is usually carried out in the emergency department of the hospital. The psychiatrist may ask the assistance of an emergency room physician or a gynecologist in carrying out such an examination. The report of this examination is usually prepared in two parts: the first part describes the factual findings from the physical examination; the second part includes the physician's conclusion and impressions with regard to the occurrence of rape, the degree of violence, the degree of struggle and resistance, and if possible, the psychological status of the patient. A physical examination in such cases should include scanning of the entire body for cuts, bruises, scrapes, and debris. The pelvic examination should note lacerations, bruises, bleeding, discharges, and the presence of foreign material such as hair, debris, and semen. The laboratory tests usually include the preparation of two dry slides of vaginal secretion (air dried), one slide preserved in an ethyl alcohol bottle, one wet mount to be checked by the examining doctor, a swab for Transgrow culture medium, a VDRL test, and a pregnancy test. Special attention should be paid to the neurological portion of the physical examination if the patient manifests confusion, intoxication, psychosis, or severe depression. Depressed adolescents should be checked for physical signs of infectious mononucleosis.

Laboratory Tests

In addition to the routine laboratory tests (complete blood count [CBC], urine analysis, SMA-18, and VDRL) required by most hospitals, urine samples should be tested for the presence of marijuana, its metabolites, and other chemicals abused by adolescents such as opiates, cocaine, methaqualone (Quaaludes), barbiturates, nicotine, and various tranquilizers. Adolescents with acute brain syndrome or acute psychosis require a neurological work-up including an electroencephalogram (EEG), a computed tomographic (CT) scan, a lumbar puncture, and magnetic resonance imaging (MRI) to rule out head trauma, central nervous system (CNS) infection, tumor, or encephalopathies.

Pregnancy tests should be ordered for most adolescent females. Monospot tests are helpful in ruling out infectious mononucleosis.

Specialized Tests in Psychiatry

Biochemical studies of the brain and their relationship to mental disorders have led to an extensive search for laboratory markers that can be used in the diagnosis and prediction of treatment of these disorders. More than a dozen laboratory tests, mostly for affective disorders, have found some clinical applicability in psychiatry (Greden, 1985). However, the sensitivity and specificity of these tests remain low. It is possible that with a better classification system of psychiatric disorders and more stringent criteria for the selection of patients these tests may become more psychiatrically useful.

Only a few studies of hospitalized adolescents have investigated the biochemical and electrophysiological parameters of depression by using such tests as the dexamethasone suppression test (DST), the thyrotropin-releasing hormone (TRH) stimulation test, urinary 3-methoxy-4-hydroxyphenethylene glycol (MHPG), and polysomnography. Our data from a study of more than 100 hospitalized adolescents (Khan, 1987) indicate that the DST is a sensitive laboratory aid in the diagnosis of depression. The DST has positive findings in about 70% of the adolescents with major depression. False-positive DST findings occur in about 18% of the cases. False-positive DST results have also been reported in various medical conditions such as Cushing's disease, undercontrolled diabetes, temporal lobe epilepsy, major physical illness, pregnancy, acute withdrawal from alcohol, anorexia nervosa, severe weight loss, and the use of medications such as phenytoin sodium, barbiturates, and meprobamate.

The results of TRH stimulation tests in several studies of adults with major depression are quite variable and range from 20% to 77%. The importance of the TRH test in distinguishing groups of depressed patients remains controversial since most investigators believe that only a minority of patients with unipolar depression show a blunted response (Prange et al., 1977; Loosen et al., 1977). The TRH-induced thyroid-stimulating hormone (TSH) response is also reduced in males, in acute starvation, in chronic renal failure, in Klinefelter's syndrome, in anorexia nervosa, in alcoholism, and with increasing age. In our study (Khan, 1987) although about one third of the adolescents with major depression showed a blunted response to TRH tests, this finding was not significant when compared with the result of the nondepressed group, which also showed a blunted response.

A great deal of research on affective disorders has been motivated by the monoamine hypothesis, which states that affective disorders are due to functional changes in CNS monoamine neurotransmitters. This hypothesis has found support in the pharmacological use of reserpine, tricyclic antidepressants, and monoamine oxidase inhibitors, which affect catecholamines and indolamines. However, measurements of the catecholamine precursor tyrosine, the catecholamines (dopamine and norepinephrine), and their metabolites homovanillic acid (HVA), vanillylmandelic acid (VMA), and MHPG in the blood, urine, and spinal fluid of depressed patients have yielded inconsistent results. Forty percent to 60% of the urinary MHPG originates in the CNS from the metabolism of central norepinephrine (Maas et al., 1979). Several investigators have attempted to replicate the findings of decreased urinary MHPG excretion in depressed adolescents with inconsistent results (Cytryn et al., 1974; McKnew and Cytryn, 1979). In our study of adolescents (Khan, 1987) the data indicated that urinary

MHPG beyond the normal range was not specific to major depression but was present across all diagnostic categories.

Sleep variables have been used to correctly classify 68% of adult depressed patients (Kerkhofs et al., 1985). Few studies are available on sleep parameters in depressed adolescents (Kupfer et al., 1979). Mendlewicz et al. (1984) reported no significant decrease in rapid eye movement (REM) latency in three depressed adolescents. Our data also indicate that adolescents between the ages of 13 and 17 years with major depression do not show a significant decrease in REM sleep latency as do adults with depression.

The diagnosis of anxiety and panic disorders in adolescents may at times be quite difficult. The physiological measures indicating anxiety include an increased heart rate, greater skin conduction and α-blocking on the EEG. The biochemical markers include high levels of cortisol and catecholamines (and their metabolites, especially MHPG), both in the serum and the urine. The lactate infusion test has been shown to determine the predisposition to acute panic attacks. The history of the lactate infusion test is frequently associated with Pitts and McClure (1967), who infused sodium lactate in a group of anxious patients and nonanxious controls. The majority of the anxious patients developed panic reaction by receiving lactate infusion. None of the controls developed the reaction. A solution of lactate plus calcium tended to modify and diminish the panic reaction. The authors concluded that the anxious patients metabolize lactate somewhat differently from the nonanxious and that panic attacks were induced by an alteration in the calcium balance. Liebowitz and Klein (1981) have shown that blood lactate levels rise faster and higher in patients than in controls, which suggests that lactate is being handled differently in those patients. Although all patients in the control group showed a significant reduction in ionized calcium levels with each infusion, no difference was found between patients and controls. Several lactate infusion studies are in progress to determine the underlying mechanism(s) of anxiety from lactate infusion. There are few studies of adolescents that use the lactate infusion test. This may be because adolescents rarely give a clear history of panic attacks. However, there are many borderline cases in which this diagnosis should be ruled out. In those cases, lactate infusion tests may be helpful.

Psychological Tests

It is generally quite easy to obtain information through clinical interviews for assessing the personality problems and emotional conflicts of adolescents once a good rapport has been developed with them. Adolescents do not respond well to self-administered personality inventories such as the Minnesota Multiphasic Personality Inventory (MMPI), mainly because of the large number of questions included in these inventories. Adolescents also have great difficulty in making decisions about the questions that require self-assessment. In our experience, adolescents respond fairly well to about the first 50 questions, and then they begin to respond randomly to the rest of the questions. We found that about 80% of the MMPIs administered to our hospitalized adolescents were invalid. However, shorter inventories may show a more valid assessment. Projective tests such as the children's perception test, and the Rorschack are helpful in obtaining more information about conflict areas. However, the overall interpretation of these tests by psychologists is frequently in conflict with the clinical judgement of the psychiatrist, particularly in the diagnostic categories of depression, anxiety, and schizophrenia. Psychological tests are very helpful in the assessment of shy and withdrawn adolescents who require a great deal of time to build a working relationship with a therapist. Educational evaluation and intelligence quotient (IQ) testing is necessary and important for the evaluation of the adolescent with learning disabilities.

Educational Evaluation

Most adolescent psychiatric programs provide 2 to 4 hours of daily educational instruction to the patient. The program is usually run by teachers who are trained in special education techniques. The students generally receive credit for half a day of regular school attendance for attending these programs. The majority of hospitalized adolescents have experienced some difficulty in school during the 6 months prior to admission. It is possible to divide the hospitalized adolescents into three or four groups on the basis of their educational difficulties.

Group 1 consists of those adolescents who have been doing well in school and have maintained their grades until the time of hospitalization. They are well motivated and utilize their school time well in finishing their daily assignments. This is generally a very small group.

Group 2 (usually the largest group) is composed of those adolescents who were doing well in school until about 6 months to a year prior to their hospitalization. Their grades had steadily fallen and included some failing grades (mainly resulting from incompletion of assignments). Their motivation to learn is at the lowest point of their academic career. They are not sure whether they want to return to school.

Group 3 includes adolescents from special educational backgrounds. Most of them have very poor motivation for academic achievement and have chronic behavior problems.

Group 4 includes adolescents whose academic and behavioral difficulties are long-standing but who cannot be classified as learning disabled. This is a group of emotionally disturbed adolescents who may have received mental health counseling off and on for years. Multiple factors including familial, socioeconomic, and educational difficulties contribute to their learning problems.

The educational program for adolescents is an integral part of the psychiatric treatment. The goals of educational evaluation and treatment should be consistent with the overall program. The evaluation should be completed quickly, within a few days of admission. The teachers should contact the school of each student to gather oral or written information with regard to his level of achievement, areas of excellence, deficits, classroom placement (learning disability/behavior disorders), and behavioral problems. The test results of psychological and education evaluations may be available from the schools. The hospital evaluation should include a detailed history of past academic performance and that of current functioning. One of the important aspects of psychoeducational evaluation is a determination of the motivation to learn. Many adolescents verbally claim a high level of motivation to learn, but that claim may not be supported by their behavior and performance in the classroom. An educational program should be designed in collaboration with mental health workers to help the unmotivated or poorly motivated adolescent.

It is not uncommon to find many adolescents who have remained in the regular classroom but in fact show specific learning deficits in carefully formalized testing. Such test batteries are generally administered by psychologists, but teachers themselves should assess the difficulties in the basic areas of learning.

The tests usually given to assess reading skills are those that involve vocabulary, paragraph comprehension, and matters of word attack (i.e., phonics and sound blendings). There are several standardized tests available to assess current reading levels such as the Gray Oral (1963), Gates (1962), and the Durrell Analysis of Reading Difficulties (1955).

There are not many standardized tests to assess writing skills. While assessing this skill a distinction must be made between the writing problems due to the mechanics of the writing act and a possible expressive language difficulty involving the formulation of what is to be written. Usually observation of a child doing writing work provides a great deal of insight into individual writing problems. Some of the points that should be noted during this process include the following (Peters et al., 1973):

1. Writing to dictation.
2. Reversals and inversions.
3. Confused letter approach—look for hesitancies before the upward and downward swing, getting on and off circular letters, and where in the connecting swing the child starts the letter.
4. Labored writing exists when the letters are drawn very slowly. It is usually a clumsy, crude, slow writing. The letter may be drawn nicely.
5. Spelling errors.
6. Reckless speed.

There are several screening tests for assessing the current level of mathematical skills. Many adolescents have failed to learn the basic concepts of math.

Teachers may also familiarize themselves with other educational screening tests such as the Wide Range Achievement Test—Revised. It is frequently used as an all-inclusive screening test for reading, writing, spelling, and mathematics.

Ward Evaluations

The patients are observed 24 hours a day by the nursing staff. Systematic observation of new patients helps the nursing staff plan specifics of treatment that they themselves can carry out. These observations also contribute a great deal to the overall planning of the treatment.

Several checklists are available for recording patients' behavior. Some of these were designed primarily for specific research studies such as on schizophrenia, depression, and anxiety. Others include symptoms of the more common psychiatric disorders. For examples, the Global Ward Behavior Scale includes observation of the manifestations of depression and schizophrenia. The primary function and purpose of these scales has been to utilize nursing observation to make a diagnosis and/or monitor clinical improvement with treatment. The main purpose in designing ward evaluation checklists is to identify and observe behavior and psychopathology for which specific treatment programs can be designed by the nursing staff. Ward observation should include self-care habits, peer interaction, adult interaction, use of leisure time, organized recreational activities, interest in education activities outside school hours, overall energy levels, attitude toward psychiatric treatment, mood changes, religious affiliations and commitments, and sleeping and eating habits.

Evaluation Through Individual Contact

This refers to evaluation interviews with the patient that are carried out by various staff members such as social workers, psychologists, psychiatrists, resident staff, and students. The focus of the interview varies with the background of the mental health professional. Psychiatric interviews are generally focused on the mental status examination of the adolescent. Individual interviews with adolescents may be quite awkward and unproductive. Most adolescents are very reluctant to reveal themselves. They deny their feelings of depression and anxiety; they attribute all their problems to maltreatment by their parents, teachers, or peers.

This evaluation highlights certain aspects of the mental status examination. It is important to determine the capacity of the adolescent to relate to various adults in an individual therapeutic context. The evaluation should also include some assessment of the adolescent's level and depth of insight into his problem; his understanding of the sources of stress, anxiety, or depression; and which problem areas he is willing to work on and which problem areas he avoids.

Information from this evaluation can help in the planning of specific therapeutic goals in both individual therapy sessions during hospitalization and after discharge.

Evaluation in a Group Setting

Adolescents generally relate better to their peers than to adults. They depend upon their peers for support and identity formation. An adolescent who communicates openly with his peers is likely to resolve most of his interpersonal problems through sharing and discussing them with his peers. On the other hand, a quiet and isolated adolescent tends to experience greater difficulty in resolving his normal adolescent conflicts. It is important to carry out an evaluation of every new patient in a group setting. This evaluation is done fairly easily since most adolescent programs utilize group psychotherapy and other forms of group discussion and activities as the main methods of daily treatment. The evaluation questionnaire (listed in the Appendix) should include such characteristics as openness, secretiveness, demanding and bossy behavior, attitude toward therapy staff (group leader and associates), ability to comprehend group issues, ability to discuss personal issues, and desire to help others with their personal issues. Some adolescents are able to relate better to their peers in an informal leaderless group than in a formal group led by an adult group leader. These evaluations facilitate the planning of specific treatment goals for each adolescent patient both in the hospital and after discharge.

Evaluation of Leisure Activities

Most adolescents have a great deal of free time after school hours, on weekends, and during vacations. Although some adolescents manage to keep themselves busy with schoolwork, sports, and part-time work, others seem to be less well organized and have more free time on their hands. Adolescents with emotional and behavior problems tend to be reluctant to involve themselves in organized activities. They seem, in general, to have great difficulty organizing their study and leisure time. Most of their leisure time is spent in watching television, listening to the radio, playing video games, or engaging in on-the-spur-of-the-moment activities. Many of these youngsters have poor social skills and are unable to initiate or participate in the group activities of their peer group. Some of them are not even aware of the possible social and recreational activities available in their communities.

A formal assessment of the leisure time activities of these adolescents will help in planning treatment goals relating to leisure awareness and leisure counseling. There are several types of instruments to assess different aspects of leisure activities. These instruments include inventories (McDowell, 1979), scales (Ragheb and Beard, 1980), and diagnostic batteries (Witt, 1982). Most of these instruments are designed to assess the following:

1. Type of activities carried out during leisure time.
2. Attitude toward leisure time.
3. Extent of the knowledge of leisure activities available in the community.
4. Leisure activity skills.
5. Interest in some new leisure activities.
6. Satisfaction with current leisure activities.

This evaluation is usually carried out by a recreational therapist and is very helpful in planning specific treatment goals for each patient.

Substance Abuse Evaluation

It is important to evaluate all hospitalized adolescents for substance abuse problems. The seriousness of the problem varies from early experimentation to serious drug dependency. Physical dependency is rarely seen in adolescents. Most adolescents are able to give a fairly accurate history of their substance abuse after their first few days of hospitalization. They may not, however, have much insight into the relationship between their emotional and social problems and their substance abuse. It usually takes an experienced and knowledgeable person to do an accurate assessment of the degree of drug dependency.

A detailed description of substance abuse evaluation is given in Chapter 2.

Psychiatric Diagnosis

Psychiatric diagnosis is an essential part of every psychiatric evaluation. It is usually made on the basis of information derived from the history, mental status examination, and the results of all the other tests and evaluations. Some centers utilize structured interviews for psychiatric evaluation. There are several such structured interviews that can be used for the psychiatric evaluation of adolescents.

KIDDIE Schedule for Affective Disorders and Schizophrenia

The KIDDIE Schedule for Affective Disorders and Schizophrenia (K-SADS) is a structured psychiatric interview designed for patients between the ages of 6 and 18 years and their parents. This has been revised several times to modify questions that are understood better by children and adolescents. This interview schedule is designed to elicit information that is pertinent for most DSM III diagnoses applicable to children and adolescents.

A copy of the interview schedule can be obtained from the Western Psychiatric Institute and Clinic, School of Medicine, Department of Psychiatry, Division of Child and Adolescent Psychiatry, Pittsburgh, PA.

Diagnostic Interview Schedule for Children and Adolescents

This is a semistructured interview schedule that elicits information with regard to the onset, duration, and severity of most diagnoses applicable to children and adolescents as listed in DSM III-R. It may be obtained from the Department of Psychiatry, Washington University School of Medicine, St. Louis, MO.

Structured Clinical Interview for DSM III-R

The Structured Clinical Interview for DSM III-R (SCID) is designed to enable a clinically trained interviewer to make DSM III-R diagnoses. There are three standard versions of this schedule:

1. The patient version is designed to be used for psychiatric inpatients but may also be used in other situations requiring differential diagnoses of psychotic disorders.

2. The outpatient version contains brief screening modules for psychotic disorders and is designed for various disorders generally treated in outpatient departments.

3. A nonpatient version is used in studies in which the subjects are not identified as psychiatric patients. It is useful in research and community studies.

This test is available from the Bio-Metrics Research Department, New York State Psychiatric Institute, 722 W. 168th St., New York, NY.

Child Assessment Schedule

The Child Assessment Schedule (CAS) is a semistructured interview schedule for the assessment of children and adolescents between the ages of 6 and 18 years. It is divided into three parts. Part I contains inquiries relating to the patient's friends, activities, hobbies, schools, and family. Part II records the examiner's observation of the patient. Part III obtains information about the onset and duration of the symptoms. This schedule can be obtained from the Department of Psychiatry, University of Missouri, Columbia, MO.

In addition to the aforementioned comprehensive interview schedules, there are various interview questionnaires and inventories that can be utilized to supplement the clinical interview.

Child Behavior Checklist

This checklist contains items relevant to childhood depression. On a three-point scale, parents indicate the extent to which each of the 113 items describe their child's behavior. There are several versions of this checklist: one designed for teachers, a second designed as a youth self-report form, and a third direct observation and report form.

Personality Inventory for Children

The Personality Inventory for Children (PIC) is used for the assessment of a child's personality. It is completed by the parents and consists of 600 true/false items. It can be used for children between the ages of 3 and 16 years.

TREATMENT PHASE

A comprehensive short-term psychiatric treatment program for adolescents must be supportive as well as therapeutic. It must focus on the primary conflicts that necessitated hospitalization. It must meet the developmental, educational, and recreational needs of the adolescent. It should also intervene in the family and the community so that the adolescent patient can return to a more supportive and therapeutic environment after discharge. Although hospital treatment programs vary from community to community, most have the following formal components:

1. Psychotherapy—group and individual.
2. Family therapy.
3. Educational program.
4. Mental health education for patients and families.
5. Specialized mileu treatment.
6. Community involvement.
7. Pharmacotherapy.
8. Follow-up program.

The details of these programs and therapeutic modalities are discussed in a separate chapter. The rest of this chapter discusses the philosophy, goals, and objectives of short-term hospital treatment.

The treatment phase may be divided into a general treatment phase and a specific treatment phase.

The general treatment phase begins on the first day of hospitalization and is provided to all new patients. This treatment is designed to help new patients adjust to the ward routine, reduce their emotional intensity, provide a structured environment, routinize their daily activities, and deal with here-and-now problems. At the completion of the evaluation phase when the nature and the dynamics of the problems of a new patient are better understood, the focus of the treatment is shifted to specific areas of difficulty and conflict. It is essential to recognize the importance of the general treatment phase. The success of the specific treatment phase depends upon the patient's receptive attitude, cooperation, and ability to deal with his specific problems. If a new patient is allowed to wander around and maintain a negative attitude toward treatment, no specific treatment objectives set after the evaluation phase can be achieved.

The staff should be fully aware of the objectives to be achieved during the general phase of the treatment. Since the objectives during the general phase of the treatment are the same for all new patients, there can be little confusion and misunderstanding about these objectives. However, these objectives should be clearly stated and repeated frequently to the staff. These objectives may be summarized as follows:

1. Help the new patient adjust to the daily routine of the ward (sleeping, eating, self-care, school, therapeutic and recreational activities).
2. Help new patients acknowledge that they have problems that require hospital treatment.
3. Help new patients develop a positive attitude and willingness to resolve their problems.
4. Help new patients reduce their emotional intensity (anger, anxiety, sadness, and stress) by thinking about the investigating the factors contributing to their emotional turmoil.
5. Help new patients understand how discussing and talking about their own problems and the problems of others will help them resolve their own problems.

In order to achieve these objectives, a great deal of attention must be paid to the organization and the therapeutic programs of the adolescent ward. The mileu of the ward must be supportive as well as provide the developmental, educational, and recreational needs of the adolescent. The therapeutic program should include daily group and individual therapy and at least twice-a-week family therapy. The staff should strive to create an atmosphere of support and an expectation for improvement.

The patient's progress in the achievement of the general objectives should be reviewed every couple of days by the staff. A questionnaire designed for this purpose can be used. The reason for a lack of progress should be found and corrected if possible. One reason for an initial lack of progress is that some patients take a long time to feel comfortable with their therapist and trust him enough to reveal themselves. The therapist must accordingly be able and willing to provide more therapy time for these patients. Another reason for a lack of progress is staff who overidentify with the adolescent patients and lower their expectations in therapy work while blaming the family for the patient's problems. Such an attitude promotes denial and avoidance on the part of the patient and is very destructive to therapeutic work.

It is almost impossible for the therapy staff not to develop specific hypotheses about the causes and nature of the patient's problems during the evaluation phase and direct their therapeutic efforts accordingly. This is a great temptation, and even experienced therapists succumb to it. Different patients progress at different rates during the general treatment phase. A few adolescents come to the hospital willingly and are able to progress rapidly to working on and resolving their specific conflicts. The majority of adolescents, however, are very oppositional to receiving any psychiatric help and need to work first on the objectives outlined for the general treatment phase. Unfortunately, some adolescents go through several weeks of hospital treatment without accomplishing even the general objectives in spite of the intense efforts of the milieu staff. Such adolescents do not benefit from short-term hospitalization and need to be transferred to another facility where they can stay for a longer period of time.

At the end of the evaluation phase, specific treatment objectives should be set by each member of the multidisciplinary team. This helps each discipline to be innovative, productive, and feel satisfied that its body of expert knowledge is being productively utilized. Each of the disciplines must be guided, however, by the overall goals of the hospital treatment plan, which include the following:

1. Resolution of the crisis.
2. Stabilization of acute psychopathology.
3. Intervention in the family and the community so that they can be supportive and therapeutic when the adolescent returns.

These overall objectives help each discipline to focus on the short-term goals that can be accomplished within the short period of hospitalization.

Specific Treatment Objectives Set by the Nursing Staff

These specific objectives are based on ward observation and systematic evaluation of each new patient during the evaluation phase. Typical nursing treatment objectives may include helping patients with peer and adult interaction, teaching self-care skills, and modifying daily habits of eating and sleeping. In addition, some of the objectives listed under the general treatment phase may also be included in the specific nursing treatment plan. The nursing staff should design a clear plan of action about how the specific objectives are to be achieved. For example, if the specific objective is to help an adolescent improve his personal hygiene, the specific nursing plan should include such nursing staff actions as asking the adolescent to shower daily, put on clean clothes, and wash his own laundry and should give feedback to the adolescent about the improvement in his personal care.

Specific Treatment Objectives Set by the Recreation Therapist

The overall goal of recreational therapy in an adolescent ward is to provide appropriate recreational activities for the patients. A combination of indoor games and outdoor activities are planned for adolescents who need to stay on the ward and for those who can go outside the ward. Since most hospitals do not have a gymnasium, a large room may be modified and used for gym activities. Outdoor activities may be carried out in a neighborhood recreational park or in indoor places such as a YMCA in the area. Adolescents tend to enjoy physical activities such as swimming, running, basketball, and volleyball. Indoor games like shuffleboard, table tennis, bumper pool, minature golf, or croquet can be utilized for indoor activities. There should be at least 1 hour set aside every day for recreational activities. In addition to providing general recreational activities, the recreational therapist should formulate specific treatment goals for each new patient. The leisure activity evaluation frequently helps the recreational therapist to arrive at a specific treatment goal for each new patient. Many adolescents with poor social skills get caught in a downward spiral of progressive social isolation. They need to understand the importance of socializing and participating in recreational activities with their peers. They may need to be informed about the recreational facilities in their own community. Some adolescents show no interest in social or recreational activities. They should be asked about their past interests, the type of activities they had the most fun with, and the kind of things they always wanted to do but were shy and reluctant to engage in. Such discussions with the recreational therapist help the new patient to discover new interests or revive old ones. Indoor and outdoor recreational activities help each patient to get emotionally involved and try out favorite activities.

Specific Objectives Set by Teachers

The educational program is an important part of the overall inpatient psychiatric treatment. The general objectives of the program are to help the adolescents to keep up with their regular educational workload and to complete at least a part of their academic assignment so that it is not difficult for them to integrate into school after discharge. However, the majority of patients hospitalized for short-term psychiatric treatment have already fallen behind in their academic achievement due to emotional, motivational, and learning problems. They are not interested in keeping up with their academic work. The initial evaluation should help teachers determine the achievement level of each child, the degree of motivation, and the existence of learning deficits. A report from the adolescent's regular school will usually reveal whether there are behavior problems in the classroom.

Students may be divided into four groups for tutoring purposes.

Group 1 includes children who have been doing well in academic achievement and who are motivated to continue keeping up with their school assignments. Their parents should bring their daily assignments (from their schools, perhaps on a weekly basis). The task of the teachers of this group of students is simply to help them with their school assignments, to grade their work, and to report it to their home schools.

The second group includes those adolescents who have been in the special educational system in their home schools and need special help to keep up with their schoolwork. This group also includes patients whose past educational history does not indicate specific learning problems because they have achieved good academic grades until about a year or two ago when their grades started falling. Both of these groups, however, should be motivated enough to work independently with some help from the teachers.

The third group includes patients who are completely unmotivated and have been contemplating dropping out of school. This group may require a special curriculum designed to improve their motivation to learn. Regular classroom work may drive these patients further away from learning.

The fourth group includes adolescents whose achievement has been depressed primarily because of chronic emotional and family problems. Their achievement motivation varies from day to day. They require a great deal of attention from the teachers. Therapy staff of the ward may also be called upon to help educate these adolescents.

This grouping of the students has to be kept fairly flexible. The ward population may fit into different groups from those mentioned above. Some adolescents are initially put into the wrong group and should be moved into the right group later on. Teachers have to adapt their tutoring style to fit the needs of each group.

In planning a special education curriculum for groups 3 and 4, it is important not to fill in their school hours with recreational or therapy activities. Recreational and therapy activities are usually scheduled during the day at different hours. Education is an important aspect of an adolescent's daily life and should not be replaced with other activities, especially when most of these adolescents have had negative experiences in learning. Spending school time in recreational activities on a regular basis is not likely to improve their motivation to learn. However, learning should be fun and can be presented in different forms including a recreational form. The educational program should maintain the basic parameters of learning such as thinking, problem solving, gaining new knowledge, and evaluating new concepts. Students should be expected to engage in educational activities during school hours. Motivation is best improved by selecting interesting educational material that can be completed by the student without difficulty. This gives the student a sense of accomplishment and increases his desire to learn. In addition, educational material should be presented in more interesting formats such as educational films and computer programs. Films should always be followed by student summaries, group discussions, or questionnaires that are completed by the students after watching the film. The teacher should feel free to ask child care or therapy staff to help them in educational planning and programming for certain children. In fact, such collaboration should take place on a regular basis and should focus on the problems of certain very difficult, unmotivated students.

Specific Treatment Objectives Set by Therapists

Most adolescent hospital treatment units provide several hours of daily psychological treatment by various members of the therapy staff such as social workers, psychologists, psychiatrists, and therapists. Therapy modalities generally include group therapy, individual therapy, and family therapy. The specific details of these modalities of treatment as applied to an inpatient psychiatric unit are discussed in Chapter 5. The rest of this section describes the overall goals of psychological treatment as carried out by various therapy staff.

The overall goals of psychological treatment are limited in a short-term hospital setting. Treatment rarely strives to achieve emotional insight or character change. Instead, the main treatment goals to which the majority of the therapy time is devoted are resolution of the crisis and stabilization of the patient and his family.

In daily therapy sessions, it is helpful to outline certain objectives that are achievable during the short-term therapy. The following objectives, although fairly broad, may be utilized in working with most adolescents, especially those with an adjustment disorder and mild conduct problems. Therapists may help patients to do the following:

1. Identify their problems.
2. Explore the possible causes of their problems.
3. Find better ways to deal with their problems.
4. Understand their problems in the context of their family dynamics.
5. Learn to negotiate with their families on matters on which there is disagreement.
6. Understand and accept pharmacotherapy when necessary.
7. Develop positive feelings about discussing and exploring problems in psychotherapy.

It is rarely possible to achieve these objectives during a short period of hospitalization, and most patients need to continue therapy on an outpatient basis after discharge. Sometimes it takes a great deal of effort and energy just to change the patient's negative attitude toward hospitalization and therapy. Denying personal problems and blaming their environment (i.e., family, school, peers) are common defense mechanisms among these patients. It may take great therapeutic effort and skill to break through this denial and rejection. Some patients leave the hospital still maintaining their denial. This situation is sometimes due to a lack of clarity in setting therapeutic objectives and poor communication among the therapy staff.

The specific therapy objectives should be shared by all therapy staff involved in the treatment of the adolescent and his family. The objective can be outlined by any of the therapists but should be based upon input from all the other therapists involved in treating the adolescent and his family. The list of objectives should be regarded as tentative, and new objectives may be added to the list as more information becomes available. Old objectives may be deleted once they have been achieved.

DISCHARGE PLANNING

Discharge planning should begin at the time of admission. The planner should assess whether the newly admitted patient will need further treatment after discharge and what type of treatment will be most helpful and economical for that patient. Most hospitalized adolescents need some type of treatment after short-term hospitalization. In fact, many adolescent programs include the cost of follow-up in the hospital charges and provide follow-up therapy for 10 to 12 sessions as part of the package. However, much longer treatment on an outpatient basis is frequently necessary for the majority of the patients.

Discharge planning should include contact with the schools and community agencies that have been involved with the patient and his family. The question of foster placement should be raised very early during the evaluation phase because a great deal of time and energy is required to find appropriate foster homes.

Delinquent adolescents currently under supervision or probation should be reported to the probation department. Probation officers are frequently interested in knowing about the outcome of psychiatric evaluation and treatment. In some cases, a recommendation to extend supervision or probation may be therapeutic, especially when the adolescent needs external controls but his family is ineffective in setting appropriate limits.

About 5% to 10% of hospitalized adolescents require extended care. This group of patients usually suffer from severe depression, eating disorders, borderline personalities, schizoid disorders, and/or severe family problems. Most short-term hospital programs do not keep patients more than 6 to 8 weeks. Many of these patients should be transferred to a medium-term facility once the acute crisis is resolved. Unfortunately, few communities have a well-planned and coordinated mental health care system. Most facilities work independently and have their own special rules for intake and admission. A lack of coordination between private and state facilities is common in most communities. Awareness of the peculiarities of different mental health facilities in a particular community helps the discharge planner avoid repeated frustrations in finding an appropriate facility. Most adolescents requiring extended care are either kept in general hospitals for a long time or are discharged to their own homes with outpatient follow-up care. Unfortunately, many of these patients return to the hospital within a short period of time. This process is frequently repeated several times until public and private agencies come up with resources to hospitalize such a patient in a medium-term or long-term facility.

For the majority of patients, discharge planning includes helping families find appropriate mental health professionals or agencies in their own community. During the treatment phase, the adolescent patient and his family must be made aware of the existence and nature of long-term problems and the need for continued treatment in an outpatient setting. Unfortunately, this aspect of the treatment is frequently ignored, and not enough time is spent in dealing with the resistance of the patient and his family to further treatment.

REFERENCES

Cytryn L, McKnew C, Logue M, et al: Biochemical correlates of affective disorders in children. *Arch Gen Psychiatry* 1974; 31:659–661.

Durrell DD: *Durrell Analysis of Reading Difficulty.* New York, Harcourt, Brace, & World, 1955.

Gates A, McKillop A: *Reading Diagnostic Tests.* New York, Teachers College Press, Columbia University, 1962.

Gray WS, Robinson HM: *Gray Oral Reading Test.* Indianapolis, Bobbs-Merrill Co, 1963.

Greden JF: Laboratory tests in psychiatry, in Kaplan HI, Sadock B (eds): *Comprehensive Textbook of Psychiatry,* ed 4. Baltimore, Williams & Wilkins, 1985, p 203.

Kerkhofs M, Hoffmann G, DeMartelaere V, et al: Sleep EEG recording in depressive disorders. *J Affective Disord* 1985; 9:47–53.

Khan AU: Biochemical profile of depressed adolescents. *J Am Acad Child Adolesc Psychiatry* 1987; 26:873–878.

Kupfer DJ, Coble P, Kane J, et al: Imipramine and EEG sleep in children with depressive symptoms. *Psychopharmacology* 1979; 60:117–123.

Liebowitz MR, Klein DF: Differential diagnosis and treatment of panic attacks and phobic states. *Annu Rev Med* 1981; 32:583–599.

Loosen PT, Wilson IC, et al: Thyroid stimulating hormone response after thyrotropin-releasing hormone in depressed, schizophrenic and normal women. *Psychoneuroendocrinology* 1977; 2:137–148.

Maas JW, Matlox SE, Greene NM, et al: 3-Methoxy-4-hydroxyphenethelene-glycol production by the human brain in vivo. *Science* 1979; 205:1025–1027.

McDowell CF: *The Leisure Well-being Inventory.* Eugene, OR, Lifestyle Consultants, 1979.

McKnew DH, Cytryn L: Urinary metabolites in chronically depressed children. *J Am Acad Child Adolesc Psychiatry* 1979; 18:608–615.

Mendlewicz J, Hoffmann G, Kerkhofs M, et al: Electroencephalogram and neuroendocrine parameters in pubertal and adolescent depressed children. *J Affective Disord* 1984; 6:265–272.

Peters J, Davis J, Goolsby C, et al: *Physician's Handbook: Screening for MBD.* CIBA, Medical Horizon, 1973.

Pitts F, McClure J: Lactate metabolism in anxiety neurosis. *N Engl J Med* 1967; 227:1329.

Prange AM Jr, Lipton M, Nemeroff C, et al: The roles of hormones in depression. *Life Sci* 1977; 20:1305–1318.

Ragheb MG, Beard JG: Leisure satisfaction: Concept, theory, and measurement, in Iso-Ahola SE (ed): *Social Psychological Perspective on Leisure and Recreation.* Springfield, IL, Charles C Thomas Publishers, 1980.

Witt PA: *Leisure Diagnostic Battery, 1982.* Denton, TX, N Texas State University, 1982.

2 | Hospital Treatment for Substance Abuse Disorders

There are a large number of treatment facilities for substance abuse disorders. It is, however, important to appreciate the differences among various types of facilities before referring your patient for treatment. Most inpatient treatment facilities for adolescents with substance abuse disorders may be grouped into two broad categories:

1. Free-standing centers.
2. Hospital-associated units.

The free-standing centers vary widely in the type of services they provide and the philosophy of treatment. These facilities may range from a modern well-furnished building with plenty of recreational activities to residential units with very meager resources. The philosophy of treatment is even more variable than the physical setups are because they originated from such diverse sources as religion, cult groups, and medicine. The facilities are managed and run by churches, cult groups, medical professionals, and patient groups. The substance abuser usually stays in these facilities from a couple of months to more than a year. The techniques of treatment also show extreme variations ranging from brain-washing techniques to self-exploration and analytic therapy designed for conflict resolution.

The hospital-based treatment units may be independent units situated away from the main hospital building, or they may be part of the patient floors and interdigitate with other treatment programs. Some units treat only adolescents with substance abuse problems, while others take adolescents with a dual diagnosis of severe emotional problems as well as substance abuse problems. The treatment philosophies of these hospital-based units tends to be fairly uniform and is based upon medical and psychiatric models.

Hospital treatment of adolescents with substance abuse disorders may be conceptualized in the same manner as that of adolescents with severe emotional problems. The treatment program is broken down into four phases:

1. Crisis phase.
2. Evaluation phase.
3. Treatment phase.
4. Discharge planning and follow-up.

CRISIS PHASE

Admission for substance abuse problems seems to be much less stressful for the patient and the staff than is admission for primary emotional problems. Many of these admissions are planned in advance, and most of these adolescents have undergone some treatment for substance abuse problems on an outpatient basis before hospital treatment. The patient and the family are well aware of the lack of progress or insufficient progress in the outpatient treatment program and are able to accept the hospital treatment more willingly. Some facilities do not accept adolescents who are to be admitted voluntarily in order to have a better control over their discharge. Most hospitalized adolescents in these programs seem to accept, at least to some degree, that they have a substance abuse problem but lack insight into the seriousness of their problem.

The families of these adolescents also appear less stressed and more relaxed than do the families of adolescents hospitalized primarily for emotional problems. This difference may be the result of a better understanding of the nature of substance abuse problems than of emotional problems. The substance abuse problem is fairly concrete and well identified and is much less confusing than is the array of labels assigned to emotional problems. It is not uncommon for some parents to say "Now that we have identified the problem, we can do something about it."

EVALUATION PHASE

Evaluation of substance abuse problems requires an investigation into the social, psychological, and biological factors that contribute to it. A comprehensive evaluation should include the following:

1. Extensive history obtained from different members of the family.
2. Mental status and physical examination.
3. Collateral information from school and community agencies.
4. Ward observation by the nursing staff.
5. Educational evaluation.
6. Use of leisure time evaluation.
7. Assessment of participation in group therapy sessions.
8. Assessment of participation in individual therapy sessions.
9. Laboratory Tests.
10. Specific substance abuse evaluation.
11. Psychiatric diagnosis.

The above list includes the same items listed in the evaluation of emotional problems in Chapter 1, "Hospital Treatment of Emotionally Disturbed Adolescents," thus emphasizing the importance of placing the drug abuse problem in the larger context of the psychiatric problem(s). A detailed description of each of these items has been given in Chapter 1. This section will discuss only those additional points that are helpful and relevant to the evaluation of substance abuse disorders.

History

The history is usually obtained from the family. However, parents are often unaware of the substance abuse problem of their adolescent. Many adolescents start smoking cigarettes at the beginning of their teenage years. Soon after, they may experiment with marijuana and other drugs. Most parents hear about their teenager's substance abuse from other people or from legal authorities after the adolescent has been apprehended for possession, use, or illegal activities under the influence of drugs. Generally, this knowledge comes as a surprise to most parents.

The family, however, can provide accurate information about the behavioral changes of the adolescent that are indicative of or frequently associated with substance abuse problems. The interviewer should probe for and carefully document changes in peer relationships, family relationships, academic achievement, eating and sleeping habits, weight changes, style of dress and hair, and changes in previous interests and hobbies. Of course many of these changes may reflect other psychiatric problems such as depression, an adjustment disorder, and an oppositional disorder or simply normal adolescent rebellion. Peers have a major influence on the acquisition of drug abuse. A close association with peers who are known substance abusers is generally an indicator of substance abuse by the adolescent.

The family history of substance abuse should be carefully elicited. This information can also be obtained from close relatives who are visited by the patient. Some parents may be reluctant to reveal their own past history of substance abuse. They must be informed, however, that their own past history of substance abuse has undoubtedly influenced their child's early development and is most helpful to a correct understanding of some of his current behavior. The current drinking habits and substance abuse problems of the parents should be recorded in detail, including the amount and frequency of abuse, behavior changes associated with abuse, and the amount of alcohol and other drugs available in the house and their accessibility to the children.

Mental Status Examination

Many adolescents with frequent and/or daily substance abuse problems become careless about their self-care and hygiene. They wear the same clothes for several days at a time without paying attention to the smell and cleanliness of these clothes. Similarly, habits of bathing and shaving may become irregular. Shirts and jerseys depicting the pictures and names of various rock groups often indicate an interest in drugs. Most interviewers are not familiar with various rock groups but should not hesitate to ask the adolescent about their interest in such groups.

The majority of adolescents are able to provide a fairly accurate history of their drug abuse. However, sufficient time and patience are necessary to elicit such information. The affect and mood of the patient may depend upon the amount and the type of drug used before hospitalization. The majority of adolescents using marijuana and stimulants appear somewhat depressed and dysphoric during the first week of hospitalization. The depressed affect may deepen during the second week, and it should be differentiated from major depression. However, several studies show that this depressed affect is frequently due to the withdrawal of drugs and does not constitute an underlying non–drug-related depression with heavy substance abusers. It may be necessary to wait 2 to 3 weeks to decide whether or not the depression is drug related.

These patients are able to give a fairly good account of their difficulties in school and in peer and family relationships, but they have little or no insight into the causes of these difficulties and deny that their substance abuse has created any problems. In fact, they are more likely to cite their problems with peers or with parents as being the cause of their excessive drug use.

Ward Observation

A systematic observation of the behavior of these adolescents should be made by the nursing staff, especially with regard to their relationships with peers and adults, attitude toward the treatment program, daily habits of eating and sleeping, self-care skills and hygiene, interest in various unit activities, interest in a particular type of music and clothes, and mood changes. These observations are very helpful in planning the specific goals of treatment by the nursing staff. Ward observation checklists (listed in the Appendix) are a helpful way to make these observations.

Educational Evaluation

This evaluation is carried out primarily by the teachers of the educational program of the ward. A great deal of information is generally available from the home schools of these adolescents. The teachers in the program should telephone the home school of the patient soon after admission to obtain basic information, especially with regard to classroom placement, behavior and learning problems in the classroom, and the level of functioning in various subjects. This information is extremely helpful in integrating the new patient into the educational program during the first week. Educational testing using such screening tests as the wide-range achievement test (WRAT) provides teachers with some insight into the patient's level of functioning in basic academic subjects. Adolescents suspected of having specific learning disabilities require more extensive testing by special education teachers and/or the psychologist.

Leisure Activity Evaluation

A detailed description of this evaluation is given in Chapter 1, "Hospital Treatment of Emotionally Disturbed Adolescents." The majority of these adolescents have dropped out of organized sports and have quit their hobbies. Most of their time is spent with other drug-abusing friends around sedentary activities. These adolescents have little or no insight into the relationship between their drug abuse and their current lack of interest in sports activities.

Group Therapy Participation

Group therapy is a commonly used modality of treatment in adolescent treatment units. In general, adolescents are more likely to respond to suggestions made by their peers than by adults. Peer pressure in groups is frequently utilized to modify individual behavior. It is quite difficult for a patient to deny some of his behavior in front of peers who are more likely to be aware of it than is the adult therapist. A systematic evaluation of group behavior can be carried out with the help of a group behavior checklist (listed in the Appendix). This checklist focuses on behavior characteristics such as openness/secretiveness, outgoing/submissive, and helpful/disruptive.

Individual Therapy Evaluations

In addition to difficulties in communicating with adults and mistrust of adults, two other common problems in individual therapy with adolescents are denial and projection of their problems. It is important that the adolescent understand the purpose of talking about his problems in individual therapy. It should be impressed upon him that talking about his problems helps in many ways such as getting it off of his chest, acceptance and better understanding, and finding new ways to solve the problems. The therapist should help the patient to find specific issues for therapeutic dialogues. The list of issues may be arranged on a priority basis, and issues are taken one at a time, depending on the primary concerns of the patient. This evaluation should accurately determine the knowledge and the insight of the patient into his problems and his capacity to verbalize them. Certain patients seem more comfortable with certain staff of certain age and sex and may respond in individual therapy sessions with them. Such choices may sometimes, however, be motivated by a desire to manipulate rather than a sincere desire to relate to a specific staff person. Some parents also request a specific therapist because they feel that their daughter or son converses better with that therapist. In most of these cases, such requests are motivated by the parents' own sex biases and do not reflect the wishes of their adolescent.

Very quiet and withdrawn patients are considered poor candidates for individual psychotherapy. These patients are also very quiet and withdrawn in group therapy. They can benefit from individual sessions if the goals of the therapy are limited and geared toward helping them become more expressive of their throughts and feelings. The capacity to develop transference is frequently considered an important factor in the progress and success of individual therapy in outpatient settings. In short-term therapy in a hospitalized patient, however, major consideration is given to the capacity and willingness of the patient to explore his problems and find alternate and more acceptable ways of dealing with them.

Laboratory Tests

In addition to the routine laboratory tests (complete blood count [CBC], urine analysis, VDRL) required by most hospitals, urine and blood screening tests for drugs are commonly performed. These tests may not be of any great significance since most adolescents voluntarily acknowledge the abuse of drugs. In cases of acute intoxication, blood levels of alcohol and drugs do help in determining the severity of intoxication and in planning appropriate treatment. In addition, drug screening at admission provides a baseline that is helpful in detecting suspected use of drugs during the hospitalization period or during short visits outside the hospital. Most standard urine screening tests will determine the presence of traces of barbiturates, nicotine, methaqualone (Quaalude), opiates, cocaine, and a number of other drugs commonly used as tranquilizers. These substances generally disappear from the body within a day and cannot be detected by urine screens a couple of days later. Marijuana, however, is slowly metabolized and stays in the body for a much longer period of time. Urine screens for marijuana can detect significant traces of its metabolites for at least a month after its use. Since substance-abusing adolescents are at high risk for sexually transmitted diseases and the acquired immunodeficiency syndrome (AIDS), it is important nowadays to check adolescents carefully for their presence.

Substance Abuse Evaluation

Substance abuse evaluation is frequently carried out by workers or exaddicts who have been working in the field for some time. These workers tend to create a climate of mysticism around the evaluation of substance abuse. They talk as if they possess a sixth sense and can smell or spot a substance abuser from a distance. Such an attitude is unfortunate and should be discouraged. Any evaluation of substance abuse should be based on clinical data derived from the patient, the family interview, and collateral information from community agencies and schools.

Most adolescents are able to give a fairly accurate history of their use of various substances. A few may hide or minimize their substance use, but even these patients give an accurate account of their substance use after they have settled down in the hospital mileu. They realize that the staff already suspects or is aware of their substance abuse and that hiding this problem is likely to prolong their stay in the hospital.

The interviewer should carry out a semistructured psychiatric interview. He should initially avoid those questions that are likely to result in denial. The interviewer should not begin by saying that he is going to do a substance abuse evaluation. There should be a standard psychiatric interview that first focuses on the problems that are of primary interest to the patient before focusing on determining substance abuse. The interviewer should progress from asking easily answered questions to more serious and insight-eliciting questions. Specific questions must be asked with regard to the amount, frequency, and duration of the use of various drugs and their perceived effects on the user. The interviewer should avoid making judgmental comments with regard to the amount and lethality of the drugs abused. A comprehensive evaluation should include the following:

1. Determination of the extent of drug abuse.
2. Lifestyle changes in the abuser (changes in personal life, in social and family relationships, and in academic achievement).
3. Motivation and contributing factors to the use of drugs (such as family situation, peer relationships, and school problems).
4. Insight into the problem of drug abuse.
5. Motivation to change.

The determination of the extent of the drug abuse problem is based on information derived from various sources. Information from the patient is gathered through self-assessment questionnaires and individual psychiatric interviews. Self-assessment questionnaires help patients think about their drug use and promote communication in the subsequent individual interviews. The following self-assessment substance use questionnaire has been found helpful by us and can be given to all new adolescent patients for completion.

Psychiatric Interview for Substance Abuse

The following questions are listed as sample questions for a semistructured psychiatric interview. The questions are divided into four groups.

Group A Questions

These questions are helpful in determining the amount, frequency, and duration of the use of various drugs.

* Do you smoke cigarettes?
* How many cigarettes were you smoking before you came to the hospital?
* When did you start smoking?
* Have you increased your smoking in the past 6 months?
* By how much?
* How does smoking cigarettes affect you?
* Have you tried smoking marijuana (pot, grass)?
* When did you try it for the first time?
* How did it affect you?
* How often have you smoked marijuana in the past 6 months?
* Is this an increase from before?
* By how much?
* When do you usually smoke?
* Do you generally smoke marijuana with friends or by yourself?
* Do you buy some of your own marijuana?
* Do you own some of the gadgets used to smoke pot?
* How does smoking pot affect you now?
* Do you drink beer or hard liquor?
* When did you start drinking?
* How often did you drink in the past 6 months?
* Is this an increase from before?
* By how much?
* How often have you gotten drunk or passed out?
* When do you usually drink?
* Do you generally drink with friends or by yourself?
* Do you buy your own alcohol?
* How does drinking affect you?
* Who else drinks in your family?
* How often?
* How much?
* Have you tried other drugs?

Note.—Name some drugs if the patient cannot recall their names. Patients frequently use the street names of the drugs. To be certain about which drugs are being used, ask the patient to describe its effect on him. For each of the drugs used by the patient, the interviewer should ask the same kinds of questions as listed for marijuana.

Group B Questions

This set of questions is more provocative and is designed to determine the effects of drug abuse on the lifestyle of the user:

- Do you have any close friends?
- Do most of your close friends use drugs?
- Who do you spend most of your time with (the ones that use drugs or the ones that don't)?
- Have you changed your close friends during the past year?
- Why?
- How do you get along with your parents? (Ask about the relationship with each member of the family.)
- Has there been a change in your relationship with your family in the past 6 months or the last year? (Discuss its severity.)
- How are you doing in school?
- What kind of grades did you receive last semester?
- How do these grades compare with your grades of a year ago?
- Are you not completing some of your assignments?
- Have you been skipping school?
- If yes, how often?
- Where do you go?
- Are you involved in any sports activities this year?
- How does it compare with your interest in sports a year ago?
- Do you have a job now?
- How does it compare with a year ago?
- Do you have any other interests or hobbies that you spend time on?
- How does it compare with your interests a year ago?
- Have you lost or gained any weight in the past 6 months?
- Do you sleep well?
- How many hours of sleep do you get in 24 hours?

Group C Questions

This group of questions is designed to determine the patient's motivation and contributing factors toward the use or abuse of drugs.

- Do you use drugs when you are upset, angry, or unhappy?
- Do you use drugs when you are tired?
- Do you use drugs to experience some excitement or "high" feelings?
- Do you believe that you would use drugs much less if you did not associate with your present group of friends?

- How do you feel when you have not taken drugs for a few days?
- Have people told you that you are always in a good mood after you have used drugs?
- Do you get along better with your family after you have used drugs?
- How often do you go to school after you have used drugs?
- How do the drugs affect your schoolwork?
- Have you ever been arrested for the use or possession of drugs?
- Have you ever been in a car accident while driving under the influence of drugs?
- Have you been on probation, or are there any charges pending against you?
- Have you stolen money or things to buy drugs?
- Do you lie often to avoid punishment or consequences?

Group D Questions
The following questions are designed to determine the presence of insight and personal motivation to discontinue the use of drugs:

- How does your drug use compare with that of your friends?
- Do you believe that you use drugs more than the average child of your age does?
- Do you think that there is a relationship between your drug use and the problems in the family and at school?
- Do you think that you may be dependent upon the drugs (that means that you have to use drugs to feel normal)?
- Have you tried to quit drugs for a month or more?
- What happened?
- Do you think that you can quit drugs whenever you want to?
- Do you believe that you have to give up your friends if you quit using drugs?
- How are you going to handle peer pressure if you quit drugs?
- Can you picture your lifestyle without the use of drugs?

Psychiatric Diagnosis
The diagnosis of substance abuse disorder is frequently associated with other psychiatric diagnoses in adolescent groups such as conduct disorder, oppositional disorder, impulse control disorders, and attention deficit disorders. The diagnosis of substance abuse disorder is frequently based on the type, the amount, the frequency, and the duration of the substances abused. In addition, diagnostic classifications take into consideration the psychological, social, and biological effects of the drugs and the degree of dependency on the drugs. Many professionals believe that any use of illegal psychoactive substances should be labeled as substance abuse, while others consider this to be an overzealous approach. There is also a disparity in the standards used to diagnose substance abuse between teenagers and adults. For example, alcohol and tobacco is normally consumed by a large proportion of adults, but their use by teenagers in any amount is considered illegal in most states. Besides the fact that

teenagers are not mature enough to handle the effects of even a small amount of alcohol (and other drugs), there are pervasive fears that each teenager who begins to drink is likely to progress to dependency and addiction.

There are several diagnostic classifications that have been advanced by different groups, and they are usually based on the philosophical biases of each group. Most classifications recognize that there is some use of illegal substances that is motivated primarily by curiosity and experimentation. The majority of teenagers, however, do not progress beyond such experimentation. There is, however, a substantial number of teenagers (and some preteens) who become regular users of illegal drugs, and some subsequently become dependent and addicted. It is frequently very difficult to distinguish between adolescents who are experimenting, those who have become regular users, and those who have become dependent. The criteria for classifying drug users has changed in the past decades and will continue to change depending upon the availability of the drug and the proportion of the teenage population involved.

The American Medical Association has suggested four categories of drug abuse:

1. Drug experimentation.
2. Drug use (further subdivided into recreational and regular use categories).
3. Drug abuse.
4. Drug dependency.

The second report of the National Commission on Marijuana and Drug Abuse (1973) identified five patterns of drug abuse:

1. Drug experimentation.
2. Social and recreational use.
3. Circumstantial and situational drug use.
4. Intensified drug use.
5. Compulsive drug use.

Nizama and Jerga (1978) take into consideration various psychosocial factors that are associated with the progressive abuse of drugs. They divide progressive substance abuse into 11 substages:

1. Curiosity.
2. Initiation.
3. Pleasure.
4. Group identification.
5. Group prestige.
6. Family isolation.
7. Psychopathic behavior.
8. Ritualistic behavior.
9. Dependency and tolerance.
10. General physical deterioration.
11. Severe sociopathic personality destruction.

MacDonald (1984) divides substance abuse into five progressive stages:

Stage 0.—Curiosity.
Stage 1.—Learning the mood swing.
Stage 2.—Seeking the mood swing.
Stage 3.—Preoccupation with the mood swing.
Stage 4.—Doing drugs to feel okay.

The American Psychiatric Association's diagnostic classification (DSM III R) divides psychoactive substance abuse into three classifications:

1. Psychoactive substance use.
2. Psychoactive substance abuse.
3. Psychoactive substance dependency.

We find it very difficult to classify teenage substance abuse into clear-cut categories as suggested by these different classifications. Substance abuse by teenagers is very erratic, and the frequency of abuse may vary greatly between the summer vacation and the school months. A clear-cut pattern may be difficult to identify. The following classification of stages has been helpful in diagnosis, prognosis, and treatment.

STAGES OF SUBSTANCE ABUSE

Stage 1, Experimental Stage

Motivation
The primary motivation for the use of drugs during this stage is curiosity. However, other important reasons include peer pressure, a strong desire to be accepted by peers, an inclination to go along with peers, and a fear to be rejected or be called "chicken" by peers.

Types of Drugs Used
The types of drugs tried during this stage are few and the less addictive types. However, the availability and cost of different drugs in a community frequently determine their choice. The most commonly abused drugs during this stage are alcohol and marijuana. The use of LSD and stimulants is also quite common during this stage.

Frequency of Drug Abuse
Drug abuse is occasional or once in a while. No consistent or regular pattern of use is present. There is no increase in drug use in the past 3 to 6 months.

Lifestyle Changes
These include changes in personal life, in social and family relationships, and in academic achievement. The changes in personal life refer to personal interests, hobbies, sports, work habits, and sleeping and eating habits. These changes should be

carefully documented and distinguished from changes due to normal adolescent rebellion. Drug abuse during this stage has no adverse effects on personal, social, educational, and family relationships.

Prognosis

Most adolescents do not increase their use of drugs beyond this stage. However, the presence of chronic problems such as learning disabilities, conduct disorders, family problems, and drug-abusing parents predispose adolescents for greater abuse of drugs.

Treatment

These adolescents should receive detailed knowledge about the adverse effects of various drugs and the psychosocial consequences of the continued use of drugs.

Stage 2, Frequent Abuse of Drugs

Motivation

There are two common motivations to continue the use of drugs after the experimentation stage.

Seeking euphoria.—There is a group of adolescents that tends to seek excitement, irrespective of the sources from which it may arise. Drugs and delinquent behavior such as fighting, stealing, and gang activities are all sources of excitement for these adolescents.

Avoidance of dysphoria (tension reduction).—This group of adolescents uses drugs primarily to reduce tension, frustration, anger, unhappiness and depression (for example, the use of drugs after an argument in the family or with a teacher or coach or to allay constant fatigue and tiredness).

Types of Drugs Used

The types of drugs used in this stage are pretty much the same ones that have been tried during the experimental stage. However, experimentation with more addictive drugs (i.e., cocaine, narcotics) may begin during this stage. The user does not depend on friends for the supply of drugs and begins to spend his own money to buy drugs and its paraphernalia.

Frequency of Drug Abuse

The frequency increases from occasional use to more frequent use such as on most weekends and holidays.

Lifestyle Changes

Drug abuse begins to affect all areas of functioning including personal life, social and family relationships, and academic achievement. Changes in interests, hobbies, self-care, style of clothes, and type of music may reflect the living style of the drug subculture. The user may want to drop out of sports activities and quit part-time work. House rules are frequently broken, which leads to frequent family arguments.

Prognosis

A few adolescents at this stage are able to quit drug abuse on their own, usually after experiencing severe consequences that "wakes them up" and "turns them around." Others maintain their drug abuse at this level at the cost of lower school grades, dropping out of sports, and having chronically strained relationship with their families. In the evaluation of these adolescents it is important to differentiate the chronic personal, family, and educational problems caused by drug abuse from the chronic problems existing before the beginning of drug abuse. However, chronic problems existing before drug abuse become worse after the onset of drug abuse.

Treatment

This group of adolescents requires fairly intensive treatment to help them quit their frequent use of drugs and to prevent them from progressing to stage 3. The modality of group therapy is frequently used to create insight into the psychosocial consequences of their drug abuse. The users should also learn about their specific reasons and motivations for using drugs. Alternate ways are explored by each user to meet the same needs without the use of drugs.

Stage 3, Dependency Stage

Motivation

Progression from stage 2 to stage 3 is frequently accidental and is possibly based on genetic and psychosocial predispositions. The abuser experiences dysphoria, irritability, low frustration tolerance, unhappiness, suicidal ideation, and occasional physical symptoms while not under the influence of drugs. The drugs are used just to feel "normal" (without dysphoria).

Types of Drugs Used

In addition to the previous drugs, the user is now pretty much open to trying any new drugs that are available. Intravenous use of drugs increases.

Frequency of Drug Abuse

Abuse of drugs increases from frequent use to daily use. The user may be under the influence of drugs during most of the waking hours.

Lifestyle Changes

All areas of functioning are adversely affected: skipping school or completely dropping out of school, quitting jobs, spending time exclusively with drug-abusing friends, severely strained relationship with the family, increased delinquency and stealing.

Prognosis

The prognosis is generally poor without professional help. An abuser may continue a very unproductive and delinquent lifestyle for years in the absence of professional help. Some are incarcerated in juvenile detention facilities as a consequence of severe delinquent activities. Overdosing and death are not uncommon.

Treatment

Initial hospitalization and long-term follow-up therapy after discharge are the treatments of choice.

TREATMENT PROGRAM

Most hospital programs for short-term treatment of substance abuse focus on intoxicated or heavy abusers of drugs and alcohol. The treatment is primarily designed to detoxify these individuals. These programs also offer psychological services to improve self-esteem and to regain a sense of responsibility. Most adolescents hospitalized in these programs rarely manifest severe withdrawal symptoms. However, withdrawal symptoms of mild to moderate degrees are frequently manifested by mood changes such as dysphoria and irritability, boredom, restlessness, impulsivity, and sleep and appetite problems. These symptoms are generally managed by a structured mileau program and the enforcement of regular habits of sleeping, eating, exercise, and recreation. Treatment with medication is rarely found necessary. However, each adolescent patient should be evaluated and observed carefully for any symptoms of severe excitement or delirium. It is generally better to treat suspected symptoms of delirium (autonomic hyperactivity such as tachycardia, sweating, and high blood pressure) fairly early to avoid possible life-threatening symptoms.

Theoretical Background

A large number of theories have been advanced to explain the social, psychological, and biological factors that contribute to the development, maintenance, and cessation of substance abuse. The interested reader may refer to several monographs that have summarized the existing points of views in this field (*Theories of Drug Abuse,* edited by Lettieri et al., 1980). The frequent questions that have been addressed by most theorists and planners of treatment programs relate to the following (Lettieri et al., 1980):

1. Why people begin taking drugs (initiation).
2. Why people maintain their drug taking behavior (continuation).
3. How or why drug taking behavior escalates to heavy abuse (escalation).
4. Why or how people stop taking drugs (cessation).
5. What accounts for the resumption of the drug-dependent behavior after stopping (relapse).

The following factors have been identified by various theorists to explain some of the aforementioned questions:

1. Degree of access to narcotic drugs.—It is necessary for the drugs to be available before a prone person can become addicted to them. The societies that limit and control the availability of drugs usually have fewer individuals who are heavy substance abusers or who are dependent on drugs.

2. Personality factors.—Most theories emphasize the specific personality characteristics of individuals who are more prone to abuse drugs. Such persons are described as motivationally immature; lacking a sense of responsibility, reliance, and initiative; possessing low frustration tolerance; and being unable to defer gratification. Greaves (1974) characterized these individuals as markedly lacking in pleasurable sensory awareness. They have lost their childlike ability to create natural euphoria through active play and recreation.

3. Beliefs.—Beliefs and internal thoughts play a major role in the development of drug dependency (Gold, 1980). The cognitive approach to treating drug-dependent behavior points out that drug abuse begins with conflict as a predisposing factor. The conflict leads to anxiety that is interpreted by the abuser as powerlessness in altering the environment to reduce anxiety. Drugs such as heroin and benzodiazepines reduce anxiety and temporarily provide better control over self.

4. Genetic factors.—These have been investigated as predisposing factors, especially for alcohol abuse. For example, it has been shown that Orientals are less likely to develop alcohol dependency because three quarters of Orientals develop a cutaneous flush and unpleasant reactions with only small amounts of alcohol (Wolff, 1973; Ewing et al., 1974; Seto et al., 1978). This finding may be related to a high frequency of atypical liver alcohol dehydrogenase among Japanese (Stamatoyannoupoulas et al., 1975). Similarly, women, in general, show higher levels of blood alcohol after ingesting a given amount of alcohol than do men (Jones and Jones, 1976).

5. Maintenance or a relapse of the drug-dependent behavior.—During the abstaining period there is an increase in anxiety, conflict, and depression or an intense desire to repeat a satisfying experience while abusing drugs. Having experienced the gratification of a supportive drug-induced pattern of ego functioning, the user may attempt to repeat this uniquely satisfying experience for defensive purposes, as a solution to conflict, or for primary delight.

Treatment Philosophy

Adolescents involved in heavy substance abuse have multiple problems relating to their personality, their attitude toward school, difficulties in peer relationships, and their family. A comprehensive treatment program must address all these social, psychological, and family problems in addition to the substance abuse behavior. The treatment philosophy and various components of treatments designed for short-term hospitalization of an emotionally disturbed adolescent also work well with adolescents who have severe substance abuse problems. However, a greater emphasis is placed on substance abuse behavior. We will describe here just those aspects of each treatment component that relate to the substance abuse problem. The reader should refer to Chapter 1, "Hospital Treatment for Emotionally Disturbed Adolescents," for a comprehensive review of the overall philosophy of treatment and a description of the various components of the treatment program.

Specific Treatment Objectives Set by the Nursing and Child Care Staff

Preoccupation with substance abuse becomes a way of life for substance-abusing adolescents. This is reflected in all areas of daily living, including the type of music they listen to, the type of clothes they wear, their recreational interests, peer relationships, self-care, and eating and sleeping habits. Most adolescent units monitor the music that these adolescents listen to. Any musical tapes with lyrics pertaining to substance use, explicit sex, or violence are censored. The unit staff should be able to point out the relationship between the type of music and the substance abuse habits. Similarly, T-shirts and clothes depicting drug symbols or muscial groups frequently associated with drug abuse are also censored on these units. The patient should not be allowed to boast about his substance abuse activities as a way of impressing his peers. The mileau staff should constantly question each patient about his preoccupation with his substance abuse and confront him with his behavior when it is related to such preoccupation.

Educational Program

This program is an essential part of the mileau and is usually divided into two categories: formal education and mental health education.

Formal education.—Almost all adolescents with substance abuse problems fall behind in their academic achievements. In fact, the beginning of the achievement problems can frequently be traced back to the onset of heavy substance abuse. An initial educational evaluation is necessary to determine the level of academic achievement and the degree of motivation to learn. The educational program is designed on the same basis as described in Chapter 1 on the program for emotionally disturbed children.

Mental health education.—There is a specific emphasis on substance abuse education through special films, lectures, and discussions. This information is organized and delivered by the staff on a regular basis. The details of several educational modules on substance abuse are given in Chapter 11 on the treatment program.

In addition these adolescents should receive mental health education on subjects such as self-esteem, assertiveness, controlling anger, and expressing their feelings and thoughts. (Refer to Chapter 11 for details.)

Group Therapy

Group therapy is a very important modality of treatment for adolescents. The details of the theory and the process have been described extensively in Chapter 3. However, group discussion is focused primarily around the substance abuse and all the social and psychological problems associated with the substance abuse. The group leader spells out the task of the group as dealing with the problems of substance abuse. Each group session begins with a brief statement about the task of the group. Then the leader asks for a brief go-around. Each member of the group states the type of problem he has been working on or would like to discuss in the group. At the end of the go-around the leader chooses some common themes for discussion by the whole group. Since most of the social and psychological problems of these groups are related to the basic problem of substance abuse, the leader can skillfully draw out individual members to discuss their specific problems and relate them to the common problems.

Most adolescents tend to blame their parents, schools, or community for their problems. They rarely recognize that in most cases it is their own substance abuse and consequent changes in their behavior that have caused the strained relationship with their parents and teachers rather than the other way around. Even those adolescents whose serious problems at home have driven them to drugs and drinking should not go unchallenged. A discussion of personal choices in the face of serious stress is always helpful to these patients and facilitates their assuming personal responsibility for their actions.

Most of these groups start out with a few adolescents dominating the group and bragging about their substance abuse activities. The group leader does not need to stop this discussion, but he should gently turn the discussion around from mere bragging to more insightful thinking. The leader should recognize that there is a great deal of curiosity and excitement associated with substance abuse and that most adolescents experiment with drugs because of these factors. The leader can ask different members to discuss the reasons and motivations for their early experimentation with drugs. The later sessions frequently deal with the consequences of substance abuse such as falling grades in school, dropping out of sports, lack of interest in hobbies, exclusive association with other drug abusers, poor self-care and hygiene, strained relationship with family members, trouble with the law, and dependency on drugs.

The concept of dependency should be focused on and heavily stressed by the group leaders. Some leaders utilized the disease concept to explain drug dependency. However, most adolescents do not feel sick and find it difficult to comprehend this concept of substance abuse. They are more likely to understand the concept in psychological terms. The leader should utilize the cigarette dependency experiences of the individual members. Questions such as why some substances cause dependency and why it is difficult to quit them are discussed in simple physiological and pathological terms. It is important that each member of the group devise his own individual plan of quitting drugs. All these plans must include necessary changes in their basic lifestyle, peer group, and leisure activities.

TREATMENT PHILOSOPHY OF NARCOTICS ANONYMOUS

This philosophy of treatment is essentially similar to the philosophy espoused by Alcoholics Anonymous (AA). The style of the meeting is also pretty much the same as that of AA. Members are encouraged, with the support of the group, to verbalize their difficulties in abstaining from drugs. Groups usually start out with confessions by each member about their past substance abuse, what brought them to the hospital, and for how many days they have been free of drugs in the hospital. The members talk about their cravings for drugs and how they deal with this craving. A great deal of emotional support is expressed by members to those who are experiencing difficulty in staying off drugs.

It is emphasized that drug addiction is a serious problem that is beyond the voluntary control of the addict. The addict cannot trust himself or his willpower to control his addiction. He must believe that he is powerless to control his substance abuse. He must trust in God and seek His help in staying drug free. The 12 steps suggested by AA and Narcotics Anonymous are listed below:

1. We admitted that we were powerless to stop our addiction, that our lives had become unmanageable.
2. We have come to believe that a power greater than ourselves can restore us to sanity.
3. We made a decision to turn our will and our lives over to the care of God as we understand Him.
4. We made a searching and fearless moral inventory of ourselves.
5. We admitted to God, to ourselves, and to another human being the exact nature of our wrongs.
6. We were entirely ready to have God remove all these defects of character.
7. We humbly ask Him to remove our shortcomings.
8. We made a list of all persons we had harmed and became willing to make amends to them all.
9. We made direct amends to such people wherever possible, except when to do so would injure them or others.
10. We continued to take personal inventory and, when we were wrong, promptly admitted it.
11. We sought through prayer and meditation to improve our conscious contact with God, as we understand Him, praying only for knowledge of His will for us and the power to carry that out.
12. Having had a spiritual awaking as a result of these steps, we tried to carry this message to addicts and to practice these principles in all our affairs.

Many inpatient substance abuse programs for adolescents utilize these 12 steps in a progressive manner for recovery from addiction. Patients learn and discuss one step at a time. Many adolescent patients find it very difficult to whole-heartedly invest and believe in these 12 steps in the treatment of their substance abuse. The main problem seems to be related to the dynamics of their developmental stage. During the early teen years, adolescents progress from total dependency upon their parents to at least a partial independence. This newly found freedom is challenged by the basic philosophy of Narcotics Anonymous. Many adolescents may in fact start substance abuse in defiance of adult authority and to exert more self-independence through substance abuse.

REFERENCES

Ewing JA, Rouse BA, Pellizar ED: Alcohol sensitivity and ethnic background. *Am J Psychiatry* 1974; 131:206–210.

Greaves G: Towards an existential theory of drug dependence. *J Nerv Ment Dis* 1974; 159:263–274.

Jones BM, Jones MK: Male and female intoxication levels for three alcohol doses, or do women really get higher than men. *Alcohol Rep* 1976; 5:11–24.

Lettieri D, Sayers M, Pearson H: *Theories on Drug Abuse.* Washington, DC, NIDA Research Monograph no. 30, 1980.

Macdonald DI: *Drugs, Drinking, and Adolescents,* ed 2. Chicago, Year Book Medical Publishers, 1989.

National Commission on Marijuana and Drug Abuse: Second Report, stock no. 5266-00003. Government Printing Office, 1973.

Nizama M: Jerga utilizada por los consumidores de drogos. *Rev Sanid* 1978; 39:175–191.

Seto A, Tricomi S, Goodwin D, et al: Biochemical correlates of ethanol induced flushing in Orientals. *J Stud Alcohol* 1978; 39:1–11.

Stamatoyannoupoulos G, Chen SH, Fukui M: Liver alcohol dehydrogenase in Japanese: High population frequency of atypical form and its possible role in alcohol sensitivity. *Am J Hum Genet* 1975; 27:789–796.

Wolff PhH: Vasomotor sensitivity to alcohol in diverse Mongoloid population. *Am J Hum Genet* 1973; 25:193–199.

3

Inpatient Psychotherapy Program

The specific therapeutic modalities commonly used in inpatient settings include group psychotherapy, individual psychotherapy, and family therapy. These therapeutic interventions have been used in and adapted to the special circumstances of inpatient units. Our discussion of these therapies will focus primarily on these adaptations.

GROUP PSYCHOTHERAPY

As a treatment modality for an adolescent inpatient unit, group psychotherapy is a very effective therapeutic tool. Most adolescents have difficulty in communicating with adults. They find it easier to talk about their problems in a group of mutually supportive peers. A working adolescent group can easily influence its members and modify some of their abnormal behavior through confrontation, mirroring, and example setting.

Types of Group Therapy

In most short-term hospitalization programs adolescents stay from 4 to 6 weeks. The group therapy program must therefore be designed to accommodate the short stay and the rapid turnover of patients. Groups have to be opened-ended to accommodate the addition of new patients and the loss of old patients. Goals have to be carefully specified so that they can be accomplished within the time frame of short-term group therapy. A homogeneous or problem-specific selection of patients for group therapy is generally impossible to achieve because of the diversity. Consequently, all patients are included in group therapy. Some therapists, however, avoid including blatantly psychotic and other very disruptive patients.

Short-term therapy groups may be classified into four or five general types (Poey, 1985):

1. Crisis groups offer multiple sources of support to members in crisis, advise

them in practical problem solving, focus heavily on solving reality problems, and motivate members to try out new action-oriented coping strategies. These groups are used for the families of adolescents who are in crisis at the time of hospitalization. Parent group meetings once a week provide a great deal of support to parents and help them through this crisis. Similarly, groups of siblings of patients may experience a crisis of their own and may be grouped in a special psychotherapy group to deal with their problems.

2. Marathon groups provide accelerated interaction techniques in the space of a day or two. Family marathon groups that include hospitalized adolescents are quite successful in dealing with severe interaction problems and with poor communication in the family. Families of patients are invited to spend a weekend with the hospitalized adolescent and the staff of the unit. The program is carefully structured to provide adequate time for supervised interaction, discussion, and recreation.

3. Process groups are frequently used in inpatient units to deal with unit problems that seem to be getting out of hand. The unit staff request such group sessions when they feel that the patients are out of control. Such group sessions are also helpful when there are specific unit problems that are escalating and not being resolved by explanations or confrontations. For example, difficulties such as scapegoating, general defiance, and misuse of equipment are general issues that concern several patients and the staff and can thus be dealt with quite effectively in these process groups. These groups are a sort of minimarathon and may last for several hours until the resolution of the identified problem is achieved.

4. Topic-focused groups (specialized groups) are focused on specific themes. They include patients who are working on a common problem such as incest, rape, adoption, assertiveness, or self-esteem. Attendance is generally voluntary, so only highly motivated youngsters join topic-focused groups, thereby deriving maximum benefits from sessions of such groups.

5. Brief open-ended inpatient groups will be the main topic of subsequent discussion.

Uniqueness of Adolescents as Patients

Although adolescents relate better to each other than to adults and learn a great deal from each other, their problems are also caused by peer influence. Adolescent patients frequently have such problems in common as substance abuse, antisocial activities, early sexual activities, rebellious attitude toward parents and adult authority figures, dropping out of school, and joining the adult work force in order to achieve economic independence and self-sufficiency.

Most adolescents feel that their problems are unique ones that adults do not understand. They are especially sensitive to criticism since they have been frequently and abundantly criticized by the members of their family, teachers, and other adults.

The majority of disturbed adolescents deny having any problems. They are quick to find rationalizations for their unacceptable behavior. For example, house rules are violated because the rules are overly strict; home chores are not done because they have other important things to do; homework may pile up because it is too much or not important enough to finish. Adolescents are also quick to blame adults for their problems. They tend to think that it is someone else who has created difficulties for them. "Everything would be fine if they (parents) would leave me alone" is a common cliché among deliquent adolescents.

Most adolescents are fairly active and restless. They are not content with sitting around and talking. They are generally more comfortable when they are active and busy in some activities. Many find it difficult to tolerate an hour-long therapy session. They have a tendency to band together in a group against adult authority. They generally have difficulty in organizing their thoughts and expressing them in a coherent manner. After a few therapy sessions, an adolescent may declare that all of his problems are resolved and that he has no need for more therapy. However, a cursory inquiry often reveals that, in reality, nothing has changed. It may be a lack of comprehension or magical thinking on the part of the adolescent that convinces him that all his problems are gone. Adolescents are frequently impatient with adults who try to take a more comprehensive approach and who explain things carefully and in detail.

Transference and countertransference problems are common in therapy with adolescents; however, not every negative or positive feeling of the patient toward the therapist is to be considered transference. A sudden and unexpected outburst of apparently irrational anger may or may not be related to the current issue in therapy. The adolescent may be angry because he perceives his therapist as one of the authority figures whom he resents. Overly dependent adolescents tend to demand and expect more favors from their therapist and may become angry when such favors are denied. Sexual feelings and fantasies are quite common toward a therapist of the opposite sex.

Goals of Short-Term Inpatient Group Therapy

Most therapists emphasize that the goals for short-term group therapy should be specific, few in number, conscious, explicit, and agreed upon by both the therapist and the participants. Furthermore, whatever goals are established and agreed upon must be related in a meaningful way to the size of the group and the duration and frequency of group sessions. Without clear goals, both the therapist and group members may wander aimlessly. Most mental health professionals are trained to deal with whatever occurs in the therapy session. This competency de-emphasizes planning and goal setting in therapy. Effective short-term group therapy requires goal setting in advance. The goals, however, should be realistic and not overly ambitious. Therapists may set group goals (for the group as a whole to work at) as well as individual goals for each patient, depending upon the unique nature of each individual problem. Group goals include the following:

1. Positive experience.—Most adolescents require further therapy after their discharge from the hospital. If their first introduction to therapy is negative, they are not likely to engage in subsequent therapy. The group leader can help ensure that each adolescent in the group has a chance to discuss his problems and that none is scapegoated or unduly pressured. Each group member must feel supported and respected for his opinion or ideas.

2. Discussion of common problems.—Most hospitalized adolescents have many problems in common, although of varying intensity. These problems include strained relationships with parents, struggle for independence, peer pressure, substance abuse, sexual intimacy, and school problems. The group leader should develop strategies to help the group discuss these issues during the period of hospitalization. In addition, there are many common problems that most adolescents experience during their teenage years. For example, the leader may focus on such specific developmental issues as the following:

- Autonomy.—Issues involving dependency/independency conflicts in relation to authority figures.
- Identity formation.—To focus on self-exploration and identity solidification by revealing one's thoughts, feelings, and opinions while being open to feedback.
- Interpersonal skills.—Focus on learning about presenter/listener and responder skills so that one can interact with more control, confidence, and less self-consciousness.
- Assertiveness.—To focus on the adolescent's tendency to relate either defiantly aggressively or compliantly passively and to replace these dysfunctional extremes with an ability to relate assertively.
- Intimacy.—To focus on the ability to be close with other persons rather than distant and isolated.

3. Improving peer interaction.—Most disturbed adolescents tend to gravitate to peer groups that are considered by others as "losers and druggies." These kids are unable to relate to other kids who are high achievers and athletic and possess high aspirations in life. The hospitalized population of adolescents contains some high achievers who are rejected by the losers. Group therapy is probably the best modality to increase awareness, understanding, and tolerance of differences among these groups of teenagers.

Selection and Preparation of Patients

It is generally impossible to run a voluntary group in an inpatient unit. Most adolescents are likely to refuse participation, at least initially, in any treatment program. Group therapy is a very important therapeutic tool, and most adolescents are likely to benefit from it. An optimum number for each group is about eight to ten patients. Each group should contain a fair proportion of male and female adolescents. Age distribution may at times be an issue for some programs. Sometimes younger adolescents tend to be dominated by older adolescents. However, a combination of older and younger adolescents generally works well because older adolescents frequently have unresolved issues from younger years while the younger adolescents may learn to avoid some of the problems of the older adolescents. If the younger adolescents form the majority of the unit population, a separate group of these adolescents may be more productive than mixing them up with a few older adolescents.

Inclusion of acutely psychotic adolescents in groups is very disruptive because they tend to make apparently irrelevant and inappropriate comments in response to their hallucinations and delusions. Such adolescents should be assigned to other tasks and should not be included in group therapy until their hallucinations are under some control with medication. Similarly, adolescents with severe attention-deficit disorder with hyperactivity find it difficult to sit in a group for an hour without becoming restless and distractible. They tend to make comments that are superficial, impulsive, and disruptive of group discussions. These youngsters generally perform better in groups after receiving hyperactivity-reducing and attention span–increasing medication.

Preparing each new patient to participate in group therapy makes it more beneficial and productive. The group leader or coleaders should interview each new patient and discuss group therapy programs as being an essential and required part of the total treatment. The leader may investigate the past experiences of the patient in individual or group therapy. The goals of group therapy are reviewed briefly with an emphasis on helping each other. Some adolescents indicate that they are not comfortable in expressing their feelings in front of others. They should be assured that they will not be forced to say things that they do not want to say. They should be advised to listen first to what others have to say and to express their feelings and ideas when they feel ready. The rapid turnover of patients is rarely a problem in such groups. There are many discharges and admissions within a short period of time. If about half of the members of each group have been in the group for more than 2 weeks it seems that they are able to integrate new members without much difficulty, and group discussion maintains continuity. It may be necessary for the therapist to repeat introductory remarks about the goals of group therapy every other session.

Leadership

Who should lead the group? Leadership of the group generally depends upon the availability and interest of the therapy staff. Adequate training and experience, however, are necessary prerequisites for leadership. The requirements of the American Group Psychotherapy Association for leaders are fairly stringent and are provided by the Association as guidelines. Hospitals in or near large urban areas and university centers generally have an abundance of qualified therapists who can serve as group leaders. Other hospitals tend to have less-qualified people available to lead such groups. Every effort should be made to have new leaders adequately trained. The requirements for group leaders should conform to the standards of the American Society for Group Psychotherapy. Inexperienced therapists frequently become frustrated and tend to overuse restrictions and control as a way of managing groups. It is perferable to have a cotherapist of equal experience and status. The leader and coleader should discuss the group process frequently so that they both have a similar understanding of the group process. The best time for discussion of the group process appears to be soon after the group meeting. The group leader and coleader should get together for 15 to 20 minutes to discuss the group process and events of that day.

Role of the Therapist

In a short-term group, therapists may utilize a variety of theoretical orientations such as psychoanalytic, cognitive, behavioral, and interpersonal. Despite various theoretical assumptions and treatment strategies, several technical characteristics are common to most short-term therapy approaches. Butcher and Koss (1978) have noted the following common issues that most short-term group therapists need to focus on:

1. Therapeutic management of time limitation.
2. Limitation of the therapy goals.
3. Focusing the therapeutic content on the present.
4. Directive approach by the therapist.
5. Rapid early assessment.
6. Promptness of intervention.
7. Selectability on the part of the therapist.
8. Ventilation and cartharsis as an important element in the group process.
9. A quickly established interpersonal relationship from which to obtain therapeutic leverage.
10. Appropriate selection of patients.

Pekala et al. (1985), through their experience with short-term problem-solving group therapy with hospitalized psychiatric patients, make the following suggestions about the therapist's role:

1. Supportive.—This includes being warm, friendly, and a good listener and responding to the needs and problems of patients in a genuine empathetic manner.
2. Provide structure.—Structure is designed primarily to promote and speed up the group process. Structure includes the format of the group meetings and a list of clear goals.
3. Seeking or requesting information.—The therapist should not hesitate to ask questions (in a nonthreatening, noncritical manner) that will clarify a problem.
4. Giving of pertinent information.—Young patients are frequently unaware of information relating to their hospitalization and treatment. They should be encouraged to question each other and the therapist.
5. Restating.—The therapist should restate a problem presented by a patient in a clearer and better-defined manner, or he may encourage another member of the group to do so.
6. Summarizing.—A long-winded description of the problem is frequently confusing to the adolescent. Summarization helps the patient and other members understand the problem better.
7. Refocusing.—Many patients are quite tangential and circumstantial in discussing their problems. They feel overwhelmed by the number of problems they experience and rapidly jump from one problem to another.
8. Giving positive feedback.—Patients appreciate a positive nod or gesture from the therapist when they try their best to help themselves and others.
9. Interpersonal observation.—Make patients aware of the opinions and feelings of other members in the group through feedback.

10. Reframing.—Take the meaning associated with a symptom, interpersonal observation, or interaction and relabel it in a less ego-dystonic way.
11. Positive connotation.—A variant of reframing, positive connotation accentuate the positive aspects of a given symptom or interpersonal interaction while altering the meaning associated with it.
12. Prompting.—Encourage members to discuss and express their opinions involving all members.
13. Gatekeeping.—This includes preventing certain members from talking while giving less-verbose members permission to talk.
14. Interpersonal inquiries.—When the therapist makes a summarizing restatement, he should ask the person whether what he said is consistent with what the patient meant. The use of such queries helps prevent mind reading and serves to clarify the interpersonal dialogue.

Yalom (1970) views the therapist as a social engineer and a model setter. As a social engineer, the therapist helps to develop a pattern of interaction and free communication. As a model setter, the therapist behaves in a forthright, nondefensive, nonjudgmental manner and accepts and appreciates other's strengths as well as their problem areas. Yalom views the group as an open system and regards the major role of the therapist as that of a manager of internal and external boundaries. The management of external boundaries involves relating the therapy to the outside world. The management of internal boundaries includes monitoring the relationship between the task of the group and its structure and ensuring that the form of the group is appropriate to its function. The therapist works as a mediator between the group members on the one hand and the consciously agreed upon primary work tasks and goals on the other hand.

A group therapist must frequently choose one of two possible poles:

- Activity/passivity.
- Common theme problems/individual problems.
- Then-and-there problems/here-and-now problems.

A therapist who focuses on "then-and-there" problems usually examines problems experienced by the patient outside the group therapy setting, including the reasons for hospitalization, and difficulties with family, friends, and other individuals. Arguments against discussing such issues are that the data presented by a patient are usually inaccurate and that the patient has had considerable time to consider the various possible solutions.

The "here-and-now" approach involves focusing on the interaction among the group members. The anger, hostility, rejection, criticism, love, and tenderness toward each other expressed in the group are real feelings and can be dealt with in the here-and-now context. The underlying assumption in this approach is that the person's present style of interaction has a past history and that the resolution of problems in the present interaction will improve difficulties in other areas. The utilization of this approach is difficult in a group of adolescents. Adolescents tend to be a homogeneous group and build up supportive relationships with each other fairly quickly. There is not enough variety of interaction among a group of adolescents to sustain group therapy for more than a few sessions. They frequently avoid confronting each other and refrain from expressing negative feelings toward each other. Adolescents are dependent upon their families and view their interaction with their families as the primary problem.

In a short-term group each individual member needs to express his unique individual problems and find some resolutions with the help of the other members. There are, however, many common problems that can be discussed by all members of the group.

There are differences among therapists with regard to adopting an active role in short-term group therapy. Some therapists feel guilty after controlling the group and subsequently become passive and withdrawn. They express constant doubts that anything meaningful can happen in such a short-term group. "It is only a Band-Aid approach." Some therapists identify with a "favorite child" or a "star pupil" and will insist on doing in-depth psychotherapy with this favorite patient. In countertransference, the therapist may express anger toward a member who is particularly resistant to the groups' rapid movement or who participates in scapegoating the other members. Many such leaders are likely to burn out quickly. In spite of these differences, most clinicians agree that the therapist in a short-term group should be active, directive, managerial, and flexible in his approach.

Curative Factors in Group Therapy

Several research studies have asked patients what helped them during the period of group therapy. Markovitz and Smith (1983) used Yalom's curative factor Q-Sort technique (1975) to compare various curative factors suggested by different studies. Q-Sort was scored by ranking each statement from 1 to 6, 6 being the most helpful. Table 3–1 shows the comparison ranking of curative factors suggested by different authors. Cohesiveness consistently ranked among the top four factors. Catharsis and self-understanding ranked high in two studies (Yalom, 1975; Markovitz and Smith, 1983).

Altruism ranked in the top four in the studies of Markovitz and Smith (1983) and Maxmen (1973). Factors that ranked high in only one out of the three studies are interpersonal learning (Markovitz and Smith), instillation of hope (Maxmen) and universality (Maxmen).

The following description of some of these factors will help clarify their meaning:

1. Cohesiveness.—Group cohesiveness develops when each member begins to feel as an important member of the group. The problems of each member become the problems of the group, and each member makes an honest effort to help resolve the problem. Such cohesiveness is difficult to develop in a short-term group. However, adolescent groups are likely to develop some degree of cohesiveness much quicker than adult groups are. Therapists can promote cohesiveness by emphasizing the equal importance of each member's problems, promoting participation by all members, and resolving negative and angry feelings among the members.

TABLE 3–1

Comparison of Curative Factor Ratings

No.	Yalom (1975)	Maxmen (1973)	Markovitz & Smith (1983)
1.	Interpersonal input	Instillation of hope	Catharsis
2.	Catharsis	Group cohesiveness	Group cohesiveness
3.	Group cohesion	Altruism	Altruism
4.	Self-understanding	Universality	Interpersonal output and self-understanding
5.	Interpersonal output	Interpersonal output	—
6.	Existential awareness	Existential awareness	Interpersonal input
7.	Universality	Interpersonal input	Instillation of hope
8.	Instillation of hope	Catharsis	Universality
9.	Altruism	Self-understanding	Existential awareness
10.	Family re-enactment	Guidance	Guidance
11.	Guidance	Family re-enactment	Family re-enactment
12.	Identification	Identification	Identification

2. Catharsis.—Open expression of sad feelings and bursts of crying are not uncommon in group therapy sessions. Adolescents, especially males, are frequently uncomfortable in dealing with such emotions. A great deal of support and understanding is provided by allowing sufficient time for a crying member to get himself together. Catharsis of angry feelings is less well tolerated by group members and should be allowed only for brief periods of time, even if not disruptive of the group process. Anger is frequently replaced by feelings of guilt and inadequacy (inability to control one's feelings). A discussion of such feelings later in the group sessions are therapeutic.

3. Altruism.—Patients frequently enter therapy with the belief that not only are they unable to help themselves but they have little to offer to others. Low self-esteem is very common among adolescents. For an adolescent to learn that he is able to be helpful to others in spite of serious problems of his own is very refreshing and elevates his own self-esteem.

4. Instillation of hope.—Adolescents with problems tend to feel hopeless about the resolution of their problems. This is probably the first time in their short life that they have encountered problems that they may consider unique and unsolvable. A successful solution of similar problems of peers may instill the hope that the adolescent's problems may not be unsolvable afterall.

5. Universality.—The patient often feels that his problems are unique and different from the problems of everybody else. Adolescents during the first week of hospitalization frequently verbalize such thoughts: "I don't have anything in common with those kids"; "They all use drugs and fight with their parents, I get along fine with my parents." Such verbalizations are generally defensive and give adolescents an excuse not to discuss their own problems for fear of rejection and criticism. Focusing on common problems in group discussions helps to reduce defensive attitudes and promotes acceptance of the universality of problems.

6. Imparting of information.—Peers provide a great deal of information to each

other about their problems, symptoms, and emotional difficulties. The group leader in a short-term group should not feel reluctant to explain and elaborate on some of the issues in which the group as a whole is less knowledgeable.

7. Corrective recapitulation of the primary family group.—Adolescent inpatient groups frequently present an opportunity for a corrective experience relating to sibling relationships, fascination and love of peers, and parental authority (represented by the group leader). Older adolescents may treat younger adolescents as their "spoiled, obnoxious younger siblings," while younger adolescents may rebel against the authority of the older adolescents. Such interactions are quite frequent in group sessions and can be discussed as transference relationships.

8. Development of socializing techniques.—Most adolescents spend a great deal of time with peers. Nonetheless, the majority of time feel that they have great difficulty in making new friends or approaching a new boy or girl that they are attracted to. Some feel that they are rejected and isolated by their peer groups through no fault of their own. Such concerns can be discussed and tested in group/peer interaction.

9. Imitative behavior.—Therapy group members often model themselves upon some traits of other members as well as those of the therapist. Adolescent groups often contain some members who exhibit aggressive behavior and an extremely negative attitude toward therapy. New members with antisocial tendencies are likely to imitate aggressive adolescents as they mistakenly view them as leaders. The leader must keep aggressive behavior and negative attitudes at a minimum level in the group through direct and indirect interventions. The therapist should emphasize that such behaviors and attitudes are not therapeutic and that they only disrupt the group process and waste time. However, discussion can be focused on the underlying causes of such behavior as anger, rebellion toward authority figures, and hopelessness.

10. Existential factors.—The ultimate concerns of existence such as death, freedom, isolation, and meaningfulness of life are quite common in adult therapy groups. However, adolescent groups appear to be rarely or only minimally concerned with such issues. Even for suicidal adolescents, death is not conceptualized as the finality of existence. Problems in existence are frequently seen as struggles with adults and peers. Freedom, responsibility, and willfulness are minimally developed concepts in most disturbed adolescents.

Frequency and Duration of Group Therapy

Because of the short period of hospitalization, if group therapy is likely to make an impact, it should be quite frequent, such as daily or at least three or four times a week. This means that most adolescents who stay from 4 to 5 weeks are likely to attend 20 to 25 sessions. Daily therapy sessions can maintain the continuity of the issues from day to day, and the unfinished business of the previous day can be quickly brought out for discussion the next day. The duration of each session should not exceed an hour because most adolescents find it difficult to sustain their attention or interest in discussion for longer periods. Taking a break in the middle of the session is generally disruptive to the flow of group discussion.

Structure of Therapy Sessions

Because of the short life of the inpatient groups and the fairly rapid turnover of the patients, it is necessary to develop a structure that will help achieve the specific goals within the allotted time. Yalom (1983) emphasizes a "here-and-now" strategy for these groups and structures the sessions as if they were part of one long single session. He suggests the following structure:

1. Orientation and preparation.
2. Agenda go-around.
3. Work on the agendas.
4. Ending meeting.

The therapist spends a few minutes (3 to 5 minutes) introducing new members and reminding the group of the basic structure and the purpose of the group. After the orientation the therapist allows each member to state what kind of problems they have been working on and what they would like to work on in that particular session. This routine helps therapists to make contact with each member and to obtain a bird's-eye view of the work possible in that session. Of course, many patients are not able to clearly verbalize what the issues are and need help to define them more clearly. After the first few sessions this phase of agenda go-around moves very quickly, and less than 10 to 15 minutes are spent in going around eight to ten members. The third phase begins by combining several common agendas and transforming them into here-and-now terms (interpersonal terms). Therapists should work on as many agendas as possible in a single session. The group ends with some feedback from the group about the agenda of the next meeting.

There are some problems in applying this approach to adolescent inpatient groups. For example, the participation of the adolescent patient in discussing combined agendas is frequently minimal. The therapist has to encourage and ask questions to motivate all members to participate in the group discussion. It is extremely difficult for adolescents to understand problems in interpersonal terms and deal with them in the context of group interactions. Most of them believe that their problems are caused by their parents. Focusing discussion on their ability to change and bring about changes in their environment should be viewed as a major therapeutic goal. It is helpful for the therapist to state that the group consists of them and not their parents. They must work to change themselves in order to acquire the ability to change or influence their environment.

The issues of peer interaction, fascinations, love or fears, sexual intimacies, substance abuse, identity problems, lack of future direction, depression, and anger are plentiful in adolescent groups and can be worked with on an ongoing basis. For example, group leaders may decide on the basis of their observations and the verbalizations of the members that identity problems are major common problems in a particular group. He can share his observation with the group and ask them to work on this problem during the span of a few sessions. The group leader should give some information on the normal development of identity. However, such didactic material should be kept to a minimum, and the members' own experiences and feelings should be used as basis for a group discussion on identity formation.

Setting Boundaries and Control Within the Group

The initial question in these groups is "How do you transform a group of adolescents who are negative and defiant toward their treatment into a working group?" The majority of hospitalized adolescents are initially very negative toward the treatment program. They view the hospital staff as allies of their parents and therefore not sympathetic to their viewpoint. This negative attitude is expressed through active disruption of the group or through the passive defiance of nonparticipation in the group. Most disruptions appear to be related to the authority of the leader. Some may defy the leader's authority in an active, hostile manner by making loud negative comments about the group, by interrupting the leader, by dominating the group, or by seductive gestures to members of the opposite sex in the group. Passive resistance against authority is expressed by bringing in books, comics, radios, and knitting work. An adolescent may claim that attending group therapy is a waste of time, especially when he needs to spend more time with books. These issues are not likely to be resolved by group discussion, and most adolescents tend to side with expressions of rebellion against authority. Confronting the group with its negative attitude and behavior and its anger toward the authority of the leader is generally not effective. In a long-term group, such attitudes and behavior can be interpreted and worked through as transference problems. But in short-term groups, such interpretations make little sense to the group. The leader needs to be very supportive and to work with the positive attributes of the group to build a cohesive working group and to help them see their problems in interpersonal terms.

Before any therapeutic work can be accomplished, the leader must work on what is called "shaping up the group." One way to deal with these disruptions is to apply the same code of conduct in the group that exists in the unit milieu. This externalizes authority outside the group since the leader simply follows the rules set by the milieu. The leader announces in the initial session and repeats on a periodic basis that he is bound by the code of conduct of the milieu and that group members will suffer the consequences if they violate the milieu code. Some leaders may choose to have a nurse or a child-care worker sit in the group for the initial session and administer the milieu punishments (checks for swearing, for holding hands, etc.). Group attendance is mandatory, and appropriate punishments are meted out for skipping any important part of the treatment program. Nonetheless, testing of limits may be expected to continue for some time before the group members settle down to work on their problems. Some leaders are extremely skillful with their wit and humor and can very effectively deal with adolescent rebellion without the use of threats or punishments.

Once the group has shaped up, it is easier to proceed with the usual format and structure suggested above. New group members are easily integrated by the rest of the group.

Effectiveness of Short-Term Group Therapy

Budman et al. (1981) reported significant positive changes in an uncontrolled study of brief dynamic group psychotherapy with a health maintenance organization (HMO) population. The group members evaluated themselves as improved on target problems, reported significant growth in interpersonal functioning, and became much less symptomatic. Similar subjective postgroup outcomes have been reported by clients in 18 groups that averaged 11 sessions each at the University of Massachusetts Mental Health Services (Poey, 1985). The majority of the members in each group reported direct target symptom relief and significant re-establishment of their psychic equilibrium.

Specialized Groups (Focused Groups)

There are many issues among hospitalized adolescents that can be dealt with in small specialized groups. Problems such as adoption, physical abuse, sexual abuse, stress management, medication groups, and substance abuse problems can form the basis of small groups. Problems are shared by each member of the group, and group discussion is focused on understanding and adjusting to these problems. Group work in these groups focuses on strengthening the members' adaptive ego functions and "uncovering the repressed positive ego." Some superego material is also appropriate, especially when severe superego functioning is inhibiting the healthy ego processes. Much less attention, however, is directed toward primitive or id material. Psychodynamically speaking, past histories are used only to help understand present focal problems. The groups are time limited. The number of sessions is decided in advance by the leader and the group members. Participation is voluntary, but members must continue to attend once they have started the group. These groups share the following characteristics:

1. There is a similarity of problems, which speeds up the group process.
2. Mutual support is generated by such groups.
3. Comfort is derived from recognizing the universality of negative feelings.
4. Members are encouraged to give advice and comfort to one another.
5. Catharsis is very common.

Although there are few controlled studies of the effectiveness of focused groups, a great deal of clinical experience suggests that such groups are frequently very therapeutic. A few examples of such groups follow.

Sexual Abuse Groups

A history of sex abuse is quite frequent in female adolescents. The problems most frequently encountered in women with a history of incest include impaired self-esteem, negative identity formation, difficulty in intimate relationships, and sexual dysfunctions. Issues of secrecy, shame, and stigma are not dealt with fully in individual psychotherapy. In such groups, members are offered a chance to relive the past but then to put it behind them and go on with their lives.

Herman and Schatzow (1984) described the stages of an incest group that lasted ten sessions:

I. Introduction.
II. Goal definition and story telling, which included:
   A. Recall of sexual events including a great deal of catharsis.
   B. Decreased isolation and improved relationships among the members and between members and the outside world.
   C. Improved self-esteem.
   D. Increased ability to reveal secrets—sharing sexual abuse secrets with a close acquaintance or family member.

The authors noticed that the feelings of sheer terror expressed in the early sessions gradually gave way to expressions of courage, the hurt gave way to anger, and feelings of helplessness gave way to desires to take the initiative. Many members began to recognize that, although they had been defenseless as children, they were no longer defenseless as adults.

The factors related to these changes include the following:

1. The social aspects of the group reduce feelings of isolation and loneliness.
2. Ventilation of feelings provides some relief of pain.
3. Information shared in these groups often provides group members with a new cognitive framework in which to understand the traumatic experience.

Eating Disorder Groups

These groups include adolescents with anorexia nervosa, bulimia, overweight problems, or underweight problems. The several studies of group psychotherapy with such patients have reported positive outcomes (Polivy, 1981; Lieb and Thompson, 1984). Theoretically, these groups are expected to be helpful for patients with eating disorders who tend to be isolated and avoid communication with other people or staff members in inpatient units. Lieb and Thompson (1984) noticed that adolescents with anorexia nervosa were reluctant to form an inpatient group and were reserved during the initial sessions of the group. Their resistance and isolation dramatically lessened as the sessions progressed, and a fairly strong group alliance developed. The group focused on their knowledge of their disorder, their strategies of dieting, exercising, and their parents' responses to their weight loss. The main topic of discussion gradually drifted away from weight control problems to concerns about becoming women. They viewed their food intake as a way of controlling their maturation. They also realized that each of them had a family that stressed high achievement and that their weight loss was partially an expression of anger and frustration toward their family and friends. The authors felt that these patients suffered from a sense of isolation and aloneness. They lacked assertiveness and felt their problems were unique. They also shared a number of misconceptions about body image, nutrition, and sexuality. These issues were effectively dealt with in short-term group psychotherapy.

FAMILY THERAPY

Hospitalization of an adolescent is frequently the result of a severe family crisis. The family usually exhausts all its internal resources before making such a decision. At this time the family is very eager for and responsive to professional direction and counseling. The initial state of crisis is soon replaced by a period of guilt and sympathy. The family feels guilty about temporarily excluding one member of the family. The hospitalization of the adolescent may be compared with incarceration and punishment. These ambivalent feelings on the part of the family are accentuated by the hospitalized adolescent who constantly complains about the environment of the hospital, the rules and restrictions, the presence of other "crazy kids" with whom the adolescent claims he has nothing in common, the bad food, etc. This is a very difficult period for the family. Some families succumb to their guilt and take the adolescent out of the hospital. This frequently happens when the family is not provided with sufficient emotional support and direction. Other parents are easily conned by the emotional appeals of the adolescent and may take him home. Occasionally a family may take their teenager out of the hospital despite a great deal of support from the professional staff. The situation in these families usually settles down for a few days before the next crisis brings the adolescent back to the hospital. Such families may make several visits to the emergency department of the hospital before the adolescent is finally hospitalized.

The family should be warned at the time of admission that most adolescents do not admit to their problems and frequently try to convince their parents about the futility of hospital treatment. A thorough assessment of the family should be made within a few days after the hospitalization. The assessment should focus on the reasons for the breakdown of the family system. It is frequently possible to divide families into two types:

1. Families who can generally identify some specific events or a point in time related to the onset of the problems. Their problems are usually of short duration, and the occurrence of a crisis is relatively recent.

2. Families in which the onset is insidious and the problems of long duration. These families usually experience frequent crises off and on. It is the worsening of the old problems and the increasing intensity and magnitude of the crisis that pre-cipitates the current hospitalization. The identifiable causes frequently include the following:

- Change in the relationship of parents.
- Parental separation or divorce.
- Change in the lifestyle of a single parent such as a new boyfriend or girlfriend or a new job.
- Moving or changing schools.
- Change in peer groups.
- Psychiatric disorders.
- Developmental conflict.

Intense strivings for independence and peer affiliation are commonly part of the adolescent's problem behavior. These strivings, however, are not generally within the normal range and are considered excessive or abnormal by the standards of the community. Families with long-term problems can trace these family problems back over many years. The patient was a problem child and grew up to be a problem adolescent.

As the guilt over hospitalization decreases, the family begins to assess the problems more realistically. The goals of family therapy during the period of adolescent hospitalization are generally very limited. Depending upon the availability of therapy time, most families are not seen more than four or five times during the 4 or 5 weeks of hospitalization. Family therapists may find the following goals helpful in their work:

1. Helping the family understand the problems of the hospitalized adolescent in the context of the family system. Even the clearly identifiable psychiatric disorders such as major depression and schizophrenia have a nonbiological component that influences the illness. These disorders are not caused by abnormal interactions in the family per se but do certainly influence family life. The family should not feel guilty over causing these disorders but should spend their energy in learning about their abnormal interactions and normalizing them as much as possible.

2. Reintegration of alienated adolescents. Problem adolescents frequently alienate themselves from their families. There is little normal communication within the family. Most of the communciation between the adolescent and the family consists of angry exchanges and disciplinary commands. Efforts should be made to initiate a normal dialogue between the family and the alienated adolescent.

3. Negotiating house rules. This should be accomplished before the adolescent returns home. The emphasis should be on the process of negotiating rather than agreeing on some house rules. Hospitalized adolescents tend to agree rather quickly on abiding by the rules suggested by the parents in the hope of being discharged early. The family therapist may ask the family and the adolescent to prepare their separate lists of house rules. This list may then form the basis for negotiation in the family sessions.

4. Family communication outside the therapy sessions such as during visiting hours, a weekend pass, or a family outing provide opportunities for improved family communication. It should be emphasized that in these informal contacts the family should focus on improving communication.

Family Therapy After Discharge

Most families need continuing family counseling after the adolescent is discharged from the hospital. This is essential to maintain the therapeutic gains achieved during hospitalization. Arrangements for continuing family therapy in community facilities should be made before the patient is discharged. Some families who feel that the teenager is not ready to be discharged, may be quite apprehensive and may need a great deal of support from the therapy staff.

Theoretical Considerations

The multiple theories and techniques of family therapy frequently create confusion for new trainees. Most theories, however, have in common a set of basic principles proven to be therapeutic through long clinical experience. In the pioneering days of family therapy, Nathan Ackerman (1958) laid the foundations of psychodynamic family therapy. Other authors such as Bateson et al. (1956) and Jackson (1965) hold an interactionalist view of family therapy. They regard family therapy as a series of communicational interactions that create constructive or disruptive family patterns. Treatment using this approach focuses on interrupting and redirecting these interactions to alter the family system. A lack of genuine emotional expression in the family is seen as the root cause of problems in many families. Satir (1972) and others have developed techniques that enhance emotional communication within the family system. Structuralists (Minuchin, 1974) view the family as a system of boundaries and have suggested methods of entering the system and adjusting those boundaries. The systems approach has had a profound influence on most family therapists. The system theory assumes that the family is a set of units or elements that are actively interrelated or operate in some sense as a bounded unit. Members of a family not only interact with each other but are interrelated and interdependent. The family system is influenced by the actions of one member, who in turn is influenced by the reactions of the other members.

Families undergo recognizable and predictable developmental stages (Carter and McGoldrick, 1980) in a manner analogous to the way in which an individual develops and with all the problems inherent in the developmental process. The birth of children, children leaving home for college, marriage, and new jobs present challenges to each family, some of whom adjust easily while others get stuck and require help to get back on the track.

No one member of the family is blamed for the breakdown or dysfunction of the family system. Each member is assigned equal responsibility in the system theory. This concept of causality is variously referred to as circular causality or equicausality.

Families are assumed to be open systems interacting with their environment. The importance of societal influences on the development of families has been emphasized by several authors (Keniston, 1965; Coles, 1977; Garbarino, 1977). These authors recognize the difficulties that society imposes upon the families of today. Keniston disputes the myth of the family's ability to insulate itself from outside pressures and societal expectations. Indeed, he suggests that society, and not the family, educates children today. Melvin Kohn (1977) points out the vulnerability of the family system and believes that family systems are deeply affected by societal expectations, regardless of their position in society.

Engaging the Severely Dysfunctional Family

Some hospitalized adolescents come from severely chaotic families. Most members of these families are preoccupied with their own problems such as severe drug abuse and alcoholism and have little or no regard for the adolescent's problems.

These families are very difficult to engage in any treatment process. Weitzman (1985) has suggested the following special considerations in treating these families:

1. Reduce the intensity of family therapy. Many of these familes present symptoms of intense emotional charge such as incest, violence, alcoholism, suicide, and severe behavior problems. Encouraging family members to interact around these issues can be extremely volatile and may increase destructive behavior to intolerable levels. Experiential techniques and confrontations are initially avoided for the same reasons. These families need support and understanding from the family therapist.

2. Use a parenting role in families that require a great deal of control and structure. The therapist may have to assume a strong parenting role, often acting as advisor, limit setter, mediator, and authority figure. These roles are gradually turned over to the family as they are able to function with greater organization and internal structure.

3. Avoid defocusing too rapidly. Many family therapists insist on defocusing on the identified patient and discuss problems entirely in the context of the family system. Too rapid defocusing robs the family of their defenses and disorganizes their thinking and emotional responses.

4. Examine biological factors. Many of these families are genetically at risk to develop mental disorders. Therapists may utilize the educational approach to help these families understand the contribution of genetic and environmental factors in the development of mental disorders. Similarly, the role of medications as well as environmental factors in the treatment of mental disorders need to be discussed clearly.

5. Structure the interview. Help the family define the problems and create an atmosphere of problem solving. Any member of the family losing emotional control or anticipating a loss of control should be temporarily excused from the family session.

6. Anticipate the impact of intervention. Prematurely attempting to change well-established transactions may lead to uncooperativeness and dropout of the family from therapy. The therapist should not push for changes the family does not want or considers harmful.

7. Devise realistic goals. Many families have no goals they want to achieve as a family. The therapist can help them devise realistic goals that can be achieved in family therapy.

8. Normalize the crisis. Most of these families experience frequent crises. Their sole goal in life becomes to survive these crises. Therapists should guide the family through crises and help them look beyond.

INDIVIDUAL PSYCHOTHERAPY

The role of the individual therapist in short-term hospitalization is frequently confusing. A hospitalized adolescent has a great deal of individual contact with milieu staff such as nurses and child-care workers. Most of these individual contacts with milieu staff occur around a discussion of the issues immediately facing the adolescent such as peer problems, discipline, unhappy visits with the family, or a disturbing telephone call. Most milieu staff deal with these issues by sympathetic listening and providing some direction as necessary. It is the job of the individual therapist to become aware of these day-to-day problems and to deal with them in the context of the patient's past history, his relationship with his family and peers, and his coping style and to bring about more permanent changes in the adolescent's ability to handle problems. The individual therapist is also aware of the patient's basic conflicts and focuses his therapy on resolving these conflicts.

Most hospitalized adolescents have experienced some type of counseling previously, although the experience has not always been a positive one. There is a great deal of pressure on hospitalized adolescents to work on their problems before discharge. This helps them engage in therapy more quickly than in an outpatient clinic. The issues in the initial sessions are frequently related to adjustment problems in the hospital milieu. Many adolescents have great difficulty in following ward rules and in getting along with certain peers and certain adult staff. They experience a great deal of frustration in not having freedom of movement and play. Once the adjustment to the ward milieu improves, other issues relating to family and peers arise. These, however, may be the main issues that precipitated hospitalization. It is not possible to resolve all of these issues in the short period of hospitalization. However, the therapist may help adolescents focus on the main issues and understand the multiple factors contributing to the presence of conflicts. The therapist should focus on those ingredients that make a therapy session productive and helpful for patients. For example, adolescents may need to understand the meaning and purpose of talking in therapy and the importance of focusing on problem-solving techniques. Overall, inpatient therapy can be considered a success if the adolescent desires and seeks further therapy after he is discharged.

There are several models of brief psychotherapy that can be successfully utilized in short-term hospitalization.

Brief Psychotherapy

There are numerous publications about short-term dynamic psychotherapy. The 1950s marked the appearance of the initial publications indicating that brief psychiatric interventions were helpful to a selected group of neurotic patients. By the 1970s the results of several research studies had been published and provided further documentation to the efficacy of individual dynamic psychotherapy (Sifneos, 1972). A great deal of interest has lately been focused on short-term therapy. The reasons for this interest as suggested by Reich and Neenan (1986) include the following:

1. Recent evidence that psychotherapy is efficacious. Smith and Glass (1977) demonstrated that the typical client is better off than 75% of the untreated individuals.
2. The realization that most psychotherapy as it is actually practiced is quite short-term. For example, Garfield (1978) found that the median number of visits in most settings was 5 to 6. Similarly, psychiatrists in private practice tended to see their patients for an average of 12.8 visits.

3. The effect of psychotherapy on the utilization of other medical resources. In a review of the research, Jones and Vischi (1979) indicated that outpatient psychotherapy reduced medical care utilization by a median of 20% in organized health care settings. The length of treatment did not seem to proportionately enhance the benefit (Mumford et al., 1984).

4. Increased awareness of medical consumers and health insurance providers who consider short-term psychotherapy a cost-effective, efficacious method of performing psychotherapy.

Brief psychotherapy is carried out to achieve a specified goal within a delimited amount of time. Most therapists limit brief therapy to 15 or fewer sessions.

Selection Criteria

Earlier therapists tended to set stringent criteria for the selection of patients. However, with more experience with different types of patients the selection criteria have become less stringent and now include the majority of patients with only a few exceptions such as psychotics (Davanlo, 1980; Liebovich, 1983). Most therapists emphasize in their selection criteria the motivation to change and the ability of the patient to specify those problems they wish to focus on in therapy. Other important but not essential criteria include good interpersonal relations, psychological sophistication, having had some meaningful interpersonal experience, having achieved success in at least one area of their lives, and the ability to interact effectively with a therapist.

Diagnostic categories should not influence the selection criteria. It is more important to determine the central issue underlying the patient's problems than the *DSM-III* diagnosis as the selection criterion for brief psychotherapy. Most investigators agree that the issues that respond best to brief psychotherapy include unresolved multiple conflicts, morbid grief, loss or separation issues, phobias, crisis situations, and developmental conflicts. The more completely the central issues is understood, the better able is the therapist to provide appropriate interventions.

Technical Issues

Most therapists agree that brief psychotherapy should include the following ingredients:

1. Helping patients find important areas of immediate concern or conflict.
2. Enabling the patient to clarify the problem and to become aware of potential options for coping with it.
3. Establishing and utilizing a therapeutic alliance (working together).
4. Maintaining a focus on problems during the course of therapy.
5. Using problem-solving techniques.

Most therapists avoid dealing with the issue of transference. It is argued that, because no free association is being used, the therapist has limited access to the patient's fantasies. Therefore, if the transference neurosis is allowed to take place, the therapist will be unable to analyze it. Malan (1963) recommends interpretation of transference and points out to the patients how they characteristically relate to significant people in their lives. The interpretation may increase the probability of the patient recognizing and modifying maladaptive behavior.

Termination

The ending phase of brief therapy is as important as the beginning or the middle. The end phase should include a review of the therapy with regard to what has been accomplished and should deal with fears of the loss of support and guidance. Therapists should emphasize that it may take months before the patient experiences the full benefit of therapy.

Development Approach

The implications of the developmental approach for brief psychotherapy are great. First of all, the basic thesis, implicit and explicit in the writings of adult developmentalists, is that people are always in motion or have the potential for motion (action and change). Therefore, the role of the brief therapist with most patients need not be one of providing the energy for change but rather of freeing the individual to return to a state of action. Furthermore, changes need not take place under the watchful eye of the therapist because the working-through process occurs naturally if and when the patient resumes his development.

Cognitive Approach

The therapist may respond to a patient's verbal and/or behavioral contents by focusing either on cognition (understanding, problem solving, and making causal relationships) or on feelings. Focusing on the cognitive processes leads the patient to understand his problems in cognitive terms and helps him solve his problems through logical thinking. The therapist directs the patient to identify his problems in terms of individual, familial, and environmental causes. These causes are analyzed one by one to determine their significance and the amount of contribution of each to the patient's problems. The therapist then helps the patient to find ways to deal with the causal factors.

This approach is not to be considered just an intellectual exercise between the patient and the therapist. Feelings are associated with all cognitive contents to a greater or lesser degree. The therapist may appeal to the patient's cognition to understand his irrational feelings. However, understanding feelings in a logical manner is generally very difficult for most patients. This task is usually reserved for the later stages of therapy when the patient has developed enough skills to think about his problems in a logical manner.

We find that the cognitive approach or the problem-solving approach is a more successful technique for inexperienced therapists and recommend that medical students use it with their patients. Most new therapists find it difficult to handle the moderate emotional responses of their patients such as crying, laughing, or being irritated or angry. They do quite well, however, with the cognitive approach.

The Role of the Therapist

It is only in recent years that economic, social, and political factors have converged in a manner that makes it urgent for most psychotherapists to consider giving treatment quickly, efficiently, and cost-effectively. A significant characteristic of all brief therapies is relatively high levels of therapist activities. A passive and waiting stance on the part of the therapist whereby the patient eventually finds the "solution" to his problems results in a protracted process. Thus, brief psychodynamic therapists make frequent and often empathetic interpretations. More behaviorally oriented brief therapists require various types of self-monitoring and homework by their clients (Wilson, 1981). A therapist used to doing long-term psychotherapy may feel rushed and under a great deal of pressure in doing brief psychotherapy. It is important that brief psychotherapy be carried out with mutual understanding between the patient and the therapist regarding the goals and objectives to be achieved in the short period of allotted therapeutic time.

Who Should Do Individual Therapy in the Inpatient Setting

Individual therapy may be provided by any member of the mental health discipline. The therapist who has been working with an adolescent prior to hospitalization is frequently asked to continue individual therapy after the adolescent is hospitalized. This practice is fraught with several problems. Most nonpsychiatrists are reluctant to hospitalize their patients since it implies a loss of control over the management of their patients. It may represent their failure or inability to sustain a patient outside the hospital. Therapists who are not familiar with inpatient work tend to side with adolescents with regard to discipline. They may see the hospital staff as overly punitive and convey those sentiments to their patients. Frequently the therapeutic goals of an outside therapist conflict with the goals of the milieu staff. The therapist frequently feels left out because most day-to-day issues in the milieu may not be conveyed to the therapist. The therapist who works with a team on a daily basis is perhaps a better choice to provide therapy in the hospital setting.

REFERENCES

Ackerman N: *The Psychodynamics of Family Life*. New York, Basic Books Inc Publishers, 1958.

Bateson G, Jackson D, Haley J, et al: Towards a theory of schizophrenia. *Behav Sci* 1956; 22:251–264.

Budman S, Randall M, Denby A: Outcome in short-term group psychotherapy. *Group* 1981; 5:37–51.

Butcher JN, Koss MP: Research on brief and crisis-oriented therapies, in Bergin AE, Garfield SL (eds): *Handbook of Psychotherapy and Behavior Change*. New York, John Wiley & Sons Inc, 1978, pp 725–767.

Carter E, McGoldrick M: *The Family Life Cycle*. New York, Gardner Press, 1980.

Coles R: Privileged American Children. *Pediatrics* 1977; 60:381–382.

Davanlo H: *Short-term Dynamic Psychotherapy*. New York, Jason Aronson, 1980.

Garbarino J: The price of privacy in the social dynamics of child abuse. *Child Welfare* 1977; 56:565–575.

Garfield S: Research on client variables in psychotherapy, in Garfield S, Bergin A (eds): *Handbook of Psychotherapy and Behavior Change,* ed 3. New York, John Wiley & Sons Inc, 1978.

Herman J, Schatzow E: Time-limited group therapy for women with a history of incest. *Int J Group Psychother* 1984; 34:605–616.

Jackson D: The study of the family. *Family Process* 1965; 4:1–20.

Jones K, Vischi T: Impact of alcohol, drug abuse and mental health treatment on medical care utilization: A review of the literature. *Med Care* 1979; 17(suppl):11–82.

Keniston K: *The Uncommitted: Alienated Youths in American Society*. New York, Harcourt, Brace & World, 1965.

Kohn ML: *Class and Conformity: A Study of the Values,* ed 2. Chicago, University of Chicago Press, 1977.

Leibovich M: Shy short-term psychotherapy for borderline. *Psychother Psychosom* 1983; 39:1–9.

Lieb R, Thompson T: Group psychotherapy for four anorexia nervosa inpatients. *Int J Group Psychother* 1984; 34:639–642.

Malan DH: *A Study of Brief Psychotherapy*. New York, Plenum Press, 1963.

Markovitz R, Smith J: Patient's perceptions of curative factors in short-term group therapy. *Int J Group Psychother* 1983; 33:21–39.

Maxmen J: Group psychotherapy as viewed by hospitalized patients. *Arch Gen Psychiatry* 1973; 28:404–408.

Minuchin S: *Families in Family Therapy*. Cambridge, Harvard University Press, 1974.

Mumford E, Schlesinger J, Glass G, et al: A new look at evidence about reduced cost of medical utilization following mental health treatment. *Am J Psychiatry* 1984; 141:1145–1158.

Pekala R, Siegel J, Farrar D: The problem-solving support group: Structured group therapy with psychiatric inpatients. *Int J Group Psychother* 1985; 35:391–409.

Poey K: Guidelines for the practice of dynamic group therapy. *Int J Group Psychother* 1985; 35:331–354.

Polivy J: Group therapy as an adjunct treatment for anorexia nervosa. *J Psychiatr Treat Eval* 1981; 3:279–283.

Reich J, Neenan A: Principles common to different short-term psychotherapies. *Am J Psychother* 1986; 40:62–69.

Satir V: *People Making*. Palo Alto, CA, Science & Behavior Books, 1972.

Sifneos PE: *Short-term Psychotherapy and Emotional Crisis*. Cambridge, Harvard University Press, 1972.

Smith ML, Glass G: Meta-analysis of psychotherapy outcome studies. *Am Psychol* 1977; 32:754–760.

Weitzman J: Engaging the severely dysfunctional family in treatment: Basic considerations. *Fam Process* 1985; 24:473–485.

Wilson GT: Behavior therapy as a short-term therapeutic approach, in Dugman SH (ed): *Forms of Brief Therapy*. New York, Guilford, 1981.

Yalom ID: *The Theory and Practice of Group Psychotherapy*. New York, Basic Books Inc Publishers, 1970, pp 83–108.

Yalom ID: *Inpatient Group Therapy*. New York, Basic Books Inc Publishers, 1983.

Yalom ID: *The Theory and Practice of Group Psychotherapy*. New York, Basic Books Inc Publishers, 1975.

4

Organization of the Inpatient Milieu

Ideally, the environment of the hospital psychiatric unit should conform to the normal conditions of daily living. The daily activities should include time for formal education, recreation, peer and adult interaction, sufficient time for rest, sleep and exercise, and promotion of specific individual interests and hobbies. The adults supervising the adolescents should be sensitive, loving, understanding, respecting, consistent, and compassionate.

In addition, a hospital psychiatric unit is a very complex organization with multiple levels of administrative structures with conflicting economic, social, and therapeutic goals. The unit staff, whose primary allegiance is to the patient, is expected to communicate with the families and the community agencies in order to induce a more favorable environment for the patient to return to after hospital treatment. The large number of personnel involved in providing around-the-clock service are expected to maintain continuity of care. Communication between the staff on different shifts becomes a horrendous problem. The daily program of therapy, education, recreation, and rest is organized so that the patients do not become too tired, bored, or burdened. The daily schedule becomes quite complex when special times have to be set aside for showers, laundry, medical appointments, special consultations, evaluations, and separate treatment for each patient.

The daily routine of the psychiatric unit must also be a therapeutic one for the emotionally disturbed adolescents. The majority of the adolescent patients come from disturbed home situations and have had chaotic lifestyles. Their daily activities often contained little or no time for formal education, for sufficient rest and exercise, for healthy meals, and for proper recreation. Their interaction with adults, especially with their parents, has been minimal and mostly negative (consisting of arguments, fights, and conflicts). It is therefore understandable that any effort to impose an organized lifestyle on these patients will be met with great resistance.

The adjustment of new patients to the unit program is greatly influenced by the example set by their peers. The rebellious attitude of some patients can have a detrimental influence on newcomers, especially if the newcomers have a negative and rebellious attitude toward treatment. The patients in the unit are at different stages of improvement, change, and progress, and group rebellions are rare. However, some "hard-core" groups do form, and they resist change. Caudill (1957) pointed out that small patient cliques or groups are formed in mental hospitals. Some of these groups resist institutional values and avoid constructive adaptation to the dominant institutional culture. These groups create most of the rebellious, negative, and aggressive activities in the unit. In addition to these negative groups there are positive groups that are not resistant to treatment and that exert informal pressure on other patients to conform to staff values, socialize new patients, and provide an understanding of the treatment goals. It is thus important to promote such positive groups in the milieu and discourage the formation of negative groups.

Patient councils or patient governments are important groups that provide a forum for the patients to express their dissatisfaction. Patients should run such council meetings by themselves without much interruption or direction by the unit staff. These meetings should be held on a daily basis, preferably in the morning or the evening. The patients should discuss their responsibilities in the program (such as cleaning chores in their bedrooms and in the general areas of the unit), negotiate rules with the staff, express needs, and make suggestions for improving the program. The patient council should elect a chairman to conduct the meeting in an orderly manner. The chairman should also serve as a liaison person between the patients and the representative of the unit staff. The representative of the unit staff should be invited to attend patient council meetings as an exofficio member. Every request made by the patients through their council meetings should be discussed with the rest of the unit staff and an appropriate action taken. The staff representative should explain to the patients in detail the underlying reasons for the staff's action on any particular request.

Since the organization of the unit milieu on the principles of "a therapeutic community" maximizes the effectiveness of the treatment program, the following brief description of a therapeutic community and its application to the adolescent inpatient program is provided to help the reader to design a therapeutic community for an adolescent inpatient unit.

THERAPEUTIC COMMUNITY

Thomas F. Main (1946) coined the term *therapeutic community* to describe the social organization of a psychiatric hospital or institution. This concept has been developed extensively by several other authors, especially Maxwell Jones (1976) who has contributed greatly toward its popularization and implementation. Jones defines the therapeutic community as the social organization of the hospital or psychiatric unit that promotes therapeutic changes in the patients. The social organization includes both the staff and the patients. Natural social relationships are utilized to bring about the therapeutic changes. The terms *therapeutic milieu, therapeutic community,* and *milieu therapy* have different theoretical connotations, but in practice they are frequently used synonymously.

In the organization of a therapeutic community attention must be paid to all aspects of a program for it to be maximally effective, for example:

1. Space utilization of the inpatient unit.
2. The role of the patient.
3. Relationships between the patients and the staff.
4. The lines of authority and decision making.
5. Communication among the staff, between the staff and the patients, and among the patients.

The type and organization of the space for a psychiatric unit are very important for the success of the program. The construction of the unit should allow maximum interaction between patients and staff. There should be a large space sufficient to accommodate organized play activities, school, and large meetings. A separate space for smaller-scale activities should also exist. Several medium-sized rooms for group and family therapies are necessary. The location of the staff offices and the staff lounge should be isolated from the main activity area of the unit. Most hospital units are not well-suited for adolescent psychiatric programs. They are usually designed for maximum bedroom space and the quick accessibility of the nursing staff to the bedrooms. There are many good designs for an inpatient adolescent psychiatric unit.

The ideal role for the patient is to acknowledge the presence of problems and to seek help from the staff and other patients to resolve these problems. This role, however, is almost nonexistent among new patients, at least during the initial period after hospitalization. The psychiatric unit must be designed to provide extensive support for new patients, to improve their cooperation, and to facilitate their integration into the unit. The more cooperative patients should be asked to introduce new patients to their peers and to give some information about the unit's routine and daily program. The support of the adult staff helps to increase patient participation. Several studies indicate that the amount of improvement parallels the degree of patient participation. A.W. Clark (1964) used a participation scale to monitor the progress of patients in an inpatient unit. The participation scale included the following six observations:

1. Getting on well with the staff.
2. Doing their share of jobs.
3. Getting on well with other patients.
4. Joining in social and recreational facilities.
5. Thinking that being in the unit is worthwhile.
6. Liking the unit.

Adolescent patients have a variety of attitudes toward the unit staff depending upon their relationships with other adults and authority figures. Some patients are very negative and rebellious and detest all authority, while others are overly cooperative, pleasing, and at times clinging. However, adolescents with conduct problems understand authority well, and they usually get along fairly well with the adults in the unit staff in the hope of avoiding problems and getting a few breaks here and there during their stay on the unit. Their relationship with adults is, however, very superficial. The staff also has a variety of attitudes toward the adolescent patients. Some tend to view adolescent patients as "just kids," while others may treat them more like adults. These differences in attitudes are frequently based on their own past experiences and their relationships with their own teenage children. It is important, however, that the developmental difficulties of these patients during their adolescent years be given proper consideration so that they never be treated as just kids but as individuals who are experiencing great difficulty in becoming adults. They do not want to be treated like children, even if they behave like them. It is always difficult to give up child-level responsibilities and assume adult responsibilities. The unit staff must maintain their role as adults, provide role models, supply guidance, and respect patients' feelings. Giving adolescents appropriate responsibilities with clear instructions and guidance promotes their self-esteem and helps them assimilate adult roles.

Adolescent patients are frequently very sensitive to the hierarchy of authority and begin to respond differentially to different staff, depending upon the amount of authority or decision-making power they perceive a particular staff member has. It is important, however, that all patients understand that all the major decisions are made by the staff team involved in their treatment. It is equally important that patients not be able to create divisiveness among the staff. This, unfortunately, is fairly common in adolescent units. Staff members may identify with the adolescent or may have a transference relationship based on their feelings toward their own children. A staff-patient relationship based on these factors may create a lack of objectivity in the staff and reduce its therapeutic effectiveness. Such relationships should be pointed out and routinely discussed in staff treatment planning meetings.

Communication among the staff is probably the most difficult and serious problem that exists in all short-term psychiatric units where the average length of a patient's stay is about 3 to 4 weeks. The evaluation, treatment and discharge planning move fairly rapidly. There is never enough time for all members of the therapy team to meet frequently enough to share information and make decisions. Although some decisions can be delayed until the opportunity for a team discussion arises, many treatment decisions are made by only one member of the team because an acute situation has arisen that requires an immediate decision.

Since the psychiatrists are in charge of the patients care, they are more likely to make decisions that will affect the care of the patients. They are also more prone to be criticized by other team members for not discussing matters with the team before making their decisions. The decisions that affect the treatment of a patient are best communicated verbally but should at least be indicated in the progress notes of the patient so that the other members of the team become aware of the changes and change their own actions accordingly. Progress notes are also a very important method of communication among the various members of the staff working on different shifts.

Occasionally some staff may complain about too much communication: "All we do is have meetings and spend little time with patients." Such sentiments are very unhealthy and usually develop because the team meetings deteriorate into aimless discussions. Team discussions should center around the attainment of specific goals and objectives for each patient. The objectives should be specific enough to be accomplishable by each discipline within its level of training and experience.

Miscommunications are also very common occurrences in the adolescent units and are often deliberately intended by the adolescent patient to either misdirect the staff or to line up the staff against their parents. Such distorted communications are passed onto the unit staff who may act on them without verifying them with the parents. For example, an adolescent reported to the nursing staff that his mother was going to take him out of the hospital that evening. The nursing staff called the psychiatrist and other team members to write the discharge order and set up a plan for aftercare. In fact, the adolescent himself had called his mother and had asked her to take him out of the hospital. Although the mother did not agree with his request, he continued to insist that he was going to leave that evening. The verbalizations of adolescent patients are frequently repeated by various members of the team as if they were factual without verifying the information with the family. Miscommunications among the staff may also be based on their misinterpretation of a particular event. Interpersonal relationships greatly influence the degree of communication among the staff. Communication is easier among people who work together with a spirit of cooperation. However, personal feelings of anger and dislike toward each other may severely interfere with communication.

Problems in the social structure of the unit induce stresses, both in the staff and the patients. Stanton and Schwartz (1954) identified some of the following common problems:

1. Intrastaff conflicts.
2. Overlapping lines of authority.
3. Institutional change.
4. Lack of clarity of role definition.
5. Conflicting values and inadequate communication of values between patients and staff.

Intrastaff conflicts are common in hospital settings. The therapy team in a psychiatric unit includes different professionals with various levels of training and clinical backgrounds. It is not uncommon for these professionals to jockey around for greater influence and power. The power struggle is usually expressed around issues related to patient care. An effective way of influencing patient care is through knowledge and sound opinions. However, some staff create a power struggle through a specific concern that they always express about every patient, whether it is appropriate or not. For example, in recent years, it has become fashionable to raise the issue of sexual and physical abuse in every psychiatric case. Some staff, struggling for power, dominate the discussion of a case with this concern and ignore all other factors contributing to the psychiatric disorder. Since in most states of the United States reporting suspected child abuse is mandatory, any discussion of child abuse forces other members of the team to pay attention to such verbalizations. Such power struggles may at times be dissipated by recognition of the contribution of a particular member of the team to the overall discussion of the case. However, it should be pointed out that psychiatric disorders are multidetermined and that each factor in the etiology should be weighed and judged separately for its contribution to the overall etiology of the disorder. The discussion of the case must include all possible factors: the biological, the social, and the psychological.

Some of the power struggles result from dissatisfaction with one's status and resentment of other professionals who are better paid. This struggle is perhaps universal and is not unique to psychiatric units. However, such resentment of higher-paid professionals may surface more easily in a psychiatric unit where the roles of the members of the psychiatric team are somewhat blurred and overlap with each other. Each member of the team may see himself doing the same work or even better work than the higher-paid staff and may consequently resent their status and authority.

DEVELOPING A DAILY SCHEDULE

The daily schedule should consist of a carefully formulated mix of therapeutic, recreational, and educational activities. There should be at least 3 hours of therapeutic activities (such as group psychotherapy, mental health education and discussion, individual psychotherapy, family therapy, and process groups), 3 hours of formal education, and 3 to 4 hours of recreational activities. Short break and rest periods are interspersed throughout the day. A structured program is necessary because most disturbed adolescents have a difficult time organizing their leisure activities. In the absence of planned activities one is likely to observe a lot of horseplay, mischievious activities, arguments, and fights. Free times are frequently used by adolescents to listen to music, smoke, play games, snack, or make telephone calls. These times should be kept short (10 to 20 minutes). Most adolescents do not require rest during the day. They are likely to take naps if confined to their bedrooms during rest periods, and this may result in difficulty falling asleep at night. It is better to spend rest periods in quiet recreational activities such as arts and crafts. The planning of the recreational activities depends on the type of facilities available in and around the hospital. Availability of a gymnasium and a swimming pool are ideal. However, community facilities can be utilized for those patients who are permitted to go out of the hospital. Therapeutic activities such as individual therapy and family therapy are scheduled at different times by different therapists, and a definite time slot cannot be set aside for these activities. The patients involved in these sessions should be excused from other scheduled programs for the duration of the therapy and should be returned to the ongoing activity in the program at the end of the session. However, individual and group therapy sessions should not compete with other therapeutic activities such as group psychotherapy or process groups. A daily activities schedule might look as follows:

Daily Schedule
7:00 A.M.—Wakeup time, wash up, dress, clean room, exercise.
8:00 A.M.—Breakfast.

8:30 A.M.—Patient council meeting.
9:00 A.M.—School.
10:20 A.M.—Recess/free time/snack time.
10:40 A.M.—School.
12:00 noon—Lunch/free time/rest.
1:00 P.M.—Group psychotherapy.
2:00 P.M.—Recreational activities.
3:30 P.M.—Mental health education groups.
4:30 P.M.—Rest time.
5:00 P.M.—Dinner time/free time.
6:00 P.M.—Special therapy groups.
7:00 P.M.—Patient's own projects or community projects.
9:00 P.M.—Goodnight groups.
9:30–10:30—Bedtime for each level of patients.

MILIEU RULES AND CONTROL ISSUES

It is necessary for most adolescent psychiatric units to devise a set of rules to help adolescents organize their daily activities within the hospital milieu. These rules should be associated with appropriate rewards and punishments. It should be emphasized that every behavior has a consequence: a positive or a negative one. The rules should not be too different from what most families are likely to enforce at home. Some modifications, however, are necessary because the unit is dealing with disturbed adolescents who have not been in the habit of following rules at home.

Theoretical Principles

Child-rearing practices and styles have varied throughout the ages. The autocratic style of the Middle Ages has given way to more democratic methods of raising children. Behavioral research in the past few decades has identified the underlying principles in various child-rearing practices. It is important for the milieu staff to become familiar with the following general principles involved in setting rules and giving rewards or punishment.

Behavior may be classified into two broad categories: respondent and operant. Respondent behavior is generally unlearned and is reflexive in nature. It occurs automatically in response to a specific condition. This is exemplified by such physiological responses as salivation in the mouth in the presence of food or shedding tears in response to peeling onions.

Most behavior modification in children is related to operant behavior. Operant behavior is voluntary and is learned under various conditions of reward and punishment. The conditions or consequences of a behavior response that increase the probability of its occurrence are termed *reinforcers*. Reinforcers may be some tangible reward, a smile, praise, or a hug. It is extremely important to understand the nature and the importance of various types of reinforcers. A positive reinforcement is that stimulus that occurs at the end of some behavior and increases the probability of its recurrence. A negative reinforcer is any stimulus that, by its removal, increases the probability of the recurrence of the behavior.

In positive reinforcement the behavior is strengthened by the addition of something that follows its occurrence. Positive reinforcers may be grouped into three broad categories:

1. Social reinforcers.
2. Token and tangible reinforcers.
3. Intrinsic reinforcers.

A smile, praise, affection, or approval are examples of social reinforcers. Tangible reinforcers are material items such as food, candies, toys, money, and games. Token rewards may assume the form of checkmarks, points, stars, plastic strips, or anything else that can be exchanged for tangible reinforcers. Intrinsic reinforcers refer to satisfactions inherent in performing the activity itself. These satisfactions typically involve curiosity, novelty, and pride resulting from achievement.

Reinforcers may be further classified as primary or secondary. Primary reinforcers are stimuli that have biological significance and/or satisfy a physiological need. Thus, water and food may be designated primary reinforcers. Secondary reinforcers refer to stimuli that have acquired reinforcement properties by being associated with primary reinforcers. Numerous types of stimuli can function as secondary reinforcers since any stimulus that is paired with or precedes a primary reinforcer acquires reinforcing properties. Stimuli that have been paired with more than one primary reinforcer acquire the attributes of generalized reinforcers. A good example of a generalized reinforcer is money.

Memories of past experiences and images often have a positive or negative value associated with them. When we recall our experience in a situation that has a positive connotation, we are likely to make responses that are closely related to the previous situation. In fact, just thinking about a positive experience might lead us to involve ourselves in the same experience over again. The process by which individuals evaluate their behavior in positive or negative terms and permit or restrict themselves from accepting certain rewards is referred to as self-reinforcement.

Reward and Punishment Systems

Most adolescent psychiatric units have devised elaborate systems of reward and punishment on the basis of sound behavior principles. Beyond the basic needs all the activities of daily living may be considered privileges and used as rewards. These include a later bedtime, telephone times, special recreational activities, and increased monetary allowances.

Punishments include verbal warnings, time out, sit out, room restrictions, work detail, and loss of privileges. In extreme cases of aggression, confinement to a seclusion room and arm and body restraints are used.

There should be a balance between the amount of reward and punishment that an adolescent receives. If an adolescent is constantly in trouble and seems to have no opportunity to receive any reward, the situation should be carefully analyzed and ways found that could help the youngster to receive some rewards.

A newcomer is usually placed at the entry level with only a few privileges that are gradually increased as the youngster progresses through the treatment program. Depending upon the average length of the program, the reward system is organized in four different levels in a progressive manner.

Special Therapeutic Systems

Some level systems are automatic, and patients gain more privileges with the passage of time. If they do not lose any privileges for various behaviors such as defiance, noncompliance, and aggressive and destructive behavior, they will continue to rise in the level system and reach the highest level at the end of 4 or 5 weeks. The automatic system is designed primarily to help the adolescent to abide by the rules of daily living in the unit and does not reflect positive changes in attitude or in the capacity to better handle problems or stresses. In fact, there are many adolescents who comply to the milieu just enough to advance to the higher level systems, without actually addressing their problems in therapy sessions. Some of these patients develop an attitude of "just passing time." They make up their minds to go through the motions of working in the program but do exactly what they want to do after they leave the hospital. Such individuals should be identified early, and a special contract should be made with them. Their advancement through the level system should depend upon explicit evidence that they are working on their problems. Such a system is called a *positive reinforcement system.* In this system behavior is strengthened by the addition of something that follows its occurrence. The automatic level system is suspended for such a patient, and progress through the level system is based on the occurrence of the expected behavior. Various therapists are asked to provide direct feedback to a person who keeps track of the patient's progress. In other words, this patient does not advance through the level system automatically but receives his level raises only after positive feedback from various therapists. Similarly, an absence of progress in therapeutic situations may lead to a demotion in the level system.

A negative reinforcement system is used when a youngster is under some type of punishment such as room restriction, social isolation from peers, or restriction of free time. Under these circumstances, the patient has to behave in a way that will get him out of the punishment situation. It may be a short-term situation or may last for several days or even weeks.

Flexible Reinforcement Systems

Patients with severe psychiatric problems such as psychosis, major depression, manic episodes, severe anxiety, and attention-deficit disorder with hyperactivity are less likely to meet the expectations of the milieu program. The automatic level system should be modified to meet their needs. For example, a psychotic patient may co-operate enough with the milieu to reach a level where he is entitled to go out of the unit for various group activities. However, if such a patient is still psychotic and under the influence of delusions and hallucinations, he may not be able to handle such privileges. Each new privilege for these patients should be evaluated on the basis of their psychiatric condition.

Behavior Modification Prescription

There are many situations that are not covered by a level system. There are many patients who have undergone various types of reward-and-punishment systems without much success. These patients arouse confusion and differences of opinion among the staff over managing their problems. Under these circumstances, it is helpful for a psychiatrist to write a clear behavior modification program on the order sheet of the patient's chart. A discussion with the therapy team should precede the writing to determine the need for such a prescription. The team should identify the behavior that needs to be modified. The number of behaviors should be kept to a minimum. The team should also agree on the type of consequences to be used to modify such behaviors. It is necessary to identify those consequences that have some importance to the patient and are likely to be effective. The physician's order in the patient's chart may look as follows:

Behavior: Verbal threats or aggression.
Consequences:
   1. Room Restriction for 30 minutes with a written assignment.
   2. Extra video game time if free of verbal threats for the entire day.
Behavior: Aggression and destruction of property during room restriction.
Consequences:
   1. Seclusion room for 2 hours with a written assignment.
Behavior: Violence during room seclusion, striking out at staff or hurting himself.
Consequences:
   1. Body restraints, gradually releasing restraints with visible signs of calming down; written assignment to be completed after completely out of body restraints.

Unit Guide

Most programs have prepared a written document for the patients to help them learn the rules of daily living in the psychiatric unit. The same guides are given to family members to acquaint them with the program. This document usually includes a brief introduction of the unit, reasons for admission, problems to be solved while in the unit, and discharge planning. All this is written very briefly in a positive manner to create the hope of a better life after the completion of the treatment program. In addition, the rules of daily living are spelled out clearly along with the various consequences resulting from not following the rules. A part of the document should emphasize the necessity of having rules and should describe the underlying philosophy of discipline. Some units have fairly strict policies with regard to clothes, makeup, hygiene, smoking, and the type of music allowed.

Level systems are frequently used to indicate to the patients as well as to the staff the degree of progress that the patient is making in the program. In a short-term program (4 to 6 weeks), the level system is divided into four or five levels. Each patient is started at level 1 at the time of admission and progresses slowly to level 5. Each level is divided further into steps (five to seven). Patients earn one step each day. The attainment of each higher level is accompanied by new privileges that a patient can look forward to. How the higher levels are achieved is clearly explained. For example, in the automatic level system, the higher levels are achieved automatically with the passage of time, such as one level per week if the patient continues to abide by the unit rules without discipline or consequences. In a conditional level system, the patients have to take some definite steps to earn the higher levels.

Examples of Privileges Associated With the Level System

1. Wearing their own clothing instead of hospital gowns.
2. Later bedtime.
3. Smoking privileges.
4. Telephone privileges.
5. Going out of the unit for supervised recreational activities.
6. Visits from members of the extended family such as grandparents, aunts, and uncles.
7. A pass to go out of the unit with the family.
8. A pass to go out of the unit by themselves.
9. Other token reward specified by different programs.

Examples of Disciplinary Measures

Disciplinary measures are divided into two broad categories:

1. Loss of earned privileges.
2. Loss of personal freedom, i.e., room restrictions, sit out, social isolation, etc.

Disciplinary measures resulting in the loss of earned privileges are generally preferable to the second category of discipline. However, there are many patients who are extremely rebellious and do not follow any rules. They do not accumulate any earned privileges that can be used to motivate their behavior. Their unacceptable behavior can only be modified by the disciplinary measures of the second category. These disciplinary measures are justified on the basis that these patients, especially the emotionally and behaviorally disturbed adolescents, have not internalized the rules of the society. They are in a state of rebellion and should surely and swiftly experience the consequences of breaking the rules. For example, one treatment unit described their policy as follows:

> The primary goal of the policy and practice of discipline is to promote development of our patient's inner controls and responsibility for their actions. The underlying idea of this discipline packet is that the discipline will help teach our patients where those inner controls lay within themselves and, through repeated experiences, how to tap these resources. The discipline policy has been designed on the assumption that discipline is a progression, from outside control to teaching self-control.

Disciplinary measures are used for such infractions as verbal abuse (such as swearing, name calling, and insulting), loud and noisy behavior, mouthiness, insolence, making fun of others, refusal to abide by certain rules, hoarding items in their rooms, stealing, lying, intimidation, horseplay, and fighting.

Types of discipline include the following:

1. Verbal warning.—The patient is warned by the staff about his inappropriate or unacceptable behavior. The warnings should specify the unacceptable behaviors such as "check your language, you are disrupting; check your attitude, you are threatening; you are too loud; you are uncooperative." The patient should know that such verbal warnings are based on the observation of the staff giving the warning. They may ask only later on (when they calm down) about the details of their behavior that resulted in the warning. Repeated warnings are accumulated into further consequences such as a drop in level or loss of other privileges.

2. Level drop.—It is frequently tied to misuse of privileges or unacceptable behavior such as verbal or physical aggression or threats.

3. Loss of earned privileges such as later bedtime, smoking, going out of the unit.—Such a loss of privileges usually results from misuse of the privileges themselves.

4. Sit-out.—This consists of the patient being told to sit out. The patient is expected to remove himself from the group in order to regain self-control and avoid further discipline. The decision when to return to the group is left up to the patient.

5. Hard chair.—This consists of a child being removed from the group to a chair for a period of time (15 to 30 minutes). This is used when sit-out has not been effective and the patient continues to be disruptive.

6. Room restriction.—This is usually used when it is essential to remove a patient from all unit activities for some period of time to allow the patient to be by himself and to think about the possible attitudinal changes he must make in order to join the unit activities.

7. Seclusion room.—When it is anticipated that the patient is likely to be destructive of property or may hurt himself during confinement to his room, the patient is confined in a seclusion room that is usually devoid of breakable items and has padded walls. Behavior in the seclusion room is closely monitored by the staff through frequent observations.

8. Physical restraints.—This generally results from severe violent activities directed toward peers, staff, or property.

9. Social restriction.—When two or more patients cannot get along with each other and are in constant arguments, fights, or teasing or are unacceptably intimate with each other, they may be asked to stay away from each other and have no communication in any form until they feel they can act in more socially appropriate ways with each other.

10. Social isolation.—This may be used for nonaggressive behavior that is constantly disruptive to the group and when other lesser punishments have not been effective for managing those behaviors. This consists of the patient being removed for a specified period of time to his room or to a specialized area of the unit. Seclusion

and restraint have been misused in many institutions. Most states have passed laws to include specific indications and restrictions for room seclusion and restraint of mental patients. Various psychiatric and psychological associations have published their own guidelines for such punishments. It is important to clearly document the reasons for seclusion and restraint in every case. When a patient is removed from a group for a short or a long period of time, his punishment must be accompanied by a written or verbal assignment. The patient should write the reasons for his removal from the group and should indicate alternate ways of handling his difficulties in the group.

The Illinois Mental Health Code (1987) specifies the following points for restraint and seclusion:

1. Restraint must be used only as a therapeutic measure to prevent a recipient from causing physical harm to himself or others.
2. Restraint should not be used to punish or discipline the recipient.
3. Restraint is applied only upon the written order of a physician, a clinical psychologist, or a registered nurse with supervisory responsibilities. These individuals, after personally observing and examining the recipient, must be satisfied that the use of restraint is necessary to prevent the recipient from causing physical harm to himself or others. Restraints applied by a clinical psychologist or a registered nurse must be confirmed by a physician within 2 hours by telephone or in person and must be countersigned by the physician after he has personally examined the patient within 16 hours from the time the restraint was started.
4. No order for restraint is valid for more than 16 hours. If further restraint is required, a new order must be issued by a physician.
5. In an emergency when a physician, a clinical psychologist, or a registered nurse with supervisory responsibilities is not available, any qualified person may order restraint. In such an event, an order should be obtained as soon as possible from a qualified person but no later than 8 hours after the initial employment of such restraint.
6. The person ordering the restraint must inform the facility director in writing of the use of restraints as soon as practicable.
7. The facility director must review all restraint orders daily and must inquire into the reason for the restraint by any person who routinely orders them.
8. Restraint is limited to only one restraint period in 3 consecutive days, unless specially authorized by the facility director.
9. Parents or guardians of minors must be notified of the restraint order.

Procedures

It is essential to have an adequate number of personnel on hand before initiating restraint to avoid injury to the staff or the patient. At least two extremities must be restrained at one time (usually the right arm and the left leg).

The patient is monitored, either continuously on a video monitor screen or through observation at least every 15 minutes. Vital signs are checked and documented at least hourly. The patient is offered elimination hourly or on demand. Food and water is served at appropriate times. The patient is kept in the room for a couple of hours after all the restraints are removed to monitor the absence of explosive behavior. The patient is also asked to write an assignment with regard to the circumstances leading to the restraint, his feelings about his restraint, and possible ways he could avoid similar circumstances in the future.

The Illinois Mental Health Code for seclusion (1987) is as follows:

1. Seclusion may be used only as a therapeutic measure to prevent a recipient from causing physical harm to himself or others.

2. In no event shall seclusion be utilized to punish or discipline a recipient. Seclusion is applied only upon the written order of a physician, a clinical psychologist, or a registered nurse with supervisory responsibilities. These individuals, after personally observing and examining the patient, must be satisfied that the use of seclusion is necessary to prevent the patient from causing physical harm to himself or others. Seclusion applied by a clinical psychologist or a registered nurse must be confirmed by a physician within 2 hours by telephone or in person and must be countersigned by the physician after he has personally examined the patient within 16 hours from the time the seclusion was commenced.

3. No order for seclusion is valid for more than 16 hours. If further seclusion is required, a new order must be issued by a physician.

4. The physician who orders seclusion must inform the facility director in writing of the use of seclusion as soon as possible.

5. The facility director must review all seclusion orders on a daily basis.

6. Seclusion is limited to only one seclusion period in 3 consecutive days, unless specially authorized by the facility director.

7. Parents and guardians of the minors must be informed of the seclusion order.

Elopement Precautions

Patients who are on a closed unit may be placed on elopement precautions if they have expressed intentions to run from the unit. This type of order generally requires the nursing staff to put the patient in a hospital gown and keep him under constant observation or check his whereabouts every 10 to 15 minutes. Patients continue to participate in the normal activities of the unit. They are not allowed to wear shoes, but they may wear slippers. In open units a staff member is assigned to care for such a patient. This staff member is responsible for keeping the patient within eyesight and for transporting him from one place to another when necessary.

Suicidal Precautions

Patients expressing suicidal intentions or actually carrying out suicidal acts are put on suicide precautions. This order provides for intense observation of such patients by the unit staff. The patient is put in a hospital gown. All jewelry and sharp objects are removed. The nursing staff has to observe these patients day and night, including their trips to the bathroom and shower.

UNIT PERSONNEL AND ADMINISTRATION

The location of the psychiatric unit in general hospitals imposes a certain administrative structure that is already present in the hospital setting. Usually, a vice-president of operations is assigned direct administrative responsibility for such a unit. The personnel responsible for the day-to-day operation of the unit include the following:

1. Nursing staff (R.N.s, L.P.N.s, and aides).
2. Mental health technicians.
3. Child-care workers.
4. Unit clerks.
5. Therapists.
6. Social workers.
7. Psychologists.
8. Unit administrator.
9. Recreational therapist.
10. Teachers.
11. Medical director.

The nursing staff provides primary care on a 24-hour basis. The nursing personnel include R.N.s, L.P.N.s, and nursing aides. Child-care workers and mental health technicians supplement the nursing staff. This staffing pattern in a hospital is quite different from residential treatment centers where primary care is provided by child-care workers and the nursing staff is available only for matters relating to physical health and medication. Nursing training generally includes very little exposure to child and adolescent psychiatry. New graduates from nursing schools are little equipped with the knowledge necessary to work with disturbed adolescents. Child-care workers with prior experience in working with children and adolescents are much better equipped in providing care to adolescents. It is, however, quite difficult to change the staffing patterns in general hospitals. The nursing staff forms a backbone of patient care in psychiatric units of general hospitals. This pattern is not easy to change. If it is at all possible to shift the primary care of patients to child-care workers, it is then essential to have at least one R.N. on each working shift to provide necessary medical care.

Therapeutic recreational activities are a very important part of the unit activities. They are organized primarily by a qualified recreational or occupational therapist who carries out these activities with the help of other staff such as child-care workers and nurses.

Social workers, psychologists, and psychiatrists all engage in various types of therapeutic activities such as family therapy, group and individual therapy, psychodrama, specialized groups, and cognitive therapy groups.

Inpatient Unit as an Organization

It is helpful to conceptualize the inpatient unit as an organization of personnel and patients. Although individuals from different disciplines are assigned to this unit, they all have primary affiliations to their discipline. For example, the nursing staff is organized by the director of nursing and is bound by rules and regulations set by the hospital heirarchy of nursing. Similarly, most other staff members are affiliated with their primary discipline, which is frequently represented in a general hospital. Thus, a unit may be considered a type of "matrix" organization in which different resources are deployed around a specific project (providing inpatient psychiatric treatment to emotionally disturbed adolescents).

In order to help all the individuals to work together effectively, the project has to be defined, goals and objectives specified, and the special knowledge and skills of each discipline and each individual carefully assessed in order to achieve optimal task assignments and the specific objectives and overall goals of the project. This should not of course, be a static process, and individuals should be able to shift places and roles as they become more knowledgeable and experienced in the other tasks of the project.

Role of the Medical Director

The medical director is the primary person responsible for setting the goals and specific objectives of the project. His responsibilities include the following:

1. Explain clearly in operational terms the existing goals and objectives to all staff members.

2. Revise and modify the existing goals and objectives when they are no longer efficient or applicable.

3. Work with the heads of the different services (disciplines) in modifying goals and objectives.

4. Work with the hospital or unit administrator to meet the needs of the unit.

5. Identify problems in the therapeutic activities of the unit (appropriateness, timeliness, effectiveness). Rectify problems through discussion with the therapy staff involved in those activities.

6. Periodic review of goals and objectives for the staff.

7. Communicate with community agencies the goals and objectives of hospital treatment, criteria for hospitalization, and the nature of the treatment provided.

8. Review knowledge on new treatment and therapy and share this knowledge with the staff.

9. Review the effectiveness of the therapeutic programs periodically and make changes to improve them.

10. Monitor the care provided by other attending psychiatrists. Most of this monitoring relates to the standards of care set by the medical staff and the hospital. This includes admission criteria and the type of care and treatment provided by the psychiatrists.

11. Maintain high-quality care. The medical director is usually involved in maintaining the quality of care given by the various attending psychiatrists. The criteria used to judge the quality may vary from place to place, but the following points should be emphasized:

- Criteria for admission.—Inappropriate patients or insufficient reasons to hospitalize an adolescent should be determined.
- Appropriateness of treatment.—Treatment approaches vary among psychiatrists based on their theoretical background and experience. However, blatant disparities such as a patient with a diagnosis of major depression not receiving any type of antidepressant should be questioned.
- Readmissions.—Patients readmitted soon after discharge or within a few weeks raise questions about the adequacy of the discharge planning.
- Other issues of quality assurance are frequently monitored by a specially designated staff. These issues include a history and physical examination within 24 hours after admission; an initial assessment including clear treatment goals and objectives; discharge planning; and multidisciplinary and interdisciplinary goals and objectives.

Unit Administrator

This function is frequently performed by a nursing staff member, a mental health professional such as a social worker or a psychologist, or a graduate business administrator. The responsibilities of such administrators are varied depending upon their background training and prior experience. These responsibilities include the following:

1. The basic function of the unit administrator is to provide the nuts and bolts of the unit so that an effective therapeutic program can be built upon it. This includes the personnel and supplies. The unit administrator is the basic liaison person with the hospital administration. The needs of the unit can best be communicated to the hospital administration by the unit administrator.

2. The unit administrator should be familiar with all the maintenance services of the hospital and should be able to utilize such services as needed.

3. Personnel policy and grievance procedures are monitored by the unit administrator.

4. The unit administrator may also become involved in marketing efforts such as informing other agencies of the unit's existence and planning other services for the discharged patient.

Relationship Between the Unit Administrator and Medical Director

At times the relationship between the unit administrator and the medical director can become very conflicting. This may be due to the fact that many times the responsibilities of the two individuals overlap and result in a power struggle. It is axiomatic that the unit administrator and the medical director should function together to provide the best possible care for the patients. There are, however, all sorts of variations on how two individuals can work together depending upon their predispositions, aggressivity, knowledge, and experience. These qualities cannot be legislated. A struggle for power may occur frequently and result in inefficient functioning and low morale. Although the clinical experience of psychiatric social workers or psychologists helps them to understand the problems of a psychiatric unit better, their experience rarely allows them to set up and supervise effective clinical programs in a hospital setting. The unit administrator should concern himself primarily with the basic material and personnel needs of the programs. He should provide the resources and let the medical director run the clinical program. New programs suggested by the medical director or the unit administrator should be discussed in administrative meetings and should evaluate the availability of resources and the need for the new program.

REFERENCES

Candill W: Social processes in a collective disturbance on a psychiatric ward, in Greenblatt M, Levinson D, Williams R (eds): *The Patient and the Mental Hospital.* Glencoe, IL, Free Press, 1957, pp 438–471.

Jones M: *Maturation of the Therapeutic Community.* New York, Human Sciences Press, 1976.

Stanton A, Schwartz M: *The Mental Hospital.* New York, Basic Books Inc Publishers, 1954.

State of Illinois, Department of Mental Health and Developmental Disabilities: *Mental Health and Developmental Disabilities Code, 1987.*

5

Specific Management of Various Disorders

The most common psychiatric disorders on an adolescent inpatient unit include conduct disorders, oppositional defiant disorders, substance abuse disorders, adjustment disorders, depression, and eating disorders. Many of these patients may have a second diagnosis of attention-deficit disorder (ADD) and learning disorder. Less common disorders include anxiety disorders, somatoform disorders and obsessive/compulsive disorders. Acute psychosis subsequently diagnosed as schizophrenia is infrequent. In this chapter we will highlight the common psychiatric disorders and specific issues in the management of each of these disorders.

CONDUCT DISORDERS

According to *DSM-III(R)* criteria, conduct disorders have been classified as group type, solitary aggressive type, and undifferentiated type. The essential feature of the group-type conduct problems occur mainly in group activity with peers. The solitary aggressive type of conduct disorder is characterized by aggressive physical behavior, usually toward both adults and peers, that is initiated by the person and usually not in a group activity. The undifferentiated type includes clinical features that are a mixture of the other types and that cannot be classified in either of the other two groups. Common conduct problems include aggression directed to people or animals, destruction of property, fire setting, stealing and robbery, rape and assault, homicide, truancy from school, running away from home, low frustration tolerance, increased irritability, frequent temper outbursts, and impulsive behavior.

Delinquency is generally used by law enforcement personnel to designate the behavior of adolescents who have been found guilty by a juvenile or family court of some of the aforementioned offenses. In many states, a distinction is frequently made between status offenses and other kinds of delinquent acts. Status offenses refer to behaviors such as running away, being truant from school, and drinking that kids, by virtue of their age, are not allowed to do but are legal for adults. Delinquency refers to acts such as aggression toward other people or property, theft, robbery, rape, assault, and homicide. These are the same acts for which adults would be prosecuted.

Conduct disorder problems are estimated to occur in about 9% of the males and 2% of the females under the age of 18 years. The delinquency statistics reported by the Department of Justice indicate a continuous rise in juvenile delinquency over a couple of decades. The distribution of juvenile delinquency varies, being much greater in urban areas and in low socioeconomic groups.

Etiology

Among the multiple factors theorized as contributing to the development of conduct disorders and delinquency are the following:

1. Faulty socialization by the family.
2. Lack of close interpersonal and societal affiliations.
3. An environment in which delinquency is widespread.
4. Deficiencies in affective empathy and cognitive role-taking abilities (Rotenberg, 1974). In this hypothesis, cognitive role-taking ability is defined as the ability to understand another's thoughts and behavior from the other's point of view. No active sharing of or identifying with feelings is necessary. Affective empathy involves identifying another's emotion in a particular situation, sharing that emotion at least at the pleasant/unpleasant level, and willingness to help the person who is in an unpleasant situation.
5. Containment theory (Reckless, 1967). The basic thesis of this theory is that the propensity to commit deviant acts (against the norm of the society) is inherent within everyone. Thus any juvenile is a potential delinquent. The determining factor in both conformity and deviance is the extent to which a person is prohibited from committing a deviant act. The prohibition is acquired through learning self-control (intercontainment) and via social controls (alter containment).

Multiple biological factors relating to temperament, personality, learning disability, brain damage, brain dysfunction, seizure disorder, ADD, and chromosomal patterns interact with developmental experiences to produce an aggressive predisposition. Children with a difficult temperament tend to become difficult and explosive adolescents (Thomas and Chess, 1977). Similarly, children with immature personality development continue to throw temper tantrums during their adolescent years. A fairly large proportion of juvenile delinquents have a reading disability. Critchley (1968) found that 51% of the juvenile delinquents in his sample were 3 or more years below their expected reading level. Rutter et al. (1970) found that about one quarter of the children with reading retardation showed antisocial behavior. It is not clear how reading retardation is associated with delinquent activities. Children with true reading disorders are exposed to a great many frustrations in the classroom. They develop very low self-esteem in comparison to their classmates. Their anger, aggression, and delinquent behavior may be viewed as their attempt to gain some status with their peer group.

It may also be possible that the same brain dysfunctions that cause reading disorders also predispose some of the children to aggressive behavior. Brain damage resulting from head injury, meningitis, or encephalitis frequently predisposes children to develop a low threshold for anger and aggression. Mendelson et al. (1971) studied adolescents who were diagnosed as having brain dysfunction in childhood. They exhibited more antisocial and aggressive behavior in their teen years than did normal adolescents. Brain tumors located in the limbic structures of the brain can cause uncontrollable eruptions of violent behavior. Malamud (1967) reported a study of 18 patients with tumors of the limbic area. All suffered from psychiatric disorders. Nine had tumors of the temporal lobe, and of this group 2 were aggressive and assaultive, 2 were suicidal, 1 was both aggressive and suicidal, 1 had episodes of depression, 1 had episodic uncontrollable fear, and 2 others showed secondary psychotic symptoms. Patients with tumors in other parts of the limbic system are also described as being aggressive and assaultive.

Psychomotor seizure disorder has been associated with delinquent behavior. Some authors tend to define psychomotor seizure disorder in much broader terms. For example, Lewis (1981) includes all behaviors that are unusual or out of context, confusion, distorted or absent memory about the event, and postictal physical symptoms (tiredness, falling asleep, headache) as a psychomotor symptom complex. About one fourth of the children with the aforementioned symptomotology showed abnormal electroencephalographic (EEG) findings. However, many of the aforementioned symptoms are nonspecific, and temporal lobe spikes are seen very infrequently.

ADDs are frequently associated with delinquent behavior in adolescents. Several studies of adults with antisocial behavior show a high prevalence of ADD in their childhood. Children with these disorders are at high risk for juvenile delinquency (Huessy et al., 1974). Mendelson et al. (1971) studied 83 ADD children for 2 to 5 years after the initial diagnosis. The children were 12 to 16 years old at the time of the final evaluation. The symptoms of restlessness, distractibility, impulsiveness, excitability, and aggressiveness seem to have persisted in most of the children and were associated with poor performance in school and feelings of low self-esteem. Fifty-nine percent had some contact with the police, 23% had been taken to the police station one or more times, 18% had been before the juvenile courts, and 17% had been involved with the police three or more times. In a 5-year follow-up study of ADD children, Blouin et al. (1978) found that in adolescence the hyperactive group had more conduct problems and drank more alcohol than did the children who had school problems without hyperactivity. Satterfield et al. (1982), in a 3-year follow-up study, compared 110 boys with ADD (mean age, 17.3 years) with 88 normal adolescent boys (mean age, 16.9 years). The percentage of ADD adolescents arrested at least once for a serious offense in the lower, middle, and upper socioeconomic classes was 58%, 36%, and 52%, respectively, as compared with 11%, 9%, and 2% for the similar socioeconomic groups in the control population. The percentages for multiple arrests for the same socioeconomic groups were 45%, 25%, and 28% for ADD groups as compared with 6%, 0%, and 0% for the control groups. Twenty-five percent of the ADD adolescents had been institutionalized as compared with 1 subject in the control group. All these results were very significant and indicated strong relationships between juvenile delinquency and conduct disorders and ADDs. Satterfield et al. (1987)

also noted that ADD children who received therapy (cognitive-behavioral-interpretive) in addition to methylphenidate showed a significant reduction in delinquent behavior as compared with the ADD children who were treated with medication only.

One in every 1,000 individuals have an XXY or XYY chromosome aberration. Although there are many XYY men who are perfectly normal, an individual born with an XYY or XXY kerotype is statistically more likely to be incarcerated. People with an XYY pattern seem to have less ability to restrain themselves. They exhibit extremes of emotions, so when they are happy, they are extremely happy, or when they are angry and frustrated, they are excessively angry and frustrated.

Neurological Dysfunctions

McManus et al. (1985) studied 71 incarcerated, seriously delinquent adolescents in the following ways:

1. A neurological examination to determine the presence of active neurological signs of focal or progressive neurological disease.
2. A physical and neurological examination for soft signs (PANESS).
3. The relationship between the hard and the soft signs.

Neurological examination detected three subjects (two males and one female) with a history of closed head injuries. Two of these subjects had developed seizure disorders. The third subject showed evidence of progressive neurological disease. Thus gross neurological dysfunction was uncommon in this group. The frequency of focal or localizing neurological signs was minimal (1.5%). Neurological soft signs were more prevalent in this age group than is reported in the normal population (Wolff et al., 1982). Soft signs were negatively correlated with intelligence quotient (IQ) scores and achievement scores. However, there was no significant correlation between soft signs and the severity of delinquent behavior.

Electroencephalogram

Several studies have investigated the association of EEG abnormalities with delinquent behavior. Loomis (1965) and Lewis et al. (1982) both reported about 25% of the delinquent population they studied showed abnormal EEG findings. Lewis et al. suggested that EEG abnormalities probably reflected psychomotor epilepsy and were associated with delinquent behavior.

Hsu et al. (1985) compared 120 educated juvenile delinquents (108 males and 12 females) with 113 adolescent psychiatric inpatients who had never been adjudicated for delinquency. The EEG abnormalities were classified into the following categories:

1. Borderline records were just outside the normal limits and usually contained a few scattered, slow waves.
2. Diffused records showed a mild, generalized slowing of the waking background that was excessive for age.
3. Focal abnormalities showed one major area of abnormality.

4. Paroxysmal records with epiletogenic activity in any distribution included photoparoxysmal responses.
5. Combination records with any combination of the above.

The results showed the juvenile delinquent group had EEGs that were borderline (2), diffused (3), focal (2), and paroxysmal (14); there were no combinations. These abnormalities accounted for about 18% of the total number of records. These findings, however, were not significantly different from the EEG records of a comparison group.

The relationship between psychomotor epilepsy and violent behavior is controversial. Eight subjects in this study (four males and four females) showed a preponderance of temporal lobe paroxysmal activity. None had been diagnosed previously to have seizure disorder. The pattern of behavioral manifestations were very different between males and females. Four males were subjected to severe violent outbursts. Among the four females one showed a recurrent depression with repeated self-destruction (cutting and slashing). The second female had recurrent depression with temper outbursts and destruction of property. The third female patient suffered from "spells" characterized by initial nausea and brief auditory hallucinations. The fourth female subject had symptoms of anorexia nervosa.

Psychiatric Diagnoses

Comorbidity among conduct disorder adolescents has been studied by several groups. In one study (McManus et al., 1985), 90% of the incarcerated juvenile delinquents met *DSM-III(R)* criteria for conduct disorders. In addition, all subjects received other secondary diagnoses: schizophrenia/schizotypical personality disorder, 7; major affective disorder/dysthmic disorder, 13; borderline personality disorder, 26; mental retardation, 3; other diagnoses (personality disorders, conduct disorders, substance abuse disorders), 22. Several studies have found the coexistence of depression in adolescents with conduct disorders. For example, one study (Kaplan et al., 1986) examined the presence of depression in 33 consecutive intakes to the family court. The referrals were made for either a status offense or a juvenile delinquency petition. Seventy percent were males. In this study 61% of the youths were diagnosed with clinical depression and 100% as conduct disordered based on *DSM-III* criteria, with parents reporting symptoms for an average length of 23.5 months. There was a 71% remission in major depression disorders in these youths over a 60-day period, with no new youth becoming depressed. These youngsters received social services from the court during this period but did not receive any psychotropic medication.

Risk Factors in Early Delinquency

Multiple factors contribute to juvenile delinquency. Levine et al. (1985) studied multiple forms of risk among a group of 53 delinquents (aged 11 to 16 years) who were committed for the first time to the Division of Youth Services. The group was compared with an age-matched nondelinquent group from the same region. All subjects underwent an extensive battery of tests that included physical and neurological examinations, educational screening, and neurodevelopmental screening tests (for soft neurological signs, gross and fine motor coordination, temporal sequential organization, and auditory-language skills). Parents completed extensive questionnaires that included inventories of the subjects' early life, medical, developmental, and educational history. In addition, parents filled out behavior checklists for five categories of possible problems: affective-dependent, somatic, social-aggressive, social withdrawal, and attention and activity.

The significant demographic variables included the following: breaking up of the nuclear family was more common in the delinquent group (74% vs. 26%); approximately 11% of the delinquent-cohort fathers were unemployed or imprisoned as compared with none in the comparison group. In the delinquent group there was a high level of reported medical problems, a history of socially aggressive behaviors, developmental language disabilities, and widespread delays in academic performance. There was no significant difference between the two groups on the variables of psychosomatic disorders (and enuresis, headaches, chronic pain), early social rejection, withdrawal from peers, and low birth weight. Medical examinations revealed few positive findings. Neurological examinations showed no difference between the groups with regard to the number of soft neurological signs, neuromotor functions, temporal sequential organization, or regional perceptual skills. The delinquent group showed a high prevalence of head trauma, physical injuries, and a relatively high level of maternal weight gain (greater than 15 pounds) during pregnancy. Delinquent youths tended to aggregate risks from multiple sources.

Homicidal Adolescents

Psychiatrists are frequently asked to evaluate adolescents who have committed or attempted homicide. Some of these adolescents are hospitalized for a psychiatric evaluation. Several studies indicate that the juvenile murderer is usually psychotic or suffers from a transient episode of psychosis before he carries out a murderous assault. Lewis et al. (1983) have reported a high incidence of psychosis and brain damage in homicidal adolescents. Corder et al. (1976) emphasized the homicidal influence of interpersonal and intrapsychic conflicts created by several chaotic families. They compared three groups of adolescents: group 1, those who murdered their parents; group 2, those who murdered a relative or an acquaintance; and group 3, those who murdered a stranger. They found that group 1 could be distinguished from the other two groups on the basis of a higher incidence of physical abuse and exposure to spouse abuse. Duncan and Duncan (1971) believe that abuse and excessive pressure from the parents lead to a homicidal attempt on family members.

Dewey et al. (1987) studied 72 juvenile murderers. They were classified into three groups: (1) the psychotic group included those adolescents who were clearly psychotic (with delusions, hallucinations, or grossly disorganized behavior) according to the criteria of *DSM-III;* (2) the conflict group included adolescents who were not psychotic and were engaged in interpersonal conflict such as arguments or a dispute with the victim; and (3) the crime group of adolescents appeared to have committed the homicide in the course of another crime such as robbery or rape. The results indicated that there were 5 cases (7%) with the diagnosis of psychosis, 30 cases (42%) were categorized as conflict group, and 37 cases (51%) fell in the crime group.

Female Juvenile Delinquents

Females have become increasingly more involved in delinquent behavior. Currently, women account for at least 21% of all arrests for index offenses (for example, murder, robbery, aggravated assault, and grand theft), with adolescent girls accounting for almost half of these arrests (U.S. Department of Justice, 1984).

Several authors have suggested that the family relationships of female delinquents are more disturbed than those of male delinquents are (Widom, 1978). Henggeler et al. (1987) studied 32 two-parent families who were divided into four equal-sized groups on the basis of the adolescent's delinquency status (delinquent vs. well adjusted) and the gender of the adolescent. The ages ranged from 14 to 17 years (the mean was 16). The results revealed that the families of delinquents have lower rates of facilitative information exchange and that delinquent adolescents were more dominant toward their mothers than well-adjusted adolescents were. It was also observed that the fathers of delinquents were more dominant toward their wives than were the fathers of well-adjusted adolescents. Mother-adolescent dyads and parents in families of female delinquents had higher rates of conflict than did their counterparts in the families of male delinquents. The fathers of female delinquents were more neurotic than were the fathers of male delinquents.

Management of Conduct Disorders

Historical Trends

Trends in the treatment of juvenile delinquency and conduct disorders have shifted from a purely genetic biological focus to a predominantly sociopsychological focus. The criminologists of the 19th century followed the suggestion of Lombroso (1911) who felt that criminals were degenerate biological specimens capable of transmitting criminal behavior in toto from generation to generation. The implications of the theory resulted in the isolation of criminals from the rest of society without any psychosocial treatment. At the turn of the century widespread legal reforms focused attention on juvenile delinquents. Improving the social environment combined with psychological treatment of delinquent children and their families became the main focus of treatment in the early decades of this century. Psychoanalysis was provided the main tool of psychotherapy. Various well-known individuals spent a great deal of time in treating these youngsters. Healy (1915) published *The Individual Delinquent,* which advocated improving the social and moral environment of these youngsters such as the family and the school and advocated church activities. August Aichhorn published *Wayward Youths* (1935), which advocated and described psychotherapeutic techniques with delinquent children. Using a psychoanalytic model, Aichhorn believed the primary problem leading to delinquency resided in defective ego ideals (superego). He identified three broad diagnostic groups:

1. Criminals from a sense of guilt had very harsh superegos that made them

feel very guilty for minor violations of rules. Their repeated delinquent acts were interpreted as requests for punishment to relieve their guilt.
2. A second group had nonsocial superegos that developed from identifying with the faulty values of their parents.
3. In a third group the superego was weak and almost nonexistent. They had no internal conscience to guide their social and moral behavior.

The treatment recommendations for the first group of delinquents included psychoanalysis or psychodynamic psychotherapy. The second group was considered quite difficult to treat and required social techniques in psychotherapy. The third group could not benefit from psychotherapy and required the structure of the institutions and relationships with nondelinquent adults to develop normal superego structures.

In Europe several clinicians utilized psychoanalysis and psychotherapy in the treatment of delinquents. In England Glover (1944) reported that in an outpatient program 40% of the delinquents receiving psychoanalysis and psychotherapy showed a complete remission of symptoms. These statistics were at the top of the cure rate normally expected in outpatient treatment. Friedlouder (1947) published her work with children and adolescents in a book entitled *Psychoanalytic Approach to Juvenile Delinquency*. She emphasized selecting the right cases for this type of therapy. In addition, she emphasized the necessity of environmental change for the welfare of these patients.

Anna Freud (1949) made additional contributions to the etiology of delinquency. Besides defective ego ideals, she indicated that there are other possible mechanisms that can be utilized by delinquents:

1. Excessive use of early defensive mechanisms, for example, magical thinking and projection.
2. Acting out of poorly suppressed phallic masturbation fantasies.
3. Transference from family members to other objects.

Johnson and Szurek (1952) advanced the concept of superego lacunae in the development of delinquency. They found that delinquent acts in children were sometimes attempts to fulfill and act out their parents' own forbidden but poorly repressed impulses. The parents, through their attitude and inconsistency, promoted delinquent acts in their children.

Many clinicians in the 1950s and 1960s became skeptical about psychoanalysis as the choice of treatment for delinquency (Rexford, 1966) and began doing intense parent therapy to bring about changes in the family environment. In addition, residential treatment of delinquent adolescents became a quite acceptable mode of treatment in the 1960s and 1970s (Rinsley, 1971; Masterson, 1972).

Family Therapy

Many therapists working with delinquent adolescents have felt the need of working with the families of these youngsters to bring about more durable changes in their environment. They argue that an adolescent is still very dependent upon his family and that the family is somehow implicitly or explicity allowing the adolescent to continue to maintain his delinquent behavior. Family therapists have found that all kinds of problems in a family may lead to delinquent behavior in an adolescent. These problems include marital discord, frequent arguments, fights and physical abuse in the family, inability of the parents to set effective limits, and the parents' own delinquent tendencies, which allow the adolescent to become delinquent.

Most of the therapeutic techniques advanced in the past few decades can be grouped into two broad categories: psychodynamic and behavioral. The psychodynamic approach investigates the interpersonal and intrapsychic conflicts in the adolescent and his family as they relate to the delinquent behavior. The resolution of these conflicts is expected to bring about improvement in the delinquent behavior. Behavioral approaches, on the other hand, focus on the removal or modification of reinforcers (social and psychological) in the family to bring about changes in the delinquent behavior. These two orientations have given rise to a large number of techniques in family therapy. Most therapists using the psychodynamic approach tend to evaluate the family as a whole to determine its strengths and weaknesses and the interpersonal as well as the intrapsychic conflicts in various members of the family. Symptoms in one or more members of the family are viewed as expressions of these conflicts. Thus, elimination of symptoms in one member of the family is accompanied by improvement in other members of the family and changes in their relationships. A well-organized psychodynamic approach is reflected in the systems theory, which assumes that the emotional problems manifested by one or more members of a family results from dysfunction in the family system. Thus, the therapeutic approach of this theory is to focus on the interpersonal relationships of the family and to bring about positive changes in the disturbed relationships of the various members in the family rather than focusing on the behavior of the delinquent adolescent alone.

Behavior approaches to family therapy include a cognitive approach, an operant approach, and a combination of the two. A family therapist using an operant behavioral approach identifies the problem behavior in the delinquent adolescent. He evaluates family members and other significant adults with regard to reinforcers that may be promoting delinquent behavior. Family therapy is focused on helping parents to identify the reinforcers and to change their responses toward the adolescent so that his delinquent behavior is no longer approved or rewarding. The therapy tries to achieve changes in delinquent behavior through a set of consequences (rewards and punishments).

In the cognitive approach, the family is evaluated with regard to its understanding of the problems and its ability to solve problems as they arise. The therapist helps the family to learn to communicate, to negotiate with each other, and to deal with problems.

The success of family therapy in the management of delinquent adolescents has not been well proved. It has been difficult to compare with the various types of family therapies used in the treatment of delinquent adolescents. There are many case reports of successful treatment of delinquency with psychodynamic family therapy (Rabinowitz, 1969; Schneiderman and Evans, 1975). A few studies have compared family therapy with other treatments. In one study (Everett, 1976), 50 adolescents and their families who received family therapy were compared with another 50 adolescents who received individual or group therapies. The adolescents were typically status offenders with behavior problems including truancy, running away, drug abuse, and sexual delinquency. The parents and the adolescents in the family therapy group were more cooperative and wanted to work within the time-limited family therapy. Garrigan and Bambrick (1977) compared a group of behaviorally disturbed adolescents with a similar untreated group. The treatment group received ten sessions of family therapy, with the primary focus of treatment being the changing of the disturbed relationship of various family members rather than the adolescent's behavior. The results indicated greater improvement in the treated adolescents with regard to attitude and behavior. The families also improved in their interactions and marital relationships.

Similarly, Alexander and Parson (1973) reported that the delinquent adolescent treated with the system theory approach did better than those treated with other types of therapies did (client-centered family therapy or eclectic dynamic therapy).

There are several negative reports indicating that the dynamic family therapy approach may not be very helpful in treating delinquent adolescents and their families. Druckman (1979) found that family therapy did not significantly reduce recidivism rates among treated delinquent adolescents.

Patterson and Fleischman (1970, 1973) have provided a great impetus toward the behavioral approach in family therapy. These therapists utilized behavior modification techniques, both at home and in the classroom. The techniques included the following procedures:

1. The family members were asked to study a programmed text outlining the basic principles of learning and reinforcement.
2. Next, parents were instructed in identification and recording of the child's deviant behavior.
3. The parents were then assigned to 5 weeks of training groups where the therapist and parents practiced various management techniques.
4. The parents also learned to design contingency contracts to use with their own adolescents. The contract was basically a point system in which a child earned points for nondisruptive behavior. These points could then be exchanged for rewards.

The results of this research have been published in several studies. Patterson (1974) compared behavioral measures obtained before and after therapy on 27 families of conduct disorder males. The results indicated a significant reduction in deviant behavior in adolescents, both at home and in school. Subsequent attempts at replicating Patterson's results have not shown equally good results. Bernal et al. (1980) noted that behavior management training was more effective than short-term client-centered treatment was in reducing conduct disorder. However, the long-term effects (2 years) of behavior approach family therapy were less persistent than were those of client-centered therapy. Similarly, Weathers and Lieberman (1975) noted that contingency-contracting procedures were ineffective over a long period of time. Many of the families were inclined to quit treatment before completing it.

Several studies have reported positive results with the cognitive behavior approach in which families are trained in problem-solving skills. The family is expected to define a conflict, generate all possible options, weigh the consequences for each option, and select the best possible option. Robin (1981) compared three therapy groups of behavior disorder adolescents; (1) a cognitive behavior approach therapy group, (2) an alternate short-term family therapy group, and (3) an untreated group (on the waiting list). Both treatment groups improved significantly more than the group on the waiting list did on measures of intensity of conflict, self-reported appraisal of their conflictual communication, and an audiotaped proportion of positive to negative communication behavior. The cognitive therapy group proved to be superior to the other therapy group on the last measure.

Group Therapy

This modality of treatment is generally not very successful in an outpatient setting. It was hypothesized that since delinquent adolescents have a great deal of difficulty in developing transference in individual therapy they may relate better in a group setting where the pressure to develop a one-to-one relationship is less intense. However, delinquent adolescents often promote each other's acting-out behavior in a group setting. They can quickly join each other in unacceptable and destructive activities. Therapy groups can be organized and successfully run in an inpatient setting, detention homes, and prisons where the residents are expected to follow definite rules and the rules are enforced through a system of consequences. In outpatient clinics, such restrictions are not possible, and individual adolescents are free to leave or drop out of the group therapy.

Lavin and associates (1984) organized a group therapy program with delinquent adolescents in a school setting. The group was held during a 50-minute class period once a week for 2 years. The purpose of the group was explained to the students as learning how to get along with other people. The consequences for unacceptable behavior were the same as those in any other classroom. Most of the students remained resistant to focusing on their unacceptable behavior. They frequently questioned the purpose of the group and distrusted the adult leaders. No systematic improvement in their overall behavior was documented. A detailed description of organizing and conducting group psychotherapy in an inpatient unit is given in Chapter 4. It is helpful to divide the adolescents with conduct disorders into different groups rather than including them in one group. The leaders of the group should be cognizant of the impulsive and acting-out potentials of the adolescents. Direct intervention by the group leader is frequently necessary to curtail the disruptive behavior manifested by delinquent adolescents in therapy groups.

Behavior Modification Programs

Behavior modification programs are helpful in institutional settings where the environmental control is maximal. Delinquent adolescents respond best to a great deal of external control when starting to develop self-control. These programs generally are not successful in outpatient settings. However, if such a program is started in the inpatient unit or in an institution, it may be continued at home and in the community after discharge. We frequently work on a list of acceptable behaviors in family therapy sessions. Each behavior is associated with a consequence (reward or punishment). The adolescent and his family are expected to abide by the mutually agreed upon rules after discharge. The follow-up family sessions in the outpatient settings are focused on helping the adolescent and his family to continue their mutually agreed upon contract. In most cases such programs are successful only to a small degree. Parents frequently give in to the adolescent's unacceptable demands or impose harsher consequences than were initially agreed upon. Similarly, adolescents themselves try to get away from following any house rules. It is not uncommon for some parents to bring a long list of behaviors that they want corrected. It is important to narrow down such a list to a few salient behaviors. In order for the program to be successful, it is important that the initial contract contain a minimum number of behaviors requiring correction (fewer than five) and that the consequences imposed for unacceptable behavior be reasonable. A great deal of time is spent in negotiating a reasonable contract between the parent and the hospitalized adolescent. Adolescents are likely to agree with their parents fairly quickly in the hope that they will be discharged from the hospital and thus free of all restrictions. The therapist must evaluate the negotiating capacity of the adolescent as well as his parents. If they continue to fight and argue about other things, it is an indication that they are not likely to abide by the agreed-upon behavioral consequences.

Pharmacological Treatment

Several drugs have been used in treating aggressive and violent delinquent adolescents. The use of these medications is justified on the basis of the findings of neurophysiological studies. Most of this research has been focused on the metabolism of catecholamine and serotonin. Animal studies frequently utilize electrical stimulation of the brain to induce sham rage. Norepinephrine turnover increases during such stimulation. The frequency of sham rage episodes decreases if the synthesis of norepinephrine is reduced with the use of α-methylparatyrosine, which blocks the rate-limiting enzyme tyrosine hydroxylase (Reis, 1972). Similarly, sham rage attacks decrease when norepinephrine stores are depleted with the use of reserpine. On the other hand, monoamine oxidase inhibitors (MAOIs), which increase catecholamine, also increase the frequency of sham rage episodes.

The dopamine system is equally implicated in aggressive behavior. Drugs that stimulate the dopaminergic system (for example apomorphine) increase aggression, while dopamine blockers (for example, phenothiazine) decrease aggressive episodes. Several human studies have shown an increased turnover of catecholamine in aggressive individuals. Brown et al. (1979) found increased levels of 3-methoxy-4-hydroxyphenylglycol (the primary norepinephrine metabolite in the brain) in the cerebral spinal fluid of a group of hospitalized aggressive males.

Serotonin appears to decrease aggressive behavior by inhibiting cathecholamine-induced arousal. Electrical stimulation of the raphe nuclei (serotonin system) in animals produces aggressive behavior. Drugs that block the synthesis of serotonin (for example, parachlorophenylalanine) increase aggressive behavior in animal models (Katz and Thomas, 1976). Brown et al. (1979) found low levels of serotonin metabolites (5-hydroxyindolacetic acid [5-HIAA]) in the cerebral spinal fluid of aggressive patients.

Neuroleptic Agents.—Neuroleptics, in general, block dopaminergic transmissions. They are frequently used to calm severely agitated and aggressive patients. All neuroleptic drugs have been found useful in controlling these patients. LeVann (1971) carried out a double-blind trial of haloperidol (Haldol) and chlorpromazine in a group of mentally retarded children. Haldol was found superior to chlorpromazine in reducing aggressive behavior. Barker and Fraser (1968) compared Haldol and placebo in a double-blind study of 16 aggressive children. Thirteen of the 16 children improved on 0.05 mg of haloperidol per kilogram of body weight. However, prolonged use of neuroleptics in reducing aggressive behavior has not been studied well. Prolonged use is generally avoided because of the potential of these drugs for causing serious side affects. In our own experience, we have found that a small dosage of these agents (for example, thioridazine [Mellaril], 100 mg/day) has been very helpful in reducing the aggressive episodes of very aggressive institutionalized adolescents for several years.

Antidepressants.—Several animal and human studies indicate that antidepressants tend to increase aggressive behavior (Rampling, 1978). However, many clinicians prescribe antidepressants for the treatment of aggressive and delinquent adolescents when these behaviors are considered expressions of internal distress, dissatisfaction, unhappiness, and possible depression. There are no control studies to indicate that such use of antidepressants is effective in the absence of true depression.

Rampling (1978) reported untoward aggressiveness as the side effect of antidepressants in four clinical cases. These patients were being treated with amitriptyline or imipramine for their depression. Aggression was expressed by one patient in hostile acts a few days after taking the medication. Discontinuation of treatment stopped the aggressive feelings, but these feelings returned upon resumption of the medication. The presence of depression in adolescents with conduct disorder has been reported by several studies. For example, Chiles et al. (1980) identified major affective disorders in 23% of the delinquent adolescent population in a correctional institution. Carlson and Cantwell (1980) argued that traditional methods of assessment frequently missed the diagnosis of depression in children with conduct disorder. Such depressed and delinquent children are more likely to respond to antidepressant medication than are conduct disorder children without depression.

When a family is not capable of setting limits and the patient is completely out of the family's control, community help must be sought in order to provide the necessary limits on the patient's behavior. Continuing follow-up in a day program or in outpatient clinics is necessary in most cases. A small proportion (about 8% to 10%) of the adolescents with a diagnosis of conduct disorder require long-term treatment in residential treatment centers.

Psychostimulants.—These drugs are likely to increase aggressive behavior. This potential may be secondary to increased alertness and possible paranoid thinking on the part of the abuser of these drugs. Kalant (1966) found 19 of 87 amphetamine abusers to have symptoms of increased hostility. However, the effects are different in adolescents with ADDS; their aggressive behavior decreases with the use of these stimulants.

Minor tranquilizers.—Benzodiazepines were initially reported to have a taming effect on vicious animals (Randall, 1960). However this calming effect appeared to be the result of the sedative and muscle-relaxing effects of benzodiazepines. Other studies have reported increased hostility after the use of benzodiazepine (Feldman, 1961). Since increased hostility or rage reaction occurred in some individuals, it was labeled as paradoxical rage. At present, ample evidence has accumulated to indicate that benzodiazepines arouse hostility in some individuals, but the majority of the individuals taking benzodiazepines report calming effects from this class of drugs. However, benzodiazepines have a high potential for addiction and dependency, and individuals may show temporal lobe spikes in their EEGs.

Lithium.—The use of lithium in treating conduct disorders has shown mixed results. Annell (1969) found that, in a group of 12 children with mixed diagnoses but with dominant features of episodic aggressive behavior, 11 showed improvement with lithium. In another study, Dostal and Zvolsky (1970) found a 65% reduction in outbursts of aggressive behavior in 14 mentally retarded adolescents treated with lithium for 8 months. Platt et al. (1984) compared lithium carbonate and haloperidol in a placebo-controlled, double-blind study of 61 hospitalized children who all had a *DSM-III* diagnosis of conduct disorder and were undersocialized aggressive types with a profile of highly explosive and aggressive behavior. Both drugs reduced the aggressive behavior. The effects on cognitive function were mild; however, haloperidol caused a slowing of reaction time, whereas lithium carbonate adversely affected qualitative scores on the Proteus maze tests. No significant effects were noted on short-term recognition memory and concept attainment tests.

In summary, it is important to emphasize that the diagnosis and treatment of conduct disorders are very complex. Clinicians should make an intense effort to find possible causes that may be treated or managed with appropriate medications. EEG, computed tomography (CT), or magnetic resonance imaging (MRI) should be ordered when an organic etiology is suspected. An IQ determination and educational evaluation may be necessary in many cases with a history of poor school achievement, and appropriate school placement of a conduct disorder child with learning disability problems is likely to reduce a great deal of the stress and improve conduct problems. Evaluation of the family dynamics are extremely essential.

OPPOSITIONAL DEFIANT DISORDER

Oppositional behavior is very common in the early adolescent years. It is frequently characterized by the following manifestations:

1. Violations of minor rules set by authority figures such as parents and teachers.
2. Frequent temper tantrums.
3. Continuous argumentativeness.
4. Provocative behavior.
5. Stubbornness.
6. Lack of response to reasonable persuasion.
7. Doddling.
8. Passive resistance.
9. Belligerance in the face of corrective efforts by others.

This disorder is generally differentiated from conduct disorders on the basis that these adolescents have not violated the basic rights of others—the major age-appropriate societal norms or rules. At times this distinction is difficult to make because societal norms vary from community to community and it is just a matter of degree between conduct disorders and oppositional disorders. This disorder should be differentiated from normal adolescent rebellion. Changes in physical, cognitive, and emotional development during adolescence produce complex psychological changes in the early adolescent. There is an increasing affiliation with peers and a desire to become less dependent on parents at this age. Physical development helps adolescents convince themselves that they are quite capable of performing tasks like adults and do not need their parents to do things for them. Cognitive development induces new capabilities of reasoning and thinking (formal operations). They begin to question all the established rules of conduct and morality at this age. Defiance of house rules may be their way of testing their parents if the rules are still applicable to them since they no longer consider themselves children. Emotional development, however, seems to lag behind physical and cognitive development. There is usually turmoil in the emotional development. Periods of anxiety, depression, anger, and frustration are frequent. At times an adolescent may feel extremely depressed, loses his purpose in life, and have suicidal thoughts. These emotions, however, subside quickly and easily without any lasting consequences. Frustration and anger may be expressed in self-destructive and/or aggressive activities such as car accidents, fighting, property damage, and serious drinking bouts.

For most adolescents, the stage of turmoil is brief. They quickly return to normal daily activities in the home and in the school. In some cases the turmoil may continue unabated and may even escalate to the point where the parents and other adults become concerned for the adolescent's safety. It is usually at such times that an adolescent is referred for psychiatric care.

Successful outpatient treatment at this stage depends upon participation of the adolescent patient and his family in the treatment program. Most adolescents do not perceive the need for psychiatric help and, consequently, do not participate in family or individual therapy. If the problems continue to worsen, it becomes necessary to hospitalize the adolescent. Although hospitalization creates additional stress on the adolescent patient and his family, it creates the necessary conditions for therapeutic intervention. It gives an explicit message to the adolescent, as well as to his family, that the situation has become very serious and that something needs to be done.

All the factors promoting oppositional behavior in adolescents are not known. Certainly, children with a difficult temperament have much greater problems in following rules than do children with an easy temperament. Young children with a difficult temperament frequently become stubborn, strong-willed, and argumentative. Some children whose parents are very busy and spend little time with them become self-sufficient and independent. They resent parental rules, especially if these rules infringe on their freedom to socialize with their peers. On the other hand, children who have been very close to their parents and are overly dependent on them find early adolescence somewhat difficult. They have to try harder to feel independent from their families. Some engage in severe antisocial and delinquent activities just to prove to themselves and to their peers that they are capable of performing adult misadventures and that they are not dependent upon their parents. Many of these adolescents run away from home or become very hostile toward their parents.

Most parents have some difficulty in adjusting to normal adolescent turmoil. They usually deal with the adolescent's oppositional behavior by more strict discipline. This may result in various types of restrictions such as grounding an adolescent for weeks or months or restricting their social activities. There are many adolescents who do not respond to stricter discipline and may reach a point of being constantly punished and disciplined. They and their parents constantly argue with each other. Some of them rebel against their parents by using force and aggression. Single parents are inclined to have much greater problems with their adolescents than the intact family has. This may be due to the fact that most single parents can provide much less supervision and support to their adolescent. Also, the adolescent in a broken family is frequently angry at the remaining parent and may have a disturbed relationship with that parent for quite some time.

Problems in peer relationships, disappointment in love affairs, rejection by an idealized adult such as a teacher, and academic failures can easily induce severe frustration, anxiety, or anger in most adolescents. Expression of such frustration in the form of aggressive and defiant behavior is generally interpreted by the parents as oppositional behavior. This behavior may escalate as the parents begin to put more restrictions on the defiant adolescent.

The initial evaluation should include the exploration of various contributing factors that may be related to the anger and defiant behavior of the adolescent. These factors include the following:

1. Disturbed family dynamics such as breakup of the family, divorce, separation, the mother's new boyfriend or the father's new girlfriend, and parental remarriage.
2. Disturbed communication in the family in which the adolescent does not participate in family decisions and is always told what to do by his parents.
3. Personal frustrations on the part of the adolescent resulting from problems in peer relationships and school.
4. Substance abuse problems.
5. Depression.

Hospitalization compels the adolescent to focus on his problems. After a brief initial period of denial, most adolescents are able to think about, explore, and focus on the factors contributing to their oppositional behavior. Group and family therapy are the main modalities of inpatient treatment that bring about changes in behavior. Individual therapy is much more helpful if the adolescent has a positive feeling toward his therapist and is able to utilize the support provided by the therapist.

In group therapy sessions, confrontation and support from the peer group helps the patient to acknowledge his contribution to the problem. Family sessions are helpful in clarifying the problems in the relationship between the patient and his family. The goals of family therapy in such cases frequently include the following:

1. Facilitating the communication between the parent and the adolescent.

2. Helping the family to learn to negotiate instead of arguing over every rule and expectation. This goal is achieved during several sessions. Both the adolescent patient and the parents are asked to write their own lists of rules that they feel are necessary and reasonable. The two lists are discussed item by item. The adolescent and his parents discuss the reasoning underlying their expectations and practice negotiating (which means give and take and compromise). The therapist should not try to resolve house rules differences. Instead, emphasis should be placed on reaching agreement on a few important key rules such as curfew time, schoolwork, and substance abuse.

3. Parents with a disturbed relationship should be referred to marital counseling in addition to family therapy.

4. Parents with substance abuse problems of their own may experience great difficulty in managing the substance abuse problems of their adolescents. Family counseling in this area may be necessary.

There are no clear statistics with regard to the success of hospital treatment for oppositional defiant disorders. However, our experience indicates that when outpatient therapy fails and the oppositional behavior of the adolescent escalates hospital treatment is very helpful in bringing the adolescent and family together and improving oppositional behavior. There are, however, adolescents who have been oppositional throughout their childhood and early adolescent years (usually resulting from the disturbed family relationships), who may only improve slightly during their hospitalization, and who require continuing family therapy in the outpatient clinic.

ADJUSTMENT DISORDERS

DSM-III(R) defines adjustment disorders as mild adaptive reactions to identifiable psychosocial stressors that occur within 3 months of stressors and persist for no longer than 6 months. If the symptoms of adjustment disorder persist for more than 6 months, the diagnosis should be changed to some other mental disorder.

Symptoms of adjustment disorder frequently include difficulties or problems in the daily routine activities of the children and adolescents. For example, school grades may go down, interest in sports and other extracurricular activities may diminish, and peer relationship and interaction with family members may become strained. These symptoms are frequently associated with disturbances of mood and conduct. Mood disturbances may include depression and/or anxiety. Disturbances of conduct are quite common among adolescents and include truancy, vandalism, reckless driving, and fighting. Some adolescents may withdraw from social contacts and experience physical symptoms such as headache, backache, or pain in the chest or abdomen.

The most common stressors among adolescents include parental separation; divorce; dealing with new friends of their divorced parents, stepfather, or stepmother; and breakup with a girlfriend or a boyfriend. The pressures of academic achievement do not seem to be high on the list of stressors for this generation of adolescents. Chronic illnesses beginning in childhood such as asthma, diabetes, and hemophilia create new psychological stressors during the adolescent years and frequently cause worsening of the clinical symptoms.

The coping styles of adolescents are quite different from those of adults. Their difficulties in coping are compounded by the normal developmental struggles of finding their identity. Their capacity to deal with normal stressors appears to be diminished. Adolescents may blame themselves for the separation or divorce of their parents. Rejection by a girlfriend or a boyfriend may become a major stress leading to suicidal attempts. Anger is a frequent emotional reaction that is directed toward significant adults. Disturbances of conduct such as fighting and destruction of property may be the expression of this underlying anger. The presence of a chronic illness makes many adolescents feel sorry for themselves. While normal adolescents struggle to find an identity for themselves, handicapped adolescents have a much harder time in this regard. Feelings of inadequacy and of not being a complete or satisfactory human being dominate the thoughts of chronically ill adolescents. Their self-esteem, which is governed greatly by peer reinforcement during adolescence, also suffers some loss. Some of these adolescents are plagued by low self-esteem and confused identity. They begin to deny their chronic illnesses and behave in irrational ways such as a diabetic adolescent joining his peers in an all night eating and drinking party or a hemophiliac getting into frequent fights.

Adolescence normally includes frequent crises and upheavals. Brief episodes of depression are quite common. Anna Freud (1958) regarded most adolescent reactions as prototypes of developmental disturbances. According to her, the primary cause of emotional problems in adolescents is the emergence of sexual and aggressive drives as a result of physical and endocrinological changes. The adolescent runs the risk of having his new genital urges attach themselves to his old love objects (parents and siblings). To ward off these incestual fantasies, the adolescent completely discards the previous love objects by displaying indifference toward them or by openly re-volting against their beliefs and conventions. Erikson (1956), although subscribing to a similar formulation, assigns sociological factors a much greater role in the genesis of adolescent problems. Osterrieth (1969), following Piaget's ideas on intellectual development, considers the adolescent's opposition to the values of the adult world an exercise of his newly developed powers of abstract thinking, which necessarily involves doubts and debates before the acceptance of adult life patterns.

All adolescents need to establish an identity of their own—some kind of personal answer to the age old question "Who am I?" Adolescents clearly are not all alike and do not all face the same environmental demands. The problems confronting a socioeconomically deprived youth from a broken home in a segregated urban ghetto are vastly different from the problems faced by economically favored adolescents from a loving and protective suburban family. Becoming psychologically independent of his parents is not a simple matter for an adolescent. He is likely to be ambivalent about independence. He may desire to be a free agent, but he may just as truly want the security and lack of responsibility that are associated with continuing dependence. As as result he may suffer personal conflict over his independence needs. The ease with which this conflict is resolved in the direction of greater independence usually depends to a large extent on his past and present relationship with his parents. Parents who encourage increasing autonomy as the child grows older but who still retain an interest in and some responsibility for the adolescent's decisions are likely to promote both responsibility and independence. Authoritarian parents on the other hand tend to stifle the orderly acquisition of independent behavior, while indifferent or completely permissive parents may fail to encourage the development of responsibility.

Although most adolescents sooner or later confront the need to earn a living and to make their own way as independent members of society, there are some who fall by the wayside and become alienated from society.

These adolescents may present as youths who have not adjusted to their environment and their society. This alienation from society may be expressed in various ways:

1. *Developmental estrangement.*—Keniston (1965) described a group of youths who felt that they had somehow lost touch with their real selves and who felt that much of what they did was empty, flat, and devoid of meaning.

2. *Student activism.*—Some youths extend their struggle for independence from their family to the rest of the society. They become actively involved in changing society through political protests. The student protests of the 1960s are illustrative of such activism.

3. *Cultural alienation.*—In contrast to the politically involved or socially concerned protestor, the culturally alienated youth is far too pessimistic and too firmly opposed to the system to wish to demonstrate his disapproval in any public way. His demonstrations of dissent are private: nonconforming behavior, ideology, and dress; personal experimentation with deviant behaviors; and above all, efforts to intensify his own subjective experiences. He shows a distaste for and a lack of interest in politics and society.

4. *Dropping out.*—While culturally alienated youths may be said to have dropped out spiritually and intellectually from middle-class cultures, they have not found a substitute for it. Nihilistic and pervasively pessimistic, such youths remain in but not of the familiar middle- and upper-class culture. In contrast, the social dropout physically abandons his middle-class surroundings and lives a life outside the main structures and roles of society, e.g., hippies.

Management

Many adolescents with adjustment disorders respond well to counseling in outpatient clinics. However, some adolescents do not seem to benefit from such counseling, and their symptoms continue to become worse. The worsening of the symptoms in an adolescent is frequently associated with severe emotional turmoil and a dissociation of emotional ties from his family. Many of these adolescents become dependent on their peers for emotional support. However, some of them withdraw from social contact and from their peers because they lack stable and appropriate friends.

Hospitalization is generally helpful to prevent further escalation or a downhill course of the disorder. Individual, group, and family therapy provided during hospitalization should focus on creating an insight into the relationship between the stressors and the maladaptive behavior. Efforts should be made to decrease the possible stressors through educational, family, and community interventions. In the majority of the cases, a decreased capacity to handle stressors has existed for many years as a result of physical problems and learning difficulties. Management must address these chronic stressors and their influence on current function.

MOOD DISORDERS

The psychiatric diagnosis of major depression in a hospitalized population of adolescents varies with the type of facility (Carlson, 1983). Nationwide statistics (U.S. Statistics, 1977) indicate that the percentage of depression in juvenile admissions (under 18 years of age) to state and county facilities for 1975 was 2.7% vs. 13.8% in public hospitals and 19% in private general hospitals. This disparity is probably related to the larger number of chronic (presumably schizophrenic) patients generally serviced by state and county facilities. Several other studies of single hospital admissions (King and Pittman, 1969; Hudgens, 1974) that used more accurate and refined diagnostic criteria indicate adolescent depression to be about 40% of all hospital psychiatric admissions.

Several epidemiologic studies indicate that the symptoms of depression are quite common in adolescents and probably reflect their state of development. However, the prevalence of persistent symptoms of depression is quite close to reported figures for adults. Schoenbach et al. (1983) measured depressive symptoms in 624 adolescents (aged 12 to 15 years) with the Center for Epidemiologic Studies depression scale. The occurrence of depressive symptoms without regard to duration is quite frequent in adolescents and ranged from 18% to 76% in white males, 34% to 76% in white and black females, and 41% to 85% in black males. However, the prevalence of persistent symptoms ranged from 1% to 15% in adolescent males and 2% to 13% in adolescent females.

In a general population of children on the Isle of Wight, Rutter et al. (1970) found an incidence of depression of 0.45% among adolescents aged 14 and 15 years. In an outpatient psychiatric population, Pearce (1977) found that 23% of the adolescents exhibited depressive symptoms. Twice as many girls as boys showed depressive symptoms.

Diagnosis

Currently, the diagnostic criteria for adolescents is the same as for adults. Mood disorders are divided into bipolar disorders and depressive disorders. The essential features of bipolar disorders are the presence of one or more manic or hypomanic episodes. The essential feature of a depressive disorder is the presence of one or more periods of depression without a history of either manic or hypomanic episodes. There are two bipolar disorders: bipolar 1 is characterized by the presence of one or more manic episodes frequently alternating with one or more episodes of depression; in bipolar 2 there are multiple episodes of hypomania and depression. Similarly, depressive disorders are classified into major depression and dysthymia. The presence of a depressed mood and/or loss of interest or pleasure is an essential symptom for the diagnosis of depression. The DSM III-R criteria for a diagnosis of major depression require at least five of the following nine symptoms to be present for a 2-week period and to be a change from previous functioning:

1. Depressed, dysphoric, or irritable mood present most of the day and nearly every day.
2. Markedly diminished interest or pleasure in almost all activities most of the day and nearly every day.
3. Disturbance of appetite leading to a loss of weight (more than 5% of body weight in a month) or a gain of weight.
4. Sleep disturbance causing insomnia or hypersomnia.
5. Psychomotor agitation or retardation that should be observable (not merely subjective feelings of restlessness or slowing down).
6. Loss of energy or fatigue.
7. Feelings of worthlessness or excessive inappropriate guilt.
8. Diminished ability to think or concentrate or indecisiveness.
9. Recurrent suicidal ideation or a suicidal attempt.

The above symptoms must be present most of the day nearly every day during the required 2-week period for the diagnosis of major depression.

Associated features include tearfulness, anxiety, irritability, excessive concern with physical health, delusions, and hallucinations. Age-specific features in adolescents include negativistic and antisocial behavior, substance abuse, desire or actual running away from home, withdrawal from social activities, sulkiness, and increased aggression. When delusions are present, their content usually includes persecution, somatic delusions of a fatal disease, and delusions of poverty. Hallucinations are rare but may include occasional voices berating the person for his shortcomings and sins.

Dysthymia shares similar symptoms with major depression and differs only in duration and severity. It is a chronic mood disturbance involving depression, dysphoria, or irritability for most of the day more days than not and for at least 1 year. Impairment in social relations, academic achievement, and extracurricular activities is usually mild, and most dysthymic adolescents maintain most of their activities with a diminished capacity and achievement. Delusions or hallucinations are absent.

Bipolar mood disorders are much less common in the adolescent population than in adults (0.4% vs. 1.2%). A manic episode is characterized by a distinct period of abnormally and persistently elevated, expansive, or irritable moods. In addition, at least three (four if the mood is only irritable) of the following symptoms should be present:

1. Inflated self-esteem.
2. Decreased need for sleep.
3. More talkative than usual or pressure to keep talking.
4. Flight of ideas or subjective feelings that thoughts are racing through the head.
5. Easily distracted by unimportant, irrelevant, or external stimuli.
6. Increase in psychomotor agitation.
7. Excessive involvement in pleasurable activities that have a high potential for painful consequences.

When delusions are present, their content is usually consistent with the dominant mood. Manic episodes usually begin abruptly, and a full-blown syndrome may develop within a few days. The episode may last from a few days to months but is of shorter duration than that of major depression. In rapid cycling, short periods of manic episodes alternate with brief periods of depression.

Cyclothymia is a chronic mood disturbance characterized by numerous hypermanic episodes and numerous periods of depressed mood for at least 1 year. The person is not without hypermanic or depressive symptoms for more than 2 months during this period. Hypermanic episodes are similar to manic episodes except that hypermanic episodes are of longer duration and of lesser intensity. There is usually a mild to moderate impairment in overall function.

Issues in Diagnosis

The diagnosis of depression in adolescents is fraught with controversies. Some clinicians have argued that there are insufficient data to diagnosis depression in adolescents on the basis of adult criteria. On the other hand, some researchers (Puig-Antich, 1983) feel that depression in adolescents does not differ significantly from depression in adults. However, there are many issues that create difficulties in the diagnosis of depression in adolescents. For example, the developmental aspects of adolescence introduces a major complexity in the understanding of depression. Also, difficulties in the assessment of clinical symptoms and poor interrater reliability for the diagnosis of depression in adolescents are well known.

Developmental Issues

Developmental issues include the psychological, social, and intellectual development of adolescents that may complicate the clinical picture of depression. Carlson and Kashani (1988) studied the influence of age on the manifestation of depressive symptoms. They analyzed the findings of three studies carried out on four psychiatrically referred populations: preschool, prepubertal, adolescent, and adult. They noted that some of the symptoms of depression that increase with age and become more prominent included anhedonia, hopelessness, psychomotor retardation, and definite delusions. Depressed appearance, lower self-esteem, somatic complaints, and hallucinations decrease with age. Fatigue, agitation, and anorexia show a curvilinear relationship with age, while depressed mood, poor concentration, insomnia, suicidal ideation, and suicidal attempts did not change significantly with age. Cognitive development with regard to the understanding of time perspective and the ability to project into the future have been postulated as essential for the development of feelings of hopelessness (Bemporad, 1982). Although adolescents are cognitively capable of having a fair sense of time, their feelings of hopelessness frequently lack future perspective. It is not uncommon for many adolescents to become distraught and to have feelings of hopelessness if things do not turn out according to their expectations. Simple things (from an adult perspective) such as not getting a favorite dress, missing a dance, not getting a date, or not attending a party may result in intense frustration and hopelessness.

Adolescence normally includes frequent crises and upheavals. Episodes of depression are quite common. Mood swings are often regarded as an inherent part of adolescence. The adolescent may appear uninterested in anything one moment and then preoccupied with trivia the next. He loses interest quickly, even in his most prized activities, and then frantically seeks ways to entertain himself. Depression is expressed by withdrawal, regressive activities, aggressive activity, agitation, and hypersexuality. He may alternate between overwhelming fatigue and inexhaustible energy. The fatigue is out of proportion to daily activity. He may also complain of excessive tiredness upon awakening in the morning in spite of an adequate amount of sleep.

Many depressed youngsters complain of difficulty in concentration, which may lead to problems with schoolwork and achievement. Grades may suddenly drop from A to C to the amazement of teachers and parents. A depressed adolescent may engage in various delinquent activities such as the abuse of drugs and alcohol, running away from home, and stealing. These activities seem to serve the purpose of denying and warding off feelings of depression.

Some adolescents use sexual acting out as a method of relieving their depression. They frantically seek to make meaningful contact with other youths through sexual intercourse. Quite often, this activity produces further depression and guilt.

Growing up is perceived by some adolescents as giving up the conflict-free and sheltered life of childhood. They may also become overwhelmed by society demands to join the adult world, choose a vocation, and work for a living. Some adolescents may also see the adult world as very disappointing, whereas previously they could not wait to join it. This disparity between expectation and reality may be interpreted as loss.

All adolescents suffer from some degree of depression. In fact, it may be considered a basic psychobiological affective reaction that, like anxiety, becomes abnormal only when it persists for an undue length of time and the adolescent is unable to make a developmentally appropriate adaptation to it.

The manner of handling depression depends largely on what type of activities and peer groups are available to an adolescent. Most adolescents utilize socially sanctioned although somewhat eccentric ways of dealing with their depression. Others who are unable to utilize peer contact and activities fall by the wayside and become isolated and further depressed. Such an adolescent may resort to having suicidal ideations.

Assessment of Clinical Symptoms

A great deal of opposition to the concept of depression in adolescents has been related to the criteria with which depression is diagnosed in adolescents. The DSM III criteria for major depression include fairly well defined symptoms that can be assessed in adults with a high interrater reliability. Such is not the case with adolescents. The symptoms are not clear-cut, and most psychiatrists have difficulty in agreeing with each other in the same interview setting. The National Institute of Mental Health sponsored a field trial to determine interrater reliability by using the January 15, 1988, draft of DSM III for phase I that was supplemented by a set of criteria prepared for phase II. K coefficients of agreement among clinicians for all affective disorders for adults were 0.69 for the phase I trial and 0.83 for the phase II trial. For children and adolescents the K coefficients were 0.53 for phase I and 0.30 for phase II. These results indicated that mood disorders in children and adolescents could not be reliably diagnosed.

These difficulties can be easily appreciated in the clinical assessment of the major symptoms of depression. For example, an essential feature of major depression is reported to be a depressed or irritable mood or a loss of interest in pleasure, at least for a 2-week period. This must be present most of the day and every day. Most depressed adolescents are not depressed most of the day, nor are they depressed every day. Their sad expression dissipates quickly and easily if something exciting is available for them to do or a desired friend comes to visit them. Within a few minutes after an adolescent had told me how depressed she felt all day long, I saw her laughing and giggling with a group of peers. This experience is very common in a psychiatric adolescent inpatient unit. In fact, sad and depressed feelings are less common than are feelings of anger directed toward people who have deprived them or rejected them. Most suicidal adolescents are angry at somebody and want to hurt those who have hurt them and make them feel unhappy. Thus, it is frequently difficult to validate depressed, irritable moods even if an adolescent talks about being depressed or irritable in an interview session. In a few cases, however, observational data may corroborate interview data.

Similarly, it would be very difficult to document "markedly diminished interest or pleasure in all or almost all activities most of the day, nearly every day" through observation. In a well-structured and organized psychiatric inpatient unit where therapeutic, recreational, and educational activities are provided all day long, most adolescents are able to relate to some activities with interest and pleasure. Fatigue, loss of energy, psychomotor agitation, or retardation may be complaints of some depressed adolescents but are rarely observed all day or nearly every day. Disturbances of sleep are fairly common among normal adolescents. Most normal adolescents seem to suffer from some deficit of sleep and manifest hypersomnia during vacation or in hospitals if allowed to sleep. Complaints of difficulty in falling asleep at night are frequently subjective. In our studies of sleep disorders in depressed adolescents, sleep latency is less than 30 minutes in most cases, both in the hospital bedroom as well as in the sleep laboratory.

There are, however, a few adolescents who definitely fit the *DSM-III* criteria of major depression without any question or reservation. They appear depressed, without any expression of pleasure or excitement. They lack the energy to participate in any kind of recreational activity. They walk around in the hospital fatigued and unnoticed. Psychomotor retardation and sleeping and eating problems are invariably present. This group accounts for only 8% to 10% of the larger group of adolescents diagnosed as having major depression by different clinicians.

Course of Depression

Although the course of major depression is variable, it frequently lasts several weeks to months. In our experience about 70% of the adolescents diagnosed as having major depression at admission to the hospital recover within 2 to 4 weeks without pharmacotherapy. For these reasons we do not start treatment with antidepressants until 10 to 14 days after the hospitalization, and only those adolescents who continue to experience symptoms of major depression without much improvement are treated with antidepressants. We believe that the majority of adolescents with an initial diagnosis of major depression may in fact have adjustment disorders with a depressed mood. A quick recovery from the symptoms of depression in the supportive environment of the hospital may justify the diagnosis of adjustment disorder, although identification of precipitating psychosocial stressors may not be possible in many cases.

Management of Depression

Most adolescents with major depression are hospitalized because of suicidal ideations, suicidal attempts, psychotic symptoms such as hallucinations in the form of voices telling patients to kill themselves or do something that would endanger their lives, or visual hallucinations of some deceased person asking them to join them in Heaven. Some severely depressed adolescents may also be hospitalized because they refuse treatment on an outpatient basis, become homebound, and give up participation in normal daily activities.

Milieu Treatment

The first step in the management of depressed patients is to protect them from suicidal attempts and dangerous psychotic hallucinations and delusions. The patient is kept in sight at all times by the staff. A locked unit rather than an open unit is preferable and sometimes essential for such patients. The patient is kept on suicide precautions, which are reviewed on a daily basis until the patient gives up his active suicidal thoughts and stops experiencing dangerous hallucinations. The patients may need a great deal of support from the staff as well as from other patients. The unit staff can help the patient improve his self-esteem by improving self-care and participation in therapeutic, educational, and recreational activities. Initially, only minimal participation can be expected, but these expectations are gradually increased as the depression improves. The staff should insist that the patient look clean and presentable, even if they have to help such patients wash up, comb their hair, and put on clean clothes. Similarly, the patient should be compelled to attend therapy groups. The group leader should be cognizant of severely depressed patients and provide as much support as possible without demanding his comments or verbalization in the group. However, the group leader should give the patient an opportunity to participate by asking his comments on the subject of group discussion. School time in the unit may be quite stressful for some of these patients because they have not been doing well in their courses for some time and feel very negative toward doing any academic work. However, teachers should explain the purpose of these school hours in the program and their expectations for each student while they are in the hospital. The patient must not be allowed to sit idly or fall asleep in the classroom. He must engage in some learning activity, although he may initially choose a subject of his own interest to work on. Expectations for academic achievement are gradually increased as the depression improves.

Similarly, participation in recreational activities are minimal in the initial period of hospitalization. The recreational therapist should help the patient engage in small, simple arts-and-crafts projects that can be completed easily without a great demand on the patient's time and concentration. Participation in group activities and projects is helpful, but the therapist must discuss with the patient in advance the expectations of the group and the patient's ability to keep pace with other members of the group.

Individual Therapy

The individual therapist may utilize any of the therapeutic models that he is most familiar with. In fact, there is no evidence that any one type of psychotherapy is more effective in treating depression than others are. There are, however, some basic characteristics of depression and depressed patients that must be addressed by every therapist. For example, therapists should help motivate depressed patients to participate in various unit activities. Relationships with various significant adults should be explored to determine possible or perceived rejection by and loss of such individuals. Discussion of the patient's developmental history during childhood is frequently helpful, although the therapist must also recognize that depressed patients may not have enough concentration or motivation to explore past events in the initial phases of therapy.

Cognitive Therapy

This theory of depression proposes that depression is mainly the result of a tendency on the part of the patient to view himself, the future, and the world in a negative manner. Beck (1967) termed this tendency the "negative triad—negative view of self, future, and the world." Symptoms of major depression are considered a direct consequence of this negative cognitive set. The depressed patient distorts reality and misinterprets stimuli related to the self-concept and focuses primarily on negative events in his surroundings. It is assumed that individuals who are prone to depression have acquired a psychological predisposition through earlier experiences that promote the development of negative tendencies. For example, the death or loss of a significant individual in childhood may predispose a person to view subsequent losses very traumatically and produce depression. The responses of the depressed person to his surroundings become negative, which makes other people respond negatively toward him. This further confirms the negative view of himself.

Bipolar and psychotic patients are usually unsuited for this type of therapy. Beck et al. (1979) describe cognitive therapy as an active, directive, structured psycho-educational approach. Three theoretical assumptions underlie cognitive therapy:

1. The affect and behavior of a depressed person are largely determined by the way he views the world.
2. Cognitive processes such as thoughts, beliefs, and fantasies can be self-monitored by the patient and communicated to others.
3. Modification of depressogenic cognitive sets will lead to changes in affect and behavior.

The patient and therapist establish an agenda of prioritized issues. The therapist directs the therapy sessions to accomplish the objective set in the agenda. Beck et al. (1979) have prioritized various issues and steps that can be followed in sessions as cognitive therapy progresses:

1. Step 1.—Identify and monitor dysfunctional automatic thoughts. Automatic thoughts are subvocalizations for self-statements that a person makes to himself in response to important events or situations. Depressed patients have negative and unrealistic thoughts.
2. Step 2.—Recognize the connection between thoughts, emotions, and behavior.
3. Step 3.—Evaluate the reasonableness of the automatic thoughts. The therapist and the patient discuss unreasonableness, inconsistency with available facts, and the self-defeating nature of automatic thoughts.
4. Step 4.—Substitute more reasonable thoughts for the dysfunctional automatic thoughts.
5. Step 5.—Identify and alter the dysfunctional silent assumption. Silent assumptions are basic beliefs with which the depressed person evaluates the events around him. Most of them may be depressogenic.

Cognitive therapy is designed to be short-term therapy with 15 to 20 sessions (50 minutes per session) at weekly intervals or twice a week with more depressed patients. It is suggested that steps 1 and 2 occur during sessions 1 through 4, steps 3 and 4 occur during sessions 6 through 8; and step 5 occur during sessions 8 through 12. The remaining sessions are spent preparing the patient for termination.

Psychoanalytic Psychotherapy

The psychoanalytic treatment of depression has a long history that has been enriched by several well-known clinicians. Abraham (1911/1960a) recognized several variables that contributed to predisposition to depression. They included constitutional factors related to an increased amount of oral eroticism, libidinal fixation at the oral stage, a disappointment in love before the oedipal complex, the occurrence of a childhood form of depression called "primal parathymia," and the recurrence of this childhood form of depression following disappointments in later life.

Freud published his important psychoanalytic work on depression in "Mournings and Melancholia" (1917). He noted that in melancholia the individual is full of self-incriminations that are actually directed at an introject of the lost person. This introjection of the object also accounted for the internal sense of loss and inner emptiness of the melancholic person. In later formulations of depression (1933) Freud suggested that depression may simply be due to an excessively severe superego.

Sandor Rado (1956) emphasized an abnormal relationship of the depressed individual to his adult love objects. This abnormal hostile/dependent relationship is manifested in pushing the love object to the limit of patience. When the love object is driven away, the person tries to regain the object by the suffering and self-negation manifested during the early stages of depression.

Bibring (1953) viewed depression as a primary ego state. Depression resulted from a variety of life circumstances that caused breakdowns or lowering of self-esteem. Different individuals are susceptible to different negative life events that predispose them to the lowering of self-esteem. Some individuals are more predisposed to depression because they build up very high expectations of themselves that are frequently not met, thereby leading to feelings of helplessness and hopelessness.

Psychoanalytic psychotherapy strives not only to treat the clinical symptoms of depression but also to alter the patterns of personality to prevent a recurrence of depression. The personality characteristics of depressed individuals frequently include overdependency and self-inhibition. Depressive individuals appear to derive little pleasure from their accomplishments. There are massive inhibitions that seem self-imposed to avoid the experience of pleasure. Many of these individuals have underlying feelings of shame, guilt, and unworthiness. Some depressed adolescents have very ambivalent relationships with their parents and frequently feel rejected or left out by their parents. Displacement of a perceived lack of parental love on a boyfriend or girlfriend rarely satisfies their needs. Frequent sexual relations only make them feel more guilty and ashamed. Psychoanalytic psychotherapy explores the contributing factors to the individual's depression, helps him recognize the relationship between his actions and consequences, creates insight into the underlying reasons for his actions, and helps him modify his actions with the support of transference relationships.

Brief Psychotherapies

Various models and schemes of brief psychotherapy for depression have been advanced in the past decade. A review of such therapies can be found in *Short-Term Psychotherapies for Depression,* edited by A.J. Rush (1982). There are, however, some basic points that are common to most of these therapy models. For example, in short-term therapy it is essential to establish a time limit in advance, and to maintain therapy focus on resolution of the conflict underlying the symptoms of depression the therapist should be active and direct the therapy sessions. Negative feelings toward therapy and the therapist are dealt with early and openly. Similarly, behaviors such as over-compliance, passive avoidance, excessive politeness, and intellectualizations are pointed out early as defenses and resistances. Termination of therapy is an important process and should be dealt with in several sessions before the final session.

The effectiveness of brief psychotherapies with adolescent depression has not been evaluated. However, brief psychotherapy provides a good strategy for working with hospitalized adolescents since most therapists treating adolescents in the hospital terminate their relationship with the patient at the time of discharge and usually transfer their treatment to a previous therapist or a new therapist in the community.

Pharmacotherapy

The pharmacological treatment of depression is based on the premise that a depressed patient has some biochemical abnormalities in the brain, especially in the areas that regulate the emotions. There is no agreement on the etiology of such abnormalities. Certainly, biochemical changes in the brain can be induced by environmental stimuli. Since different individuals respond differently to a given situation, it is assumed that depressed individuals are predisposed to develop depression. The predisposition may be multidetermined and is possibly caused by genetics as well as early life experiences in childhood.

The biochemical hypothesis of depression grew mostly out of studies on the mechanism of action of antidepressant drugs. The observation that tricyclic antidepressants (TCAs) prevented the reuptake of norepinephrine into nerve terminals led to further investigations into the role of monoamines in depression and subsequently to the catecholamine hypothesis of depression. This hypothesis states that depression results from a functional deficiency of catecholamine in the brain areas that regulate emotions (Schildkraut, 1965). Since the action of TCAs also includes changes in serotonin metabolism, the indolamine hypothesis of depression arose and proposes a functional deficiency of serotonin as causing depression (Coppon, 1967). A great deal of subsequent research in animals has supported both hypotheses. However, one problem that frequently challenges these hypotheses has been related to long delays in the improvement of depressive symptoms after the intake of TCAs. The TCAs begin to block the reuptake of catecholamine and indolamine right away, but most of the symptoms of depression do not show remission until 3 or more weeks after beginning treatment with TCAs. It is now fairly well accepted that these two hypotheses do not fully explain the course of depression and that additional factors must be taken into account to understand the etiology of depression.

In recent years, attention has been focused on changes in receptors in response to antidepressant treatment. The changes in receptors are slow and correspond to the 2- to 3-week delay in clinical improvement in depressive symptoms. It has been shown that tritium-labeled TCAs bind with high affinity to α-adrenergic receptors (Richards et al., 1978). Chronic treatment with TCAs seems to increase the α-adrenergic response of nerve cells to norepinephrine but reduces the overall sensitivity of α-receptors (Menkes et al., 1980; Siever et al., 1981). Similarly, the availability and sensitivity of β-adrenergic receptors is reduced with chronic treatment with TCAs (downregulation).

TCAs also influence presynaptic (5-hydroxytryptamine 1 [5-HT1] receptors) as well as postsynaptic serotonin receptors (5-HT$_2$ receptors). Studies of postmortem specimens of suicide victims show a decrease in tritiated imipramine binding sites (5-HT$_1$ receptors) and an increase in the density of postsynaptic (5-HT$_2$) receptors (Stanley et al., 1983). This finding has been termed "denervation supersensitivity" and indicates that postsynaptic neurons attempt to compensate for the reduced availability of serotonin neurotransmitter by increasing the density of receptors. Chronic treatment with TCAs decreases the density of 5-HT$_2$ receptors (Peroutka and Snyder, 1980).

The anticholinergic effects of TCAs have been considered therapeutic by some researchers (Davis and Berger, 1978). However, the peripheral anticholinergic effects of TCAs have not been correlated with the therapeutic effects. TCAs block histamine receptors immediately and produce a reduction in histamine receptor sensitivity when used over a long period of time. This antihistaminic effect of TCAs has been considered to be antidepressant in some studies (Wallach and Hedley, 1979).

In addition to the influence on monoamine receptor sites, TCAs have other effects on brain functions that may contribute to their therapeutic antidepressant effect. For example neuroendocrine changes and changes in amino acid neurotransmitters and neuropeptides have been associated with mood disorders, and these alterations are shown with antidepressant drugs (Rubin et al., 1987).

Antidepressant Drugs.—Some of the most active cerebral stimulants belong to the group of sympathomimetic amines—the central effects of epinephrine are brief and are manifested by apprehension and excitement. Ephedrine has a more prolonged central stimulant action. Amphetamines and other related drugs have been used to overcome fatigue and depression. Although sympathomimetic drugs increase alertness and allay fatigue in normal human beings, they have been found to be of little value in the treatment of clinical depression. They tend to make the depressed more restless and agitated without lifting the lowered mood.

Antidepressant drugs include TCAs, newer antidepressants, and MAOIs. The TCAs were developed in the course of the search for compounds resembling chlorpromazine. Imipramine, the first of the tricyclics, resembles chlorpromazine except for the absence of the chloride ion and the substitution of two carbon atoms for the sulfur in the center ring. Other TCAs are similar to imipramine save for a few substitutions. TCAs are well absorbed, although some degradation may occur in the gut or on passing through the liver. They are generally highly bound in plasma proteins, but a wide variation in the degree of protein binding occurs between individuals. Similarly, there are wide variations among individual patients with regard to plasma drug levels achieved from a given oral dose. For these reasons, it has become necessary to monitor drug levels and to correlate these levels with their therapeutic effects. Table 5–1 shows the recommended plasma levels of different TCAs for maximum

TABLE 5–1
Tricyclic Antidepressants: Effective Dose and Plasma Levels

Generic Name	Trade Names	Effective Dose Range (mg/day)	Effective Plasma Levels (mg/mL)
Imipramine	Tofranil, Janimine	100–300	200
Desipramine	Norpramin, Pertofrane	75–200	40–160
Nortriptyline	Pamelor, Aventyl	30–100	50–170
Protriptyline	Vivactil	15–40	—
Trimipramine	Surmontil	50–300	—
Amitriptyline	Elavil, Amitril, Endep	100–250	150–250
Doxepin	Adapin, Sinequan	75–300	150–300

TABLE 5–2
Newer Antidepressants: Effective Dose

Generic Name	Trade Name	Effective Dose (mg/day)
Amoxapine	Asendin	100–400
Maprotiline	Ludiomil	50–300
Trazodone	Desyrel	150–600
Alprazolam	Xanax	0.5–4.0
Bupropion	—	300–700
Clomipramine	—	30–300
Mianserin	—	30–150
Nomifensine	—	50–200
Zemelidine	—	150–300

therapeutic effect. TCAs are metabolized principally by ring hydroxylation and site-chain demethylation. The latter leads to active monodemethylated metabolites (secondary amines such as desipramine and nortriptyline), which invariably accumulate when patients are treated with tertiary amines (such as amitriptyline and imipramine). The plasma disappearance rate is of fairly long duration, although exceedingly variable, which suggests the feasibility of a single daily dosage.

More than half a dozen newer antidepressants have been added to the group of antidepressant drugs (Table 5–2). These drugs are significantly different from TCAs and MAOIs with regard to their chemical structures, therapeutic potency, and side effects. For example, amoxapine may induce Parkinson-like extra pyramidal symptoms and tardive dyskinesia. Amoxapine is structurally related to loxapine, an antipsychotic drug, and one of its metabolites has potent neuroleptic activity. This combination suggests that amoxapine may be more effective in psychotic depression.

Another newer antidepressant, trazodone, has been reported to cause psychosis and priapism, a painful, prolonged penile erection in males that may require surgical intervention and cause possible permanent impotence. Maprotiline has been reported to induce or lower the threshold for seizures and is contraindicated in patients with a history of seizure disorders.

MAOIs were the first of the new antidepressants to be introduced. But they have been largely displaced by TCAs, which are less toxic and more manageable. The mechanisms of their antidepressant effects have been studied mostly in relation to monoamine neurotransmitters. MAO enzymes are widely distributed and are present in practically all tissues. It is an intracellular enzyme contained in the mitochondria that catalyzes the oxidative deamination of the side chain of catecholamine and serotonin. MAO exists in two forms—MAO-A and MAO-B. MAO-A deaminates norepinephrine, serotonin, and dopamine, while MAO-B deaminates only dopamine in some species. These drugs are rarely used in the adolescent population, primarily because of their frequent noncompliance with necessary dietary restrictions during treatment with MAOs.

Lithium has been used in bipolar mood disorders and appears to be as effective in controlling manic symptoms in adolescents as in adults. Lithium is absorbed efficiently from the gastrointestinal tract. Less than 1% of the oral dose may appear in the stools. Peak concentrations in blood plasma occur 30 minutes after an oral dosage and are followed by a plateau for the next 12 to 24 hours. From one third to two thirds of a single oral dose is excreted in the urine in 6 to 12 hours. The remainder of the lithium is excreted slowly over a period of several days. The half-life of disappearance from the blood plasma is about 24 hours. Peak concentrations in cerebral spinal fluid occur later than do those in the blood plasma. The concentrations achieved in the cerebral spinal fluid remain lower than the levels in the blood plasma. Also, the distribution of lithium ions in the brain is quite uneven. The exact mechanism of action of lithium in bipolar disorders is not known. Several hypotheses have been advanced on the basis of several lines of inquiry. Lithium is freely soluble and more evenly distributed in the body water than is sodium or potassium and may substitute for each of them. Because it is physically similar to magnesium and chemically similar to calcium, it may act like the latter cations in stabilizing the structure of proteins in membranes or in replacing magnesium as a cofactor in bioenergetic processes. In the central nervous system, lithium may interfere with neuronal conduction or carbohydrate metabolism. Another possible effect is interference with various hormone-activated adenyl cyclases. Alterations in the body distribution of electrolytes and increased excretion of cyclic adenosine monophosphate (cAMP) have been described as phenomena associated with mania. Lithium is reported to decrease catecholaminergic transmission by accelerating the presynaptic turnover of amines, inhibiting their release, or decreasing receptor sensitivity.

Because lithium is distributed freely in the body water and is not metabolized, the relationship of plasma concentrations to clinical effects is much more reliable than is the case with other drugs. During an acute manic episode the range of effective plasma concentration is reported to be 0.9 to 1.4 mEq/L. Adverse actions to lithium seem to be dose related. In adult patients, these are seldom encountered below a 1.5-mEq/L plasma level. Mild to moderate toxic reactions may occur at levels from 1.5 to 2.5 mEq/L, and moderate to severe toxic reactions may be seen at levels from

2.0 to 2.5 mEq/L. Fine tremors, polyurea, and mild thirst may occur during the initial treatment of the acute manic phase and may persist throughout the therapy. Transient nausea and general discomfort may also appear during the first few days of lithium administration. Diarrhea, vomiting, drowsiness, weakness, and a lack of coordination may be early signs of lithium intoxication and require either a reduction of the dose or complete cessation. Other reported toxic effects including epileptic seizures, slurred speech, blurred vision, albuminuria, diminished thyroid function, cardiac arrhythmia, hypertension, and leukocytosis. Lithium may also produce reversal flattening, isoelectricity, and inversion of T waves in electrocardiograms (ECGs).

Drug Treatment Outcome Studies.—Geller et al. (1985) successfully treated two groups of depressed adolescents—major depression and major depression with delusional symptoms—with TCAs. Eight adolescents with major depression were treated with nortriptyline (the dosage ranged from 70 to 150 mg/day, and plasma levels ranged between 85 and 139 mg/mL). The second group of six adolescents with delusional depression were initially treated with chlorpromazine (the dosage ranged from 50 to 100 mg/day) for 3 weeks before nortriptyline was added, starting with 25 mg daily and increasing by 25 mg once a week until the nortriptyline plasma levels reached 50 to 150 mg/mL. Mean plasma chlorpromazine levels ranged from 6 to 11 mg/mL. The nortriptyline dosage ranged from 20 to 35 mg/day to reach mean levels of 75 to 137 mg/mL. None of the subjects in either group had ECG changes outside the established guidelines (PR interval of 2.1 seconds or less, a QRS interval of 0.02 seconds or less, and a heart rate under 130 beats per minute). All patients were treated for 8 weeks after the attainment of therapeutic plasma levels of nortriptyline.

Ryan et al. (1986) treated 34 adolescents with a diagnosis of major depression for a period of 6 weeks on a fixed schedule of imipramine that was titrated to a dosage of 5.0 mL/kg/day, except as limited by side effects. All patients met research diagnostic criteria for major depression. The mean dose was 246 mg/day (4.5 mg/kg/day). Plasma levels of TCAs ranged from 77 to 986 mg/mL. In spite of good indications of compliance with treatment, only 44% of the adolescents improved to the level of no or a slightly depressed mood or anhedonia, although most of the patients had less symptomatology at the end of the treatment. They noted that adolescents with associated separation anxiety disorder had significantly poorer results than did adolescents with major depression alone.

Ryan et al. (1988) tried a combination of TCAs and lithium in TCA-resistant depression in adolescents. Fourteen adolescents diagnosed as having nonbipolar depression were treated with TCAs at least for 4 to 6 weeks before the addition of lithium, which was continued for 3 weeks to 4 months. The length of combination treatment was for at least 6 weeks, except for 3 patients in whom it was shorter. The lithium dosage ranged from 600 to 1,200 mg/day. Six of the 14 patients achieved a good response. All patients tolerated TCA/lithium combinations well.

Ryan et al. (1988) also tried MAOIs in the treatment of adolescent major depression that was unresponsive to TCAs. Twenty-three such adolescents were treated with MAOIs. Treatment was started with TCAs. If there was no clinical improvement, then MAOIs were substituted, or if they had a partial response to TCAs, an MAOI was added.

All but two subjects received at least 6 weeks of TCA treatment before they were treated with MAOIs that included either phenalzine or tranylcypromine. Seventy-four percent of this group achieved a good or fair antidepressant response, and 57% had both good or fair responses and continued dietary compliance. Special attention was paid to subject selection for this treatment with MAOIs because of the risk of impulsive or accidental dietary noncompliance.

Ryan et al. (1987) examined the relative safety of a single vs. a divided dose of imipramine in adolescent major depression. Twenty-nine adolescents with major depression were treated with imipramine on a three-times-a-day (TID) dosage schedule for 3 weeks and titrating a maximal 5.0 mg/kg/day unless limited by side effects. These patients were randomly divided into two groups: 16 received their total dose at 10 P.M. after a standard divided dosage at 7 A.M. and 3 P.M. that same day and then no more imipramine during the next 24 hours. The second group of 13 continued the TID dosage. ECG and plasma TCA levels in both groups were serially examined over the next 24 hours. There were no significant differences between the two groups with regard to ECG perameters. The author suggested that a once-daily dosage for imipramine is safe in adolescents once they have attained a steady rate. They also noticed that ECG perameters could not be used to predict plasma levels because there was a wide variation in this relationship between individuals. Even within a single patient, the plasma level could change over a wide range without any change in ECG perameters.

Several studies indicate that therapeutic levels of tricyclics in adolescents are achieved when plasma levels attain the following values: amitriptyline, 150 to 250 mg/mL; nortriptyline, 50 to 170 mg/mL; imipramine, greater than 200 mg/mL; and desipramine, 40 to 160 mg/mL.

Dugas et al. (1985) treated 110 depressed children and adolescents aged 8 to 19 years with mianserin in an open pilot study in France. The average dose of mianserin was 1 mg/kg/day. The efficacy of the treatment was noticeable by the end of the first week and was maintained throughout the 60-day study. Side effects were minimal and led to withdrawal of treatment in 7 cases. Mianserin is a tetracyclic antidepressant with no side chain, and its efficacy is well established in the treatment of adult depression. Mianserin also has a tranquilizing activity similar to diazepam and an early regulating effect on sleep.

Treatment of Manic Episodes

Several studies indicate that the diagnosis of manic episodes in adolescent years is likely to be misdiagnosed as schizophrenia or schizoaffective disorder. Dwyer and Delong (1987) suggested that the family history of manic adolescents is helpful in diagnosis because of a high rate of psychopathology in the families of these adolescents. They conducted a family history study on first- and second-degree relatives of 20 probands diagnosed with childhood manic depression. The 20 probands were 17 males and 3 females aged 4 to 18 years (mean, 11.3 years). Sixty-two and one-half percent of the probands' parents gave a positive history for major affective disorders.

The treatment of adolescent manic episode is very similar to the treatment of adult manic episode and involves neuroleptics, lithium, and carbamazepines. Hsu

(1986) described three adolescents (aged 15 to 17 years) with a diagnosis of mania who did not respond well to a combination of treatment with neuroleptics and lithium. These patients were then treated with carbamazepine, 700 to 800 mg/day alone or in combination with lithium and/or neuroleptic. The rapid cycling manic episodes are better treated with carbamazepine than with lithium.

McCracken and Diamond (1988) reported on five cases of bipolar disorder in mentally retarded adolescents. They cautioned that bipolar illness in mentally retarded adolescents is commonly misdiagnosed because of difficulty in eliciting a history of mood changes and overemphasis on psychotic and pseudo-organic symptoms. The standard treatment with neuroleptic and lithium and/or carbamazepine appeared to be well tolerated and reasonably effective.

Follow-up Studies

Follow-up studies of depressed adolescents frequently report a poor prognosis (Kandel and Davies, 1986). The prognosis is especially poor if the mood disorder is associated wtih psychotic symptoms or is the bipolar type (Strober and Carlson, 1982). Garber et al. (1988) followed 20 adolescent psychiatric inpatients for about 8 years after discharge whose initial hospitalization was at the mean age of 14 years. Seven of the 11 subjects who were diagnosed as having major depression on initial admission suffered from at least one episode of major depression during the follow-up period, and 4 of these depressed subjects reported recurrent episodes of major depression. In contrast, only 1 of the 9 psychiatric controls reported having experienced an episode of major depression during this period of follow-up.

The prognosis of bipolar affective disorder in adolescents appears to be similar to that in adult-onset disorder. Gabrielle et al. (1977) compared two groups of adults with bipolar mood disorder for 3 years. Group 1 had their first episode of mood disorder before the age of 20 years, while the second group did not experience mood disorders until after the age of 45 years. The follow-up indicated that an early age of onset was not a factor in the variable course of the prognosis of the manic depressive illness.

A 15-year follow-up study comparing adolescent-onset manic episodes with adult-onset mania indicated that patients with adolescent-onset mania presented with more psychotic symptoms and greater chronicity than adult-onset patients (McGlashan, 1988). The adolescent-onset patient displayed more delusions and/or hallucinations than the adult-onset patient did. The presence of psychotic symptoms frequently led to a diagnosis of schizoaffective disorder rather than bipolar disorder. However, the long-term (5 years) outcome of the 35 adolescent-onset patients was comparable to or better than that of the 31 adult-onset patients with regard to social contacts, heterosexual contacts, and work time.

DeLong and Aldershof (1987) reviewed the long-term treatment of children and adolescents with lithium. Fifty-nine children and adolescents were diagnosed as manic depressive. The mean age at the beginning of treatment was 10.9 years, with a range of 3.1 to 20 years. There were 49 males and 10 females. Of the 59, 28 continued lithium treatment successfully from 3 months to 108 months (mean, 30.2). The benefit of the treatment was tested by periodically discontinuing lithium therapy. In 17 others, lithium therapy was discontinued after a period of successful treatment ranging from 10 months to 70 months (mean, 33.7). These children and adolescents were studied for up to 84 months (range, 12 to 84 months; mean, 41.7 months). Overall results indicated that 39 of the 59 subjects (66%) were treated successfully with lithium over the long term.

EATING DISORDERS

Most adolescents develop peculiar eating habits including a taste for junk food, binge eating, avoidance of certain foods, and dieting. These peculiarities are not considered problems unless they lead to the development of specific syndromes such as obesity, anorexia nervosa, and bulimia.

Obesity

This is rarely a reason in adolescence for hospitalization. However, obese adolescents are frequently hospitalized for emotional and behavior problems. Obesity frequently plays a substantial role in adolescent psychopathology such as low self-esteem and depression. It is important to help these adolescents to deal with their obesity because most of the overweight problems in adolescence continue into adulthood. Abraham and Nordsieck (1960) noted that 74% of obese 10- to 13-year-old boys and 72% of obese girls became obese adults as compared with 31% and 11% of nonobese boys and girls of the same age who became obese adults. Similarly, Birch (1980) found that 63% of obese boys between the ages of 10 and 13 years became obese adults as compared with 10% of nonobese boys who became obese adults. Treatment approaches to obesity include management of nutrition, exercise, and behavior changes. Most approaches seem to work for a while, but maintenance of weight loss for any long length of time is a problem. If a comprehensive approach of weight management can be started while the adolescent patient is in the hospital, it is likely that further progress will be made after discharge.

Outpatient treatment of obesity frequently involves follow-up in a clinic or a community group. There are a number of nonprofit, and for-profit community support organizations in each community such as Take Off Pounds Sensibly (TOPS), Overeaters Anonymous (OA), and Weight Watchers groups. Unfortunately, all these groups have a very high attrition rate, with more than half of the members dropping out before the end of the first year. Short-term members lose only small amounts of weight. Long-term members may lose large amounts of weight, but they tend to regain it while still staying in the groups. Most of these group meetings provide information on diet, inspirational talks by the successful members or invited guests, regular checks of weight, and social support by the members of the group. Behavior modification techniques have been added in some of these programs with variable success. It has been suggested that since the majority of adolescents attend school a program in the schools might be more helpful in helping overweight adolescents (Brownell and Kaye, 1982).

Anorexia Nervosa

This is certainly most common during the adolescent years. Its lifetime prevalence rate is estimated between 0.5% and 2.1%. There are indications that the incidence of anorexia has gradually increased in industrialized societies following World War II.

Anorexia nervosa should be distinguished from medical conditions causing starvation and weight loss and from major depression, schizophrenia, and obsessive-compulsive disorder. Although there are several common features between depression and anorexia with regard to weight loss, in depression, appetite is generally decreased, and there is no preoccupation with losing weight. In anorexia, appetite is not decreased, but there is an active resistance to eating. Paranoid schizophrenic adolescents may stop eating or eat selectively to avoid being poisoned by some imaginary enemies. The preoccupation of anorexic patients with weight, body shape, and thinness frequently appears to have the intensity of an obsessive idea, and their ritualistic behavior with regard to exercise and eating may seem to be compulsive behavior. A diagnosis of obsessive-compulsive disorder, however, is not justified in most cases.

The criteria for hospitalization of an anorexic patient are variable. Some clinicians prefer hospitalization during the early course of the disorder to prevent physical complications and to obtain better results. Other psychiatrists, however, wait until there is a sufficient loss of weight (25% to 30% of the ideal body weight), failure of outpatient therapy, and the presence of physical and metabolic complications. There are no clear-cut studies to compare the efficacy of early or later hospitalization. However, many anorexic patients do not respond to outpatient treatment and require the structured environment of the hospital to improve their eating habits.

Anderson (1986) described the hospital treatment of the anorexic as involving four stages:

1. Nutritional rehabilitation.
2. Intensive psychotherapy.
3. Maintenance.
4. Discharge and follow-up.

It is extremely important that an anorexic patient eat a well-balanced, nutritional diet. Assigning a nurse or a child-care worker to each patient to provide one-to-one care is important. This person discusses the appropriate diet with the patient and sits with the patient to encourage eating. No more than three disliked foods are allowed to be deleted from the menu. The authors feel that much of the resistance to eating and the need for tube feeding could be avoided with this kind of individual attention. In addition, a small dosage of lorazepam (1/2 mg) before mealtime often decreases the anxiety associated with eating in these patients.

An ideal weight is calculated for each patient from weight charts or tables, usually at the 50th percentile. Most patients generally do not agree with this assessment and require a great deal of discussion and assurance that they will not look fat or overweight when reaching their 50th percentile weight. Sometimes a compromise has to be made so that the weight gain is consistent with "thin/normal weight". The patient is generally not informed about the target weight until after several weeks of therapy. The early emphasis is on eating a well-balanced diet. The diet is designed to allow patients to gain about 2 to 3 lb/wk. Usually a patient is started on a 1,500- to 1,800-calorie diet, which is increased by 500 to 750 calories/wk to a maximum of about 3,000 to 5,000 calories to obtain a 2- to 3-lb weight gain per week.

Initially, no exercise is allowed except walking around in the unit. However, a graduated program of exercises is introduced within a week or two. Heavy exercise may be introduced shortly before discharge. Exercise leads to better distribution of weight throughout the body.

Frequent problems during this stage of treatment include severe resistance to eating, hiding food, vomiting, and intense exercising.

Stage 2 of intensive psychotherapy is started when the patient begins to eat regular meals and gain some weight. The obsession with losing weight and staying thin usually decreases with weight gain. The patient's cognitive functions, comprehension, and attention generally improve. The focus in psychotherapy has to be individualized for each patient based on their history and the psychodynamics of their problems. Most patients have family conflicts that need to be resolved in family therapy sessions. Additional group therapy sessions are helpful in providing peer feedback for their body image and self-esteem. Although various theories have been advanced to explain the underlying psychological conflict in anorexia, no one single conflict appears to be specific to all patients. However, since anorexia occurs primarily during the developmental stage of puberty, conflicts are frequently related to sexual development and the dependency-independency conflict characteristic of this age.

Stage 3 of maintenance is the last phase of treatment in the hospital. The freedom and right to make decisions about diet, weight, and exercise are gradually returned to the patient. The dietician enters the picture again and helps the patient to make rational decisions. Similarly, decisions with regard to weight management and exercise are facilitated by the staff through information given and discussion. Many patients are not able to take control and begin to backslide in their diet and exercise. The patient should be confronted with this regression, and staff supervision is increased until the patient is able to internalize a better regimen. Planning for follow-up treatment is an important function of this phase.

Stage 4 treatment is carried out on an outpatient basis and may last for several years. Psychotherapy is continued on a regular weekly or more frequent basis. Family sessions may have to be held as problems become apparent in the family system with the patient's return to the home. About 30% of the hospital-treated patients relapse. Some of them may be sustained at home with more intense outpatient therapy and monitoring, while others may have to be rehospitalized.

The use of antidepressants is not helpful unless there is major depression associated with the anorexia nervosa. Similarly, there are few indications for the use of antianxiety or neuroleptic agents on a regular basis. Some patients develop gastric dilatation and feel bloated after small amounts of food. Radiologic studies may show a long emptying time. In such cases medications such as domperidone may be helpful as an antiemetic and enhancer of peristalsis.

Bulimia Nervosa

DSM-III (R) (1987) describes bulimia nervosa as a separate disorder that is characterized by recurrent episodes of binge eating (rapid consumption of large amounts of food within short periods of time) while weight gain is prevented by such means as self-induced vomiting, the use of laxatives, diuretics, dieting, fasting, or vigorous exercise. Bulimics maintain their normal weight, some may be slightly overweight, and others may be slightly underweight. These patients express consistent overconcern with body shape and weight. Their binging is usually terminated by abdominal discomfort, sleep, or induced vomiting. In some cases, vomiting itself may be desired, so the person will binge in order to vomit. Most of these patients suffer from disparaging self-criticism and a depressed mood. Studies of college freshmen indicate that 4.5% of the females and 0.4% of the males have a history of bulimia.

Several physical complications may occur depending upon the severity of the disorder. Vomiting causes an imbalance of electrolytes, especially potassium deficiency, which may lead to cardiac arrhythmia and occasionally sudden death. The acid content of the stomach causes damage to the esophagus and its sphincters. Esophageal tears and gastric ruptures may occur from the intra-abdominal pressures generated during vomiting.

Theoretical explanations of bulimic disorder range from social/cultural expectations to emotional and biological factors. The pursuit of thinness and the avoidance of fatness have become sociocultural goals in most industrialized societies. Individuals not fitting the ideal body shape feel pressured by society to modify their eating habits. Binge eating and vomiting may be a learned behavior to meet social goals. Many bulimic patients have a history of unsuccessfully trying different methods of weight management unsuccessfully before discovering and chosing binge eating and vomiting as being the most helpful. Depression itself may lead to episodes of overeating and dieting. Certainly, binge eating and vomiting may themselves cause guilt feelings and depression. It has also been suggested (Wurtman et al., 1983) that some individuals are "carbohydrate cravers." These individuals supposedly have a disturbance in their metabolic feedback mechanism. They eat multiple carbohydrate snacks, which increases their weight. They cannot avoid gaining weight by restricting food intake or increasing exercise.

Most patients with bulimia are treated in outpatient clinics. Some patients, however, are hospitalized in psychiatric units because of severe depression, medical complications, or failure of outpatient treatment. Hospital treatment generally parallels the treatment described for anorexia nervosa, including nutritional rehabilitation, intensive psychotherapy, maintenance, and follow-up. Nutritional rehabilitation is usually easier than in anorexia nervosa. Intensive psychotherapy in the form of individual, group, and family therapy is focused on resolving conflicts in the family, improving self-esteem, and understanding the relationship between binge eating, guilt feelings, and depression. Rosen and Leitenberg (1982) focused their treatment goals on reducing vomiting. They observed that bulimic patients suffer from a morbid fear of gaining weight. They are caught in a vicious circle of binge eating, anxiety, and vomiting, which reduces the anxiety. They argued that binge eating would not occur if patients could not vomit. They utilized the behavior therapy technique of "exposure and response prevention (ERP)," which has been used for the treatment of phobias and obsessive compulsive disorders (Rachman and Hodgson, 1980). The procedure required patients to eat to the point where they would usually vomit. Anxiety after binge eating progressively decreased, even though the patients could eat increasingly more food without vomiting. Johnson et al. (1984) emphasized proper eating habits, appropriate nutrition, and exercise to prevent binge eating and vomiting. The principle techniques to reach these goals included those commonly used for the treatment of obesity such as modification of eating habits, increasing exercise, cognitive restructuring, and improving self-esteem.

Medications

Several controlled studies indicate that TCAs, MAOIs, and lithium are effective in controlling the binge eating behavior of bulimic patients (Hudson et al., 1987). Pope et al. (1983) reported in a placebo-controlled trial that imipramine was superior to placebo in the treatment of bulimia. Similarly, Hughes et al. (1986) found that 68% of the chronic refractory bulimic patients improved within 10 weeks of treatment with desipramine. In a group of 32 bulimic patients a controlled trial of amitriptyline was found to be less effective than imipramine or desipramine was (Mitchell and Groat, 1984). Most authors have commented that the anticholinergic effects produced by TCAs are quite intolerable for most bulimic patients. Also, an overdose with tricyclics is not uncommon in depressed suicidal bulimic patients.

Trials of MAOIs such as phenalzine in bulimic patients have also been shown to be very efficacious, about half of the patients achieving complete remission and the other half showing some degree of improvement (Walsh et al., 1985; Kennedy et al., 1986). Side effects such as hypertension, refractory insomnia, and dietary restrictions are major problems in the use of these drugs.

Hsu (1984) found lithium carbonate to be effective in a group of 14 bulimic patients. This study, however, was uncontrolled. It is also feared that the electrolyte imbalance problems of bulimic patients may be complicated by the hyperkalemia produced by lithium. Bupropion, a newer antidepressant, was found efficacious in a group of 50 bulimic patients (Burroughs Wellcome, 1986). It is reported to have minimal anticholinergic side effects, and it possessed appetite-suppressant qualities. Unfortunately, four patients in this study developed grand mal seizures. This incidence was much higher than in trials of this drug in depression and indicates that bulimic patients may have a high potential for developing grand mal seizures.

Fluoxetine has been tried in bulimia because of its appetite-suppressing effects and possible antiobsessional properties. It has minimal side effects and a high therapeutic index. In one clinical study (Freeman, 1986) eight of the ten patients improved within a few days to a few weeks. The ninth patient showed partial improvement. The improvement was maintained by these patients for a year on follow-up.

Trazodone has been shown effective in uncontrolled trials with bulimic patients (Hudson et al., 1983). However, a few clinical case reports indicated variable effects (Wold, 1983). Similarly, uncontrolled trials of carbamazepine and sodium valproate have shown modest and variable results with bulimic patients (McElroy et al., 1987).

Several other chemicals and drugs are currently in the experimental stage of trial. Naloxone, a known opiate antagonist, has been tried in the treatment of binge eating on the assumption that the endogenous opiate system is involved in the control of eating behavior. In one study (Mitchell et al., 1986) naloxone, given as intravenous bolus followed by continuous intravenous infusion, produced a significant decrease in the amount of food consumed during a binge eating episode.

Outcome Studies of Inpatient Treatment for Anorexia Nervosa and Bulimia Nervosa

It is frequently difficult to compare outcome studies because of the differences in the severity of illness and chronicity, the duration of treatment, and follow-up therapy. A successfully treated anorexic patient in the hospital improves her eating habits, has gained some weight, and has made some changes in her attitude toward her self-esteem and body image. How long do these changes last after discharge from the hospital? What other physical and psychological morbidity are associated with anorexia nervosa?

Relapses and rehospitalizations are common for anorexic patients. Most studies indicate that the outcome improves with long-term follow-up. Morgan et al. (1983) compared three studies that have employed 4 or more years of follow-up. These three studies included the Maudsley series (Morgan and Russell, 1975), the St. Georges' series (Hsu et al., 1979), and the Bristol series (Morgan et al., 1983). The demographic characteristics of the population in the three studies were fairly similar. The outcome criteria were divided into three broad categories: good, intermediate, and poor. A good outcome meant that the patient had maintained her weight within 15% of the average weight for age, height, and sex and had regular cyclical menstrual periods. A poor outcome meant that the patient had never maintained her weight within 85% of the average weight for age, height, and sex, and menstruation was sporadic or absent. An intermediate outcome included an intermittent achievement of weight within 15% of the average weight and continuing disturbance in menstruation. With these criteria, Morgan et al. (1983) found that the outcome of the Maudsley series was 39% good, 20% intermediate, and 29% poor. The outcome of the St. Georges' series was 48% good, 30% intermediate, and 20% poor, while that of the Bristol series was 58% good, 19% intermediate, and 19% poor. It is apparent that from one third to about one fifth of these patients may continue to have serious difficulties, even after 4 years of aftercare treatment. The authors indicated that a poor prognosis was associated with disturbed relationships between the patient and the family, family hostility toward the patient, the personality difficulties of the patient, and an increased duration of illness. The factors that were not of prognostic significance included age at onset, degree of weight loss during the anorexic illness, binging, social class, a family history of mental illness, and previous psychiatric treatment.

Toner et al. (1986) compared the long-term outcome (5 to 14 years) of restricting anorexic ($n = 33$) and bulimic anorexic ($n = 27$) women in a retrospective follow-up study. They noted that bulimic anorexic patients tended to be more impulsive, extroverted, sexually active, and emotionally labile than the restricting anorexic patients. Their results indicated that bulimic and restricting anorexics did not differ in their long-term outcome. At the time of follow-up, 45% of the restricting and 30% of the bulimic anorexics were asymptomatic, 24% of the restricting and 30% of the bulimic improved, while 21% of the restricting and 33% of the bulimic remained unchanged.

Schwartz and Thompson (1981) reviewed 12 outcome studies of anorexia nervosa that had an average follow-up of more than 2 years. They included a total of 662 subjects. On follow-up, 49% of the subjects were considered cured, 31% were improved (meaning that they had achieved stable weights but had continued to have marked weight fluctuations), and 18% showed no marked change in their original symptoms and continued to have serious anorexia. Data on the presence of psychiatric symptoms and life adjustment was sporadic in different studies. The available information on 407 patients indicated that 46% of the patients had significant psychiatric symptoms and problems in life adjustment (social, marital, and vocational). Overall mortality from self-starvation was 6%.

William Swift (1982) reviewed seven outcome studies of anorexia of early age of onset. However, most of these studies included some subjects who were in their mid and late adolescence. Several of the studies indicated a very optimistic outcome at follow-up of more than 2 years. For example, Minuchin et al. (1978) reported an 86% recovery rate; only 6% remained unimproved and 4% relapsed. Similarly, Cantwell et al. (1977) found that 76% of their population at follow-up (mean duration, 4.9 years) were within 15% of their average weight. These studies were counterbalanced by several studies of pessimistic outcomes with much lower recovery rates. Swift (1982) concluded that an early age at onset of anorexia does not seem to have a more favorable outcome than a late age at onset of anorexia.

Bulimia was designated a separate diagnostic entity in 1980 with the publication of *DSM-III*. There are few follow-up studies with the strict diagnostic criteria outlined in *DSM-III*. There are several retrospective reports of clinical cases treated over short periods of time. Abraham and Mira (1983) reported a 29% to 42% cure rate (absence of binging and vomiting) in a group of 43 normal-weight bulimics followed over a period of 14 to 72 months. However, 20% to 55% were rated as unchanged. Lacey (1983) evaluated 30 bulimics 2 years after short-term (10 week) outpatient treatment. Twenty of these patients were symptom free, while 8 of the patients had only occasional symptoms of binging and vomiting.

Norman and Herzog (1986) followed 18 normal-weight bulimics at 1- and 3-year intervals. The mean age was 28 years, and the mean duration of illness was 7.6 years. These patients were treated with individual, group, and pharmacotherapy. Progress was assessed with the Eating Attitude Test, Social Adjustment Scale, Self-Report, and the Hopkins Symptom Checklist. Eating attitude and depressive symptoms improved significantly at year 1. There was no significant improvement on self-report at year 1. At year 3 significant improvement on the symptom checklist was evident. They also noticed that the bulimics whose eating attitudes and behaviors were within the normal range within 1 year (50%) maintained this improvement over 3 years.

On the other hand, those patients whose attitude did not fall within the normal range within 1 year were not likely to improve after 3 years. These patients were more chronic and suffered from severe psychiatric symptomatology.

Swift et al. (1987) evaluated the course of bulimia in 30 normal-weight bulimics who were hospitalized. The mean duration of hospitalization was 24.2 (±9.2) days. All patients were treated in an outpatient clinic after discharge. In a retrospective follow-up (2 to 5 years after discharge), 27% of the patients were still actively engaged in treatment. Thirty percent of the patients were rehospitalized since the first admission, some more than once. The mean duration of outpatient treatment posthospitalization was 17.5 ± 12.7 months (range, 1 to 48 months). At follow-up 26 of the 30 patients continued to meet the diagnostic criteria for bulimia. These patients regularly binged and vomited. However, the frequency of binging and vomiting had markedly decreased since the first hospitalization. Eight patients (27%) were considered to have a good symptomatic outcome (binging and vomiting less than monthly, no cathartic diuretic abuse), 12 patients (40%) had an intermediate outcome (binging and/or vomiting more frequently than once a month, no cathartic diuretic abuse at follow-up), and 10 patients (33%) had a poor outcome (binging or vomiting on a daily basis or ongoing cathartic diuretic abuse at follow-up). Of the remaining 4 patients, 2 were completely asymptomatic, and the other 2 were pregnant and did not have bulimic symptoms. The authors concluded that bulimia is a chronic but tractable disorder. Symptomatology persists over an extended period of time. The outcome of treatment is heterogeneous, with some patients becoming symptom free and others remaining severely affected. The factors contributing to better outcome are not yet clear.

ANXIETY DISORDERS

Adolescents with anxiety disorders are not hospitalized unless they develop severe separation anxiety disorder, school phobia, or severe avoidant disorders. DSM III-R classifies anxiety disorder in children and adolescents into the following categories:

1. Separation anxiety disorder.
2. Avoidant disorder.
3. Overanxious disorder.

Separation Anxiety Disorder

The essential feature of this disorder includes excessive anxiety for at least 2 weeks about separation from those to whom the child is attached. Other features include the following:

1. Unrealistic worry about possible harm befalling the person when the attachment figure is not around.
2. Persistent reluctance to leave the attachment figure or the home.
3. Persistent reluctance to go to sleep without being near the attachment figure.
4. Persistent avoidance of being alone.

5. Complaints of physical symptoms such as headaches, nausea, and stomach-ache in anticipation of separation.
6. Complaints of excessive distress in anticipation of separation from the home or the attachment figure.

The disorder may persist for several years with remissions and exacerbations and may at times become very incapacitating when an adolescent stops going to school, becomes homebound, or refuses to leave home for any activity outside the home. A depressed mood is frequently present and may become persistent enough to justify an additional diagnosis of dysthymia or major depression.

Avoidant Disorder

The essential feature of this disorder is an excessive shrinking from contact with unfamiliar persons that is sufficiently severe to interfere with normal social functioning with peers. The relationship with family members and familiar figures is generally warm and satisfying. This disorder is usually discovered in some adolescents who are hospitalized for other reasons. Some of these adolescents are hospitalized after a very severe act of aggression toward peers or members of their family. Poor social skills made them a prime target for teasing by peers. They continued to ignore or avoid their peers until they could no longer tolerate the teasing and then reacted with a severe act of violence toward their peers.

Overanxious Disorder

The essential feature of this disorder is excessive or unrealistic anxiety or worry for a period of 6 months or longer. The excessive anxiety and the unrealistic concern may be related to future events, past behavior, athletic and academic achievements, and social competence. Somatic complaints such as headaches and stomachaches occur frequently. Adolescents with this disorder are usually hospitalized when the anxiety becomes very pervasive and interferes severely with the normal daily routine.

School Refusal Syndrome

In the early part of this century all children absenting themselves from school were regarded as truants. Broadwin (1932) made the first attempt to describe the behavior characteristics of these children and classified them into two groups: neurotic and truant. Johnson et al. (1941) coined the term "school phobia" for the condition of the neurotic children. The early literature (Warren, 1948) was focused on separating the school phobic from true truant children in the following manner:

1. The school phobic child is frequently a good student, while the truant is a poor student.
2. The school phobic child stays home, while the truant avoids home.

3. The school phobic child remains out of school continuously for weeks or even months at a time, while the truant tends to intermittently absent himself.
4. The parents of a school phobic child are aware of his absence, but the parents of a truant child are frequently unaware of his absence.

Cooledge et al. (1957) divided school phobia into type 1 and type 2. Type 1 corresponded to the neurotic type, and the type 2 corresponded to the truant type. Berg et al. (1969) classified school phobia into acute and chronic depending upon the child's history before the onset of the phobia. The acute school phobic child is one who has had at least 3 years of trouble-free attendance at school before the illness begins. Those with long-standing difficulties were classified as chronic school phobics. Baker and Wills (1978) studied 99 cases of school phobia and divided them into acute and chronic. Children of both groups were likely to be the eldest or the youngest in the family. Acute school phobia is more likely to occur in younger children with two or fewer siblings and in children whose mothers tended to be older. It is also more common in adolescents and seems to be precipitated by stress. Chronic school phobia is likely to occur in a child from a large family and a child with a younger mother. School phobia occurs to a greater extent in the children of agoraphobic mothers.

There are many adolescents who show school phobia for the first time without any past history. These acute cases are frequently associated with some severe stress in the family or peer relationships. It is very difficult at times to determine the underlying precipitating factors that may become apparent only after some period of therapy. These cases are clearly differentiated from the other adolescents who give a past history of periodic difficulties in attending school since childhood. Several years may pass without any difficulty until early adolescence when school phobia becomes very severe.

Since the introduction of the term "school phobia," there has been continuing controversy about this term. Several authors have argued that school phobia is a misnomer and that actually the disorder results from fear of separation from the mother or the attachment figure and not from a fear of school. They have suggested the term "school refusal." The frequency of school phobia in the general population has been reported by several studies. Leton (1962) reported that 3 per 1,000 primary grade pupils and approximately 10 per 1,000 high-school students develop school phobia. Kennedy (1965) reported a total incidence of 17 cases per 1,000 school-age children per year.

Management
Both dynamic and behavioral approaches to the treatment of school phobia emphasize an early return of these phobic adolescents to the school. This tends to break up the symbolic mother/child closeness and exerts a pressure to change. It is argued that the phobic state denies the child the experiences necessary for growth. There are, however, some differences in the manner in which the child is returned to school. Berryman (1959) suggested a step-by-step approach in which the child is introduced into school with the help of the parents and the children. A few recom-

mended that psychotherapy be started before the child is forced to go to school (Talbot, 1957). In practice, however, the flexible approach needs to be maintained. Both the child and the parents are evaluated to determine the degree of the child's anxiety and the parent's willingness to force the child to return to school. There are many children who, because of their own severe anxiety as well as their parents' unwillingness to force them, may choose to stay home. An arrangement, however, must be made with the local school district to provide home tutoring for them and gradually induce the child to return to school to get his homework and to participate in gradually increasing numbers of activities at the school.

Hospitalization provides an experience of separation from the family. Separation anxiety is dealt with in the hospital with the support of the adult staff and peer relationships. It usually takes about 2 weeks for many of these adolescents to develop some control over their separation anxiety. Their anger toward their family is processed in family sessions. Many of the parents of these adolescents are highly anxious themselves. Some feel very guilty over hospitalizing their child and try to make up by bringing all kinds of gifts and try to fulfill all the requests made by the adolescent. Some parents, especially mothers, may experience depression while the adolescent is in the hospital. Marital conflict may surface in the family for the first time. Some of these families may require referral to marital and family counselors outside the hospital. It is generally helpful to allow the adolescent to attend his own school for a few days while he is still in the hospital. Parents generally transport the adolescent to the school and back to the hospital. The anxiety and fears experienced by the adolescent in attending his own school can be dealt with better by the therapy staff in the hospital.

The presence of a history of separation anxiety in some imipramine-responsive adult phobic and anxiety states led several investigators to try imipramine in the treatment of school phobia. Klein and Klein (1973) carried out a double-blind placebo-controlled study of the effects of imipramine among 35 school phobic children between the ages of 6 and 14 years. Imipramine or placebo was given in conjunction with a behavior desensitization program for a period of 6 weeks in dosages ranging from 100 to 200 mg/day. Families were seen in weekly counseling sessions. The behavioral steps for desensitization of school phobia were as follows: the parents were instructed to maintain a firm attitude promoting school attendance; the child and the mother were instructed to get ready for school at the usual time, but no attempts were made the first week to take the child to school. The second week, the child was to get ready and go to the school building without entering the school building. This process was to be continued until the child felt comfortable enough to enter the school and stay there.

It was found that the imipramine effect could not be detected after 3 weeks of therapy but was clearly present after 6 weeks. Physical symptoms while going to school and the fear of going to school were significantly improved by imipramine treatment. However, a period of placebo treatment led to school return in almost 50% of the cases. This placebo effect and parental pressure appeared to be effective until the end of the third week, at which time no further progress was made. However, 81% of the imipramine-treated children returned to school by the end of the sixth week.

There are no controlled studies of inpatient treatment of school phobia. In our sample of inpatient cases we treated 12 adolescents between the ages of 12 and 15 years over a period of 3 years. We have utilized imipramine treatment in conjunction with the behavioral steps for desensitization. These adolescents had no difficulty in attending 3 hours of school daily in the inpatient unit. However, several of them manifested great anxiety when they were sent to their own school from the hospital. Only 5 of them were successful in entering a school building and staying there for varying periods of time. Others stayed in the automobiles of their parents in the parking lot of the school and became very anxious, to the point that they were brought back to the hospital. The anxiety experienced by these children was typical of panic attacks and was manifested by rapid breathing, palpitations, weakness, and unsteadiness. Fairly high dosages of imipramine (150 to 200 mg/day) alone or in combination with small doses of benzodiazapine were necessary to control the anxiety attacks. Benzodiazepine treatment was discontinued a few weeks later when the adolescent was able to settle down in the classroom. Relapse occurred in several cases after discharge from the hospital. The adolescents developed physical symptoms in the morning and stayed home from school. Most of these families required continuing counseling in the outpatient clinic. In 4 cases, home tutoring programs were instituted for several months to help these adolescents keep up with their schoolwork until they returned to school.

It should be emphasized that our sample represented very severe cases of separation anxiety and school phobia. All families manifested severe psychopathology. In addition, there were many other behavior problems, frequently characterized as conduct disorders. Thus, there are some indications for the hospitalization of adolescents with separation anxiety disorders and school phobia: when counseling has not been successful in the outpatient clinic and the child continues to stay away from school and when it is associated with other psychopathology such as severe behavior problems and depression.

Clinical Studies

Kashani and Orvashcel (1988) studied 150 adolescents in a community high school (aged 14 to 16 years) for the prevalence of anxiety disorders. The diagnosis was based on structured psychiatric interviews, DSM-III criteria, and a psychiatrist's review of the data. Twenty-six (17.3%) of the adolescents reported a sufficient number of anxiety symptoms on the diagnostic interview for children and adolescents to meet the criteria for at least one anxiety diagnosis. Thirteen of these 26 adolescents (8.7% of the sample) had clinically significant functional impairment requiring psychiatric intervention. Of the 13 anxiety cases, 11 met the criteria for overanxious disorder, 7 for phobic disorder, 1 for separation anxiety disorder, and none for obsessive/compulsive disorder. Eight of the adolescents met the criteria for only one anxiety diagnosis (mostly overanxious), 4 met criteria for two diagnoses (overanxious plus phobic), and 1 adolescent met the criteria for all three diagnoses (overanxious, phobic, and separation anxiety disorder).

Alessi et al. (1987) studied 61 hospitalized adolescents for panic and affective disorders according to Research Diagnostic Criteria. Ten (16%) and 15 (24%) adolescents met the criteria for definite or possible panic disorder. Among the adolescents with a definite diagnosis of panic disorder, 4 were diagnosed as having major depression, endogenous subtype; 3 as having major depression; 2 as having dysthymic disorder; and 1, no diagnosable depression. The panic symptoms among the definite panic disorder group included trembling (90%), sweating (70%), palpitations (60%), fainting (50%), choking (40%), dizziness (40%), tingling (40%), chest pain (20%), and fear of death (10%). The panic attacks were frequently accompanied by depressive disorder. Separation anxiety disorder had been previously diagnosed in 4 of the 10 cases.

Anxiety disorders in adolescents have been treated with psychological as well as pharmacological therapies. Imipramine, phenalzine, and alprazolam appear to be equally effective in treating panic attacks (Sheehan, 1984). Phenalzine may have an added advantage in the treatment of resistant symptoms. Clonazepam, a high-potency benzodiazepine, is quite effective in blocking panic attacks (Spier et al., 1986). Propranolol alone has not been found very effective in the treatment of panic attacks (Noyes et al., 1984). This may be due to the fact that panic disorder is frequently associated with depression, and antidepressant medications may be a more effective choice of treatment in such cases.

Benzodiazepine and β-blockers have been found to be more effective than placebo is in several controlled studies of adult patients with generalized anxiety disorder. However, benzodiazepines are clearly superior to β-blockers (Noyes, 1985). Antidepressants generally are not effective unless the anxiety is associated with depression. A high proportion of patients, however, may experience relapse on discontinuation of benzodiazepine treatment, although the symptoms during relapse may be much less severe than the original symptoms and many patients may not seek treatment for their relapse.

Buspirone was tried in a young adolescent with anxious disorder (Kranzler, 1980). Buspirone was found to be less sedative and has shown less abuse potential than diazepam in the treatment of overanxious disorder. In this report a 13-year, 7-month-old boy with symptoms of school refusal and generalized anxiety and some phobia about being in a crowd in the classroom was treated with buspirone. The symptoms also included sweatiness, palpitations, and "a panicky feeling." No evidence of pervasive sadness, morbid thoughts, or change in appetite was present. Treatment was started with buspirone, 2.5 mg three times a day. When no side effects appeared, the dose was increased to 5 mg three times a day. He developed some daytime drowsiness but began feeling less anxious, found school more tolerable, and slept better at night. When the dose was decreased to 5 mg twice a day, he felt less sedated but remained stable for the subsequent 4 weeks. The author suggested that buspirone might be a good substitute for diazepam in the treatment of anxiety disorder in children and adolescents, especially because of its lower potential for abuse.

SUICIDAL ADOLESCENTS

A fairly large number of admissions to the adolescent psychiatric units occur because of suicidal attempts. National statistics indicate that the current suicidal rate in the 15- to 24-year-old age group is close to 13 per 100,000 population. Although no definite data are available, a few estimates indicate that the ratio of attempted suicide to completed suicide in the adolescent population may be as high as 120:1 (Dorpat and Ripley, 1967; McIntire et al., 1977). The female adolescent attempts suicide three to five times more than the male adolescent does, but the number of successful suicides is three to four times higher in the male than in the female adolescent. Suicide rates for nonwhites are lower than those for whites, with two important exceptions: (1) nonwhite females between the ages of 15 and 19 years have a slightly higher suicide rate than do white females of the same age, and (2) there has been a striking increase in the suicide rate among nonwhite males of 15 to 24 years of age.

Several studies have failed to distinguish suicidal adolescents from groups of adolescents with other psychiatric problems. Stanley and Barter (1970), for example, found that suicidal adolescents did not differ from a matched control group with respect to family situation and peer relationships. This study, however, reported a greater incidence of parental loss in the suicidal group before the age of 12 years and more threatened parental loss through talk of divorce or separation. Topol and Reznikoff (1982) noted that suicidal adolescents experienced significantly more problems in peer and family relationships. Spirito et al. (1987) compared a group of suicidal adolescents with another group of adolescents referred for psychiatric consultation with regard to family situation, past psychiatric history, substance abuse, and physical and sexual abuse. A significant difference was found only on past psychiatric history. Suicide attempters frequently had chronic psychiatric difficulties. In our study (Khan, 1987), 40 hospitalized suicidal adolescents were compared with 40 psychiatrically hospitalized, nonsuicidal adolescents and 40 never-hospitalized adolescents from a psychiatric outpatient clinic. These three groups were compared with regard to family relationship, peer relationship, academic achievement, early loss of a parent by death or divorce, and sexual abuse. There was no significant difference among the three groups with regard to age, social class, and racial background. Females accounted for 85% of the suicidal group, 30% of the nonsuicidal hospitalized group, and 47% of the outpatient group. Similarly, the three groups did not differ with regard to family relationship, academic achievement, peer relationship, and history of sexual abuse. At least 70% of the adolescents in both hospitalized groups suffered the loss of a parent by death or divorce in their preteen years. However, the outpatient group had significantly more intact families than the two hospitalized groups did.

Clinical diagnoses according to *DSM-III* criteria are listed in Table 5–3 for all three groups. It is apparent from Table 5–3 that the suicide group is a heterogeneous group with regard to psychopathology and only about one-third of this group was clinically depressed. These findings are consistent with some previous reports. For example, Jacob (1971) noted that adolescents may attempt suicide after minor adjustment problems in the family and peer relationships. In a sample of 40 suicidal adolescents selected retrospectively from a private psychiatric practice, Crumley (1979) labeled 80% of the sample as having affective disorder. Schlebusch and Minnaar (1980), in a South African study, found conduct disorder to be their most frequent diagnosis for suicidal adolescents.

TABLE 5–3
Comparison of the Three Groups for Axis I Diagnoses*

Axis I Diagnosis	Suicidal Hospitalized Group 1 (N = 40)		Nonsuicidal Hospitalized Group 2 (N = 40)		Nonsuicidal Outpatient Group 3 (N = 40)	
	N	%	N	%	N	%
Major depressive disorder	7	17.5	3	7.5	1	2.5
Bipolar affective disorder	0	0	1	2.5	1	2.5
Cycothymic disorder	0	0	1	2.5	1	2.5
Dysthymic disorder	7	17.5	4	2.5	8	20
Schizophrenic disorder	0	0	8	10	0	20
Conduct disorder	10	25	19	47.5	15	37.5
Attention deficit disorder	0	0	0	0	2	5
Eating disorders	0	0	1	2.5	1	2.5
Anxiety disorders	0	0	1	2.5	2	5
Somatoform disorders	0	0	1	2.5	3	7.5
Impulse control disorder	1	2.5	1	2.5	1	2.5
Functional encopresis	0	0	0	0	1	2.5
Oppositional disorder	0	0	0	0	1	2.5
Adjustment disorders	15	37.5	0	0	3	7.5

* From Khan AU: *J. Am. Acad. Child Psychiatry* 1987; 26:92–96. Used with permission.

If our findings are correct, then the question arises: what makes some adolescents commit or attempt suicide under the same social and familial circumstances that are also experienced by nonsuicidal adolescents? It is not surprising that environmental and demographic factors do not distinguish suicidal adolescents from the nonsuicidal groups. A relationship with one's family and peers, the emotional meaning of loss, and the importance of precipitating circumstances are complex dimensions to quantify. A conflict with one's parents about going out or about clothes, failure on school tests, or disappointment in love are ordinary everyday events that occur in the lives of all adolescents. In fact, it would be difficult to find an adolescent who has not experienced one of these events. It would be illogical to treat these events as suicidal factors. Similarly, psychiatric diagnoses are static concepts and shed little light on the cognitive and emotional responses of adolescents in the face of a perceived overwhelming stress.

We have carried out in-depth interviews with suicidal adolescents within 48 hours after the attempt. Structured interviews were carried out to elicit the details of the circumstances preceding the suicidal attempt. The interviews were focused on determining the perception of the stress and the emotional responses leading to the suicidal attempt. Almost all suicidal adolescents reported feeling overwhelmed, helpless, and hopeless before attempting suicide. Cognitive abilities capable of weighing the consequences of their act were rarely utilized. It seemed that overwhelming emotion had taken complete hold of the adolescent and had paralyzed the cognitive ability to think through the consequences of their act. A few adolescents reported a brief period of partial amnesia just before the suicidal attempt. The circumstances reported by the suicidal adolescents that preceded the suicidal attempt did not seem very different or more serious or catastrophic than the circumstances frequently encountered by nonsuicidal adolescents. However, the adolescents in the suicidal group had the following characteristics:

1. They perceived their circumstances as extremely stressful and unbearable, which led to feelings of helplessness and hopelessness.
2. They had great difficulty in dealing with anger and could not appropriately direct their feelings to the object arousing anger such as parents and peers.
3. They tended to react impulsively without thinking through the consequences of their action.

Management

Since the majority of suicide attempters arrive in the emergency room (ER) of general hospitals and are seen first by the ER physicians, it seems necessary to have a policy in each hospital that all suicide attempters be seen by a psychiatrist in consultation. There are no clear guidelines for hospitalization of a suicidal adolescent. Most psychiatrists tend to evaluate the risk of suicide and hospitalize only those adolescents with high suicidal risk. This is an unfortunate policy and has led to major mismanagement in the treatment of suicidal adolescents. Most of the adolescents (and their families) discharged from the ER do not follow outpatient treatment recommendations. They frequently return to the ER a few months later after another suicidal attempt. The recurrence of suicidal attempts in adolescents is very high. In our experience, if the first suicidal attempt by an adolescent is not properly handled, it is likely to become a coping style when frustration is encountered, thus leading to repeated suicide attempts.

We hospitalize all suicidal adolescents, irrespective of the degree of suicidal risk, for a subsequent suicide attempt. The evaluation of risk is usually based on the mode of the suicide attempt, the amount of drugs ingested, the presence of a suicide note, calling a friend after the ingestion of pills, or sharing the suicidal intention with somebody in advance. None of these factors, unfortunately, can determine the degree of suicidal risk. In the ER or shortly after hospitalization, most suicidal adolescents minimize the seriousness of their suicide attempt. They frequently verbalize statements such as "It was a stupid thing to do," "I did not want to kill myself," or "I do not want any help, I can handle it myself." These verbalizations do not reflect insight or sudden understanding on the part of the adolescent. These are desperate attempts to con the psychiatrist and the parents and get away from hospital treatment. Such an adolescent, if discharged from the ER, will continue his denial and will most likely drop out of the outpatient treatment.

All these adolescents require inpatient psychiatric evaluation. An in-depth interview with the adolescent is necessary and should focus on the details of the circumstances leading to the suicide attempt. The interviewer should ask for details of the patient's activities during the day on which the suicide attempt occurred: What were the circumstances that were perceived by the patient as stressful? What did the patient do to deal with the stress? Were these stresses different from those encountered by the patient in the past? How were they dealt with by the patient in the past? Why did the usual mode of dealing with similar stresses in the past not work this time? When did the patient first start thinking about the suicidal attempt? What other thoughts did the patient have in conjunction with the suicidal thoughts such as thoughts about various members of his family? What were the most dominant thoughts the patient had just before getting the pills or the knife for the suicide attempt? The details of the suicide attempt must be reconstructed. Inquiries are made about time, place, whether a suicide note was written before the attempt, and the thoughts and behavior immediately after the attempt. Was the patient convinced that the suicide attempt was likely to kill him? If not, what other underlying motivations were involved. The other motivations usually include making a boyfriend or a girlfriend feel sorry and resume a relationship or getting back at one of the parents who may have denied certain privileges.

In addition to the usual diagnostic information obtained from the patient and the family, additional information on the following items is extremely helpful in planning individual treatment for each patient:

1. The patient's own perception of the stressfulness of the circumstances leading to the suicide attempt.
2. The patient's usual mode of dealing with similar stresses.
3. The patient's usual mode of dealing with anger and sadness.
4. The psychiatric diagnosis on axis I.

The presence of major depression will certainly increase the suicidal potential and require in-hospital treatment until the depression improves. The main focus of treatment for all suicidal adolescents is helping them develop a better "coping style." This focus is emphasized in milieu group and individual therapy provided in the hospital setting. The term *coping style* is used here to include various cognitive and emotional variables. The cognitive variables include identifying a problem, applying known or new approaches to solve the problem, discussing the problem with friends, and thinking through the consequences before taking serious action. The emotional variables may include identifying feelings of anger, sadness, frustration, hopelessness, and helplessness and recognizing one's own habitual emotions in problem situations and the usual mode of expressing anger, frustration, and sadness. Most suicidal adolescents are impulsive in their behavior style. They rarely use their cognitive abilities to identify and think through a solution. They manifest low frustration tolerance and are not able to bear the pain or uncomfortable feelings associated with frustrations. They do not want to live if living is going to be painful and full of frustrations. The main goal of inpatient therapy is to confront these adolescents with their faulty coping style and to help them to improve their coping abilities. Such treatment can rarely be carried out in an outpatient clinic because of denial and the lack of cooperation of most of these adolescents in treatment. Family therapy, school intervention, and community help are also necessary to help reduce sources of stress and frustration for these adolescents.

SOMATOFORM DISORDERS

Somatoform disorders are characterized by the presence of physical symptoms for which there are no demonstrable organic findings or known physiological mechanisms and a strong presumption that the symptoms are linked to psychological factors or conflicts. *DSM-III(R)* (1987) classifies these disorders into five main groups:

1. Dysmorphophobia.
2. Conversion disorder.
3. Hypochondriasis.
4. Somatization disorders.
5. Somatoform pain disorder and two residual categories, undifferentiated somatoform disorder and unspecified somatoform disorder.

Dysmorphophobia

The essential feature of this disorder is preoccupation with some imagined defect in appearance in a normal-appearing person. In some cases a slight physical abnormality may be present, but the concern expressed by a patient is grossly excessive. Adolescents are frequently concerned about their appearance, but it is only a rare case in which the concern is grossly excessive to classify the disorder as dysmorphophobia. In recent years, we have seen several female adolescents who were overly concerned about their larger breasts. They tended to attribute their depressed mood and social isolation to the large size of their breasts. This disorder should be differentiated from delusional disorder, a somatic subtype in which a belief in a defect in appearance is of delusional intensity.

Conversion Disorder

Conversion disorder is characterized by an alteration in sensory and/or motor functions and usually suggests a neurological disease such as paralysis, aphonia, coordination disturbance, akinesia, dyskinesia, blindness, tunnel vision, anosmia, anesthesia, and paresthesias.

These disorders should be distinguished from organic and factitious disorders. The factitious disorders are rare in adolescents except in some cases when an adolescent could fake an injury to avoid receiving consequences from his parents for violating some house rules. Ruling out an underlying organic etiology is at times difficult and is discussed in detail later on.

Conversion disorders result from a severe stress and psychological conflicts produced by traumatic events in the environment. Conversion symptoms usually have a symbolic meaning to the underlying conflict and provide some secondary gain to the sufferer. For example, paralysis of an arm may have a symbolic meaning of avoiding aggressively hitting another person. The term *primary gain* refers to the advantage achieved by the development of symptoms that keep the internal conflict out of conscious awareness. For example, the paralyzed arm allows the sufferer not to think about his aggressive desires to strike another person. The "secondary gain" is achieved by avoiding a particular activity that is noxious to the patient and, in addition, receiving support from the environment that otherwise might not be forthcoming. "La belle indifference" refers to the attitude of a relative lack of concern on the part of the patient about the symptoms, but it is not always characteristic of conversion disorders because some patients with severe organic illnesses may develop a stoic expression about their illness.

Hypochondriasis

The essential features of this disorder is preoccupation with the fear of having or the belief that one has a serious disease. Such a person is overly preoccupied with bodily functions and misinterprets minor physical abnormalities as severe and indicators of major illness. The person maintains his belief despite medical evidence against such belief.

Somatization Disorder

This is characterized by recurrent and multisomatic complaints of several years' duration. Such a person may seek medical attention from different physicians for the same illness. *DMS-III(R)* criteria of diagnosis require at least 13 symptoms from a list of 35 symptoms involving various organ systems such as the gastrointestinal, cardiopulmonary, neurological, sexual and reproduction, and pain symptoms. Gastrointestinal symptoms include nausea, abdominal pain, bloating, vomiting, and diarrhea. Cardiovascular symptoms may include shortness of breath when not exerting, palpitations, chest pain, and dizziness. Pseudoneurological symptoms may include amnesia and dysfunctions of voice, vision, hearing, movement, and urinary functions.

Somatoform Pain Disorder

This is characterized by preoccupation with pain in the absence of any physical findings to support an organic etiology. The pain is usually inconsistent with the known neurological distribution of pain fibers. It may mimic a known disease, but extensive diagnostic evaluation does not reveal any pathothysiology. These disorders include tension headaches, angina, sciatica, etc.

PSEUDOSEIZURES

Briquet (1859) reported that nearly three quarters of his hysterical patients suffered from convulsive attacks. Similarly, Charcot (1873, 1877) classified hysteria into two main types, convulsive and nonconvulsive, which indicated a high incidence of seizures in his hysterical patients. More recently, Reed (1975) found an incidence of pseudoseizures in hysterical patients of 9%. Pseudoseizures are fairly common among adolescents. Schneider and Rice (1979) found that 25% of the children with conversion symptoms manifested pseudoseizures. Females outnumber males in all studies of adolescents.

Pseudoseizures may include varying clinical presentations such as fainting, loss of consciousness, and the tonic movement of grand mal seizures. Generalized muscular rigidity with arching of the back and random thrashing movements of the limbs, trunk, or head is common. The convulsive movements may increase on the attempt to restrain. Some patients may become combative to get out of the restraint. Similarly, pseudoseizure patients may actively resist attempts to open their eyes. Other characteristics of grand mal seizures such as alterations of reflexes, cyanosis, response to pain stimuli, incontinency, and biting of the tongue are generally absent in pseudoseizures. Pseudoseizures may occur in patients who generally suffer from grand mal seizures. However, these seizures occur at a time when grand mal epilepsy has been well controlled for some period of time.

A routine EEG is generally not very helpful. Generalized spike-wave complexes or bursts of θ activity may sometimes appear in patients with pseudoseizures alone during anticonvulsant drug withdrawal. Fenton (1974) indicated that generalized spike-wave complexes may appear in almost 3% of apparently healthy people, possibly resulting from low convulsive thresholds. Prolonged EEG recordings or ambulatory monitoring increases the chances of recording an actual seizure. If prolonged recording is not feasible, it is often helpful to record an EEG within an hour after the occurrence of a seizure. Postictal EEG changes after a genuine seizure include transient electrical silence followed by the appearance of irregular slow waves that last for several hours before they are replaced by the regular EEG rhythm. Serum prolactin levels markedly increase after a tonic-clonic seizure but not after a pseudoseizure. However, minor epileptic attacks do not alter serum prolactin levels (Oxley et al., 1980).

A large number of factors have been described as relating to the etiology of pseudoseizures. The majority of these adolescents have a low threshold for frustration tolerance. They are highly emotional and erratic in their behavior. They may have a friend or a relative who suffers from seizure disorder. The presence of recent psychological stress, physical or sexual trauma, and conflict in peer adult relationships are frequent. A small group of adolescents with pseudoseizures may be socially withdrawn and isolated and may possibly have a borderline personality type.

Management of uncontrolled seizures requires hospitalization for definitive diagnosis and treatment. If a patient is already receiving anticonvulsant medication, treatment with it should be continued until a clear clinical diagnosis of pseudoseizures is made. A trial of placebo may be helpful to convince some families of the true nature of pseudoseizures. A diagnosis of pseudoseizures may be quite difficult in patients who have suffered from genuine seizures but also have some pseudoseizures in between genuine seizures. Psychological treatment should be the primary focus of the hospital management. A great deal of family counseling may be necessary in order to reduce the secondary gains such as excessive dependency and avoidance of uncomfortable or difficult tasks on the part of the patient. The patients will benefit from the understanding of their own adjustment problems and finding ways to overcome with therapy.

HEADACHES

Adolescents are rarely hospitalized on psychiatric units for the chief complaint of headaches. However, headache is a common symptom accompanying other psychiatric diagnoses. Proper management of this symptom is necessary in order to maintain treatment focus on the psychological factors and to avoid the development of secondary gains from the intake of frequent pain medications and staff attention for headaches.

In a follow-up study of children with headaches for 7 years Sillanpaa (1983) found that all types of headaches increased during the follow-up period. At the age of 14 years almost 75% of the adolescents had headaches at least once a month. Migraine headaches were also common in 8% of the males and 15% of the female adolescent patients.

Headaches have been classified in several ways. For example, Rothner (1983) suggested two additional classifications of headaches. The first classification is location based and is helpful in localizing the sources of pain:

1. Extracranial structures including the eyes, ears, teeth, etc.
2. Intracranial structures.
3. Vascular structures.
4. Psychological factors.

The second classification is based on the temporal profile of the headaches:

1. Acute headaches with no previous history of headaches may include all three types of headaches as described by Diamond.
2. Acute recurrent headaches may typically include migraine headaches.
3. The chronic progressive type may increase in frequency and severity over a period of about 2 months. Neurological examinations may reveal focal weakness and other signs of intracranial pathology such as tumors or hydrocephalus.
4. The chronic nonprogressive type has no associated neurological symptoms. It is frequently associated with emotional factors.

Psychological management of headaches includes relaxation and biofeedback training. The biofeedback training has been found helpful in most cases of tension headaches and in some cases of migraine headaches. Biofeedback training may be carried out for the relaxation of forehead muscles and/or temperature control of the hands. Adolescent patients generally have very little patience to complete the required training and home practice. Other relaxation techniques such as listening to tapes containing suggestions to relax and listening to soothing music are much more successful methods to help these patients relax.

ACUTE PSYCHOSIS

Adolescents are frequently hospitalized with acute symptoms of hallucinations, delusions, paranoid ideation, general agitation, lack of responsivity to reason, irrational or "odd" behavior, and bizarre thinking. Although the initial treatment for controlling the acute symptoms may be similar in most cases, it is important to differentiate the following conditions:

1. Substance abuse–induced psychosis.
2. Possible organic condition.
3. Psychiatric conditions such as schizophreniform psychosis, brief reactive psychosis, schizoaffective psychosis, mood disorders with melancholia, manic episodes, childhood pervasive developmental disorder, and delusional disorder.

Psychoactive Substance–Induced Organic Mental Disorders

These disorders are induced mainly by 13 classes of substances that are commonly abused: alcohol, amphetamines, caffeine, cocaine, cannabis, hallucinogens, inhalants, nicotine, opioids, phencyclidine (PCP), sedatives, hypnotics, and anxiolytics. A variety of clinical symptoms are produced by these drugs such as intoxication, withdrawal symptoms, delirium, delusional organic disorders, organic hallucinosis and mood disorders. The organic hallucinosis and delusional organic disorders are commonly confused with the acute phase of schizophrenia. The organic delusional syndrome and organic hallucinosis are frequently caused by stimulants, hallucinogens, PCP, and alcohol withdrawal. The organic delusional syndrome is characterized by the presence of prominent delusions and occasional hallucinations. The nature of the delusions and the associated features vary with the use of specific drugs. For example, in amphetamine abuse, paranoid ideation may be associated with hypervigilance, ideas of reference, grandiosity, psychomotor agitation, and some hallucinations such as ringing in the ears, hearing one's name called, and a sensation of insects crawling up the skin or seeing insects. In cannabis intoxication, paranoid ideation may be associated with anxiety, the sensation of slowed time, impaired judgment, and social withdrawal. Hallucinations are rare in cannabis intoxication.

Organic hallucinosis is characterized by persistent or recurrent hallucinations that may be auditory, visual, or dermatologic. Different substances tend to produce hallucinations of a particular type. For example, hallucinogens commonly cause visual hallucinations, while alcohol tends to produce auditory hallucinations. The hallucinations may be well formed, highly complex, simple, or unformed. Persons may be aware of the alien nature of the hallucinations or may believe them to be true.

Alcoholic hallucinosis is only occasionally encountered in adolescent patients. We have, however, encountered two boys in their midteens who suffered from both auditory and visual hallucinations after withdrawal from alcohol. They had been drinking in moderate quantity, mostly on weekends, from 2 to 3 years.

Delusions and hallucinations caused by amphetamines, cocaine, and PCP are indistinguishable clinically. Acute manic episodes may induce similar clinical pictures that can be distinguished by the presence of the drug metabolized in the urine.

Delusional Disorder

This disorder is characterized by the presence of a persistent and nonbizarre delusion. The type of delusional theme may include the erotomanic type, grandiose type, jealous type, persecutory type, and somatic type. This disorder should be differentiated from organic delusional syndromes and the paranoid type of schizophrenia. The person with delusional disorder shows little or no impairment in his social and occupational functioning. The negative symptoms of schizophrenia are generally absent. Auditory or visual hallucinations, if present, are not permanent in delusional disorder.

Schizophrenia

The onset of schizophrenia in the early or midadolescent years is not uncommon. Diagnostic criteria are similar to those of adults and are characterized by loose associations, delusions, hallucinations, a flat or inappropriate affect, and impaired interpersonal functioning. It may be possible to classify adolescent schizophrenics by their premorbid functions. In one group the adolescent patients are likely to have been diagnosed as having a schizoid disorder of childhood in their preteen years and suffer from acute episodes of schizophrenia with bizarre behavior. The second group may show a normal premorbid history and suffer from acute episodes of schizophrenia, usually of the paranoid or catatonic type. The first group is generally characterized and diagnosed by the presence of negative symptoms of schizophrenia. These patients rarely describe their delusions and hallucinations, but their presence may be deducted from their bizarre behavior.

Schizophreniform Disorder

It is fairly common for adolescents to receive this diagnosis instead of schizophrenia because of the relatively short duration of the prodromal phase (less than 6 months). However, the prevalence and course of this diagnosis in the adolescent population is not well known.

Brief Reactive Psychosis

It is usually induced by markedly stressful events without any of the prodomal symptoms of schizophrenia. The diagnosis of brief reactive psychosis preempts the diagnosis of schizophreniform disorder.

Mood Disorders

It is usually depression with depressive delusions and hallucinations or a manic episode with delusions of grandeur that may cause some difficulty in a differential diagnosis from the acute phase of schizophrenia. Signs of the prodromal phase of schizophrenia, a positive past history of depression or mania, and a relatively normal premorbid personality may help the differential diagnosis.

Management of Acute Psychosis

Once the diagnosis of acute psychosis is made, the following considerations are helpful in the management of these patients. There are many adolescents with acute psychosis who may be treated effectively in outpatient clinics. However, the presence of confusion, delirium, acute agitation, suicidal or homicidal thoughts, and possible organic conditions require that the patients be hospitalized, carefully investigated to determine a possible etiology, and treated for acute symptoms until he is safe to return home.

Acute episodes of psychosis frequently require treatment with antipsychotic medications to reduce agitation, aggression, hallucinations, and delusions. Suspected organic conditions should always be explored before using antipsychotic medications. In emergency situations, however, acute episodes of excitement and aggression prompted by delusions or hallucinations should be treated with oral or intramuscular neuroleptics (chlorpromazine [Thorazine] or haloperidol). Thorazine is appropriate if more sedation is required; haloperidol is much more effective in reducing aggressive and agitated behavior. Pool et al. (1976) carried out a double-blind evaluation of loxapine, haloperidol, and placebo in 75 patients with diagnoses of schizophrenia, acute or chronic with acute exacerbation. The newly hospitalized patients, within the ages of 13 and 18 years, manifested disorders of thought association and/or hallucinations at the time of admission. Results indicated marked improvement in all three groups over a period of 4 weeks. However, both antipsychotic agents (loxapine and haloperidol) showed clear superiority to placebo in relation to schizophrenic symptomatology measured by brief psychiatric rating scales, nurses' observation scales for inpatient evaluation, and the clinical global ratings of improvement. Significant differences were detected over placebo in the improvement of hallucinatory behavior, disorientation, and thought disorders. The average daily dosage was 87.5 mg for loxapine and 9.8 mg for haloperidol. The most common side effects were extrapyramidal side effects in 19 of the 26 subjects receiving loxapine and 18 of the 25 subjects receiving haloperidol. Muscle rigidity and parkinsonism were the most common extrapyramidal side effects. Sedation was more common with loxapine and occurred in 21 of the loxapine-treated subjects and 13 of the haloperidol-treated subjects.

Erickson et al. (1984) studied the effects of neuroleptics on attention problems in adolescent schizophrenics. Schizophrenic adults showed frequent errors of omission and prolonged reaction times on vigilance tests. The development of attentional skills in children is influenced by a number of biological and psychological variables. Attention skills normally improve with age, with reaction time continuing to shorten until late adolescence (Taylor, 1981). However, norms for attention skills in adolescents have not been established. The authors found that schizophrenic adolescents showed more lapses of attention as measured by errors of omission than did the other three nonpsychotic comparison groups. They were not more impulsive as measured by errors of commission than were any of the comparison groups when taking medication (0.23 mg/kg thioridazine or thiothixene, 2.2 mg/kg). Schizophrenic subjects' reaction times lengthened significantly, but errors of commission lessened slightly. The authors concluded that changes in reaction times and performance errors resulted from sedation and suggested that high-potency, less-sedating neuroleptics may be preferable in the treatment of adolescent schizophrenics.

Most of the adolescent patients are able to participate in therapy programs such as group therapy, didactic groups, and recreation after about 1 week of treatment with medication. Aftercare treatment depends upon the etiology. Adolescents with substance abuse problems may require specialized programs for chemical dependency. Schizophrenic patients need to continue medication at a lower dosage for several months before treatment is discontinued on a trial basis. Environmental management through family counseling and utilization of community resources are essential in all cases of adolescent schizophrenia for a better outcome.

REFERENCES

Abraham K: Notes on the psychoanalytic treatment of manic-depressive insanity and allied conditions, in *Selected Papers on Psychoanalysis*. New York, Basic Books Inc Publishers, 1960 (original work published in 1911).

Abraham S, Mira M: Bulimia: A study of outcome. *Int J Eating Disord* 1983; 2:175–180.

Abraham S, Nordsieck M: Relationship of excess weight in children and adults. *Public Health Rep* 1960; 75:263–273.

Aichorn A: *Wayward Youth*. New York, Viking Press, 1935.

Alessi N, Robbins D, Dilsaver S: Panic and depressive disorders among psychiatrically hospitalized adolescents. *Psychiatr Res* 1987; 20:275–283.

Alexander JF, Parson BV: Short-term behavioral intervention with delinquent families: Impact on family process and recidivism. *J Abnorm Psychol* 1973; 81:219–225.

Anderson AE: Inpatient and outpatient treatment of anorexia nervosa, in Brownell K, Foreyt J (eds): *Handbook of Eating Disorders*. New York, Basic Books Inc Publishers, 1986, pp 333–350.

Annell AC: Lithium in the treatment of children and adolescents. *Acta Psychiatr Scand Suppl* 1969; 207:19–30.

Baker H, Wills U: School phobia: Classification and treatment. *Br J Psychiatry* 1978; 132:492–499.

Barker P, Fraser I: A controlled trial of haloperidol in children. *Br J Psychiatry* 1968; 114:855–857.

Beck AT: *Depression, Clinical, Experimental and Theoretical Aspects*. New York, Harper & Row Publishers Inc, 1967.

Beck AT, Rush A, Shaw B, et al: *Cognitive Therapy of Depression: A Treatment Manual*. New York, Guilford Press, 1979.

Bemporad JR: Management of childhood depression: Developmental considerations. *Psychosomatics* 1982; 23:272–279.

Berg I, Nichols K, Pritchard C: School phobia, its classification and relationship to dependency. *J Child Psychol Psychiatry* 1969; 10:123–141.

Bernal ME, Klinnert MD, Schultz LA: Outcome evaluation of behavioral parent training and client-centered parent counseling for children with conduct problems. *J Appl Behav Anal* 1980; 13:677–691.

Berryman E: School phobia: Management problems in private practice. *Psychol Rep* 1959; 5:19–25.

Bilbring E: The mechanism of depression, in Greenacre P (ed): *Affective Disorders.* New York, International University Press, 1953.

Birch LL: Effects of peer models' food choices and eating behaviors on preschooler's food preferences. *Child Dev* 1980; 51:489–496.

Blouin A, Bornstein R, Trites R: Teenage alcohol use among hyperactive children: A 5-year follow-up study. *J Pediatr Psychol* 1978; 3:188–194.

Briquet P: *Traite Clinique et Therapeutique Del'hysteria.* Paris, JB Baillier & Fils, 1859.

Broadwin IT: A contribution to the study of truancy. *Am J Orthopsychiatry* 1932; 2:253–259.

Brown GL, Ballenger JC, Minochiello M, et al: Human aggression and its relationship to cerebrospinal fluid, 5-hydroindolacetic acid, 3-methoxy-4-hydroxyphenylglycol and homovanillic acid, in Sandler M (ed): *Psychopharmacology of Aggression.* New York, Raven Press, 1979, pp 131–148.

Brownell KD, Kaye FS: A school based behavior modification, nutrition education and physical activity program for obese children. *Am J Clin Nutr* 1982; 35:277–283.

Burroughs Wellcome Co, 3030 Cornwallis Road, Research Triangle Park, NC 27709.

Cantwell D, Sturzenberger S, Burrough J, et al: Anorexia nervosa: An affective disorder. *Arch J Psychiatry* 1977; 34:1087–1093.

Carlson, GA: Affective disorders in adolescence, in Cantwell D, Carlson GA (eds): *Affective Disorders in Childhood and Adolescence.* New York, Spectrum Publications Inc, 1983.

Carlson G, Cantwell D: Unmasking masked depression in children and adolescents. *Am J Psychiatry* 1980; 137:449–455.

Carlson G, Kashani J: Phenomenology of major depression from childhood through adulthood: Analysis of three studies. *Am J Psychiatry* 1988; 145:1222–1225.

Charcot JM: *Lecons sur les Maladies du Systeme Nerveux Faites a la Salpetriere.* Delayhaye, Paris, 1873.

Charcot JM: *Lectures on the Diseases of the Nervous System* (translated by G Sigerson). London, New Sydenham Society, 1877.

Chiles J, Miller M, Cox G: Depression in adolescent delinquent population. *Arch Gen Psychiatry* 1980; 37:1179–1184.

Cooledge J, Hahn P, Peck A: School phobia: Neurotic crisis or way of life? *Am J Orthopsychiatry* 1957; 27:296–306.

Coppen A: The biochemistry of affective disorders. *Br J Psychiatry* 1967; 113:1237–1264.

Corder B, et al: Adolescent patricide: A comparison with other adolescent murder. *Am J Psychiatry* 1976; 133:957–961.

Critchley E: Reading retardation, dyslexia, and delinquency. *Br J Psychiatry* 1968; 115:1537–1547.

Crumley FE: Adolescent suicide attempts. *JAMA* 1979; 241:2402–2407.

Davis K, Berger PA: Pharmacological investigations of the cholinergic imbalance hypotheses of movement disorders and psychosis. *Biol Psychiatry* 1978; 13:23–49.

DeLong G, Aldershof A: Long-term experience with lithium treatment in childhood: Correlation with clinical diagnosis. *J Am Acad Child Adolesc Psychiatry* 1987; 26:289–294.

Doepat J, Ripley H: Relationship between attempted suicide and committed suicide. *Comp Psychiatry* 1967; 8:74–79.

Dostal T, Zvolsky P: Antiaggressive effect of lithium salts in severe mentally retarded adolescents. *Int J Pharmacopsychiatry* 1970; 5:205–207.

Druckman JM: A family-oriented policy and treatment program for female juvenile status offenders. *J Marriage Fam* 1979; 41:627–636.

Dugas M, Mouren M, Halfon O, et al: Treatment of childhood and adolescent depression with mianserin. *Acta Psychiatr Scand Suppl* 1985; 320:48–53.

Duncan J, Duncan G: Murder in the family: A study of some homicidal adolescents. *Am J Psychiatry* 1971; 127:74–78.

Dwyer J, DeLong G: A family history of a study of twenty probands with childhood manic-depressive illness. *J Am Acad Child Adolesc Psychiatry* 1987; 26:176–180.

Erickson W, Yellin A, Hopwood J, et al: The effects of neuroleptics on attention in adolescent schizophrenics. *Biol Psychiatry* 1984; 19:745–753.

Erikson E: The problem of ego identity. *J Am Psychoanal Assoc* 1956; 4:56.

Everett C: Family assessment and intervention for early adolescent problems. *J Marriage Fam Counsel* 1976; 2:155–165.

Feldman P: An analysis of the efficacy of diazepam. *J Neuropsychiatry* 1961; 3:562–567.

Fenton GW: The straightforward EEG in psychiatric practice. *Proc R Soc Med* 1974; 67:7–15.

Freeman CD: Fluoxetine treatment for bulimia. Presented at the Second International Conference on Eating Disorders, New York, April, 1986.

Freud A: Adolescence. *Psychoanal Study Child* 1958; 13:255.

Freud A: Certain types and states of social maladjustment, in Eissler K (ed): *Searchlights on Delinquency.* New York, International Universities Press, 1949.

Freud S: Mournings and melancholia, in Strachey J (ed and trans): *The Standard Edition of the Complete Psychological works of Sigmund Freud,* vol 14. London, Hogarth Press, 1961 (original work published in 1917).

Freud S: New introductory lectures on psychoanalysis, in Strachey J (ed and trans): *The Standard Edition of the Complete Psychological Works of Sigmund Freud,* vol 22. London, Hogarth Press, 1961 (original work published in 1933).

Friedlouder K: *The Psychoanalytic Approach to Juvenile Delinquency: Theory, Case Studies, Treatment.* London, Kegan Paul, Trench, Trubner, 1947.

Gabrielle A, Carlson M, Yolanda B, et al: A comparison of outcome in adolescent and late-onset bipolar manic-depressive illness. *Am J Psychiatry* 1977; 134:919–922.

Garber J, Kriss M, Koch M, et al: Recurrent depression in adolescents: A follow-up study. *J Am Acad Child Adolesc Psychiatry* 1988; 27:49–54.

Garrigan JJ, Bambrick AF: Family therapy for disturbed children: Some experimental results in special education. *J Marriage Fam Counsel* 1977; 3:83–93.

Geller B, Cooper T, Farooki Z, et al: Dose and plasma levels of nortriptyline and chlorpromazine in delusionally depressed adolescents and for amitriptyline in nondelusionally depressed adolescents. *Am J Orthopsychiatry* 1985; 142:336–338.

Glover E: The diagnosis and treatment of delinquency. A clinical report on the work of the Institute for the Scientific Treatment of Delinquency during the five years 1937–41, in Radzinowicz L, Turner JWC (eds): *Mental Abnormality and Crime.* London, MacMillan Publishing Co Inc, 1944, pp 269–299.

Healy W: *The Individual Delinquent.* Boston, Little Brown & Co Inc, 1915.

Henggeler S, Edwards J, Borduin C: The family relations of female juvenile delinquents. *J Abnorm Child Psychol* 1987; 15:199–209.

Hudgens RW: *Psychiatric Disorders in Adolescents.* Baltimore, Williams & Wilkins, 1974, pp 38–39.

Hudson J, Harrison G, Pope H: Newer antidepressants in the treatment of bulimia nervosa. *Psychopharmacol Bull* 1987; 23:52–57.

Hudson J, Pope H, Jonas J, et al: Phenomenologic relationship of eating disorders to major affective disorder. *Psychiatry Res* 1983; 9:345–354.

Huessy H, Metoyer M, Townsend M: An 8–10 year follow-up of 84 children treated for behavioral disorder in rural Vermont. *Acta Paedopsychiatr* 1974; 10:230–235.

Hughes P, Wells A, Cunningham C, et al: Treating bulimia with desipramine: A placebo controlled double-blind study. *Arch Gen Psychiatry* 1986; 43:182–186.

Hsu LK: Lithium-resistant adolescent mania. *J. Am Acad Child Psychiatry* 1986; 25:280–283.

Hsu LK: Treatment of bulimia with lithium. *Am J Psychiatry* 1984; 141:1260–1262.

Hsu L, Wisner K, Richey E, et al: Is juvenile delinquency related to an abnormal EEG? *J Am Acad Child Psychiatry* 1985; 24:310–315.

Hsu LK, Crisp AH, Harding B: Outcome of anorexia nervosa. *Lancet* 1979; 1:61–65.

Jacob J: *Adolescent Suicide.* New York, Wiley Interscience, 1971.

Johnson A, Falstein E, Szurek S, et al: School phobia. *Am J Orthopsychiatry* 1941; 11:702–711.

Johnson AM, Szurek SA: The genesis of antisocial acting out in children and adolescents. *Psychoanal Q* 1952; 21:323–343.

Johnson WG, Schlundt D, Kelley M, et al: Exposure with response prevention and energy regulation in the treatment of bulimia. *Int J Eating Disord* 1984; 3:37–46.

Kalant O: *The Amphetamines: Toxicity and Addiction.* Springfield, Ill, Charles C Thomas Publishers, 1966.

Kandel D, Davies M: Adult sequelae of adolescent depressive symptoms. *Arch Gen Psychiatry* 1986; 43:255–262.

Kaplan SL, Grossman P, Landa B, et al: Depressive symptoms and life events in physically ill hospitalized adolescents. *J Adolesc Health Care* 1986; 7:107–111.

Kashani J, Orvashcel H: Anxiety disorders in mid-adolescence: A community sample. *Am J Psychiatry* 1988; 145:960–964.

Katz KJ, Thomas Z: Effects of para-chlorophenylalanine upon brain stimulated affective attack in the cat. *Pharmacol Biochem Behav* 1976; 48:546–556.

Keniston K: *The Uncommitted.* New York, Harcourt, Brace & World, 1965.

Kennedy S, Piran N, Garfinkel P: Isocarbioazed in the treatment of bulimia. *Am J Psychiatry* 1986; 143:1495–1496.

Kennedy WA: School phobia: Rapid treatment of fifth cases. *J Abnorm Psychol* 1965; 70:285–289.

Khan AU: Heterogeneity of suicidal adolescents. *J Am Acad Child Adolesc Psychiatry* 1987; 26:92–96.

King L, Pittman GD: A 6-year follow-up study of 65 adolescent patients: Predictive value of presenting clinical picture. *Br J Psychiatry* 1969; 115:1437–1441.

Klein RG, Klein D: School phobia, diagnostic considerations in the light of imipramine effects. *J Nerv Ment Dis* 1973; 156:199–215.

Kranzler H: Use of buspirone in an adolescent with overanxious disorder. *J Am Acad Child Adolesc Psychiatry* 1980; 27:789–790.

Lacey JH: Bulimia nervosa, binge eating and psychogenic vomiting. A controlled treatment study and long-term outcome. *Br Med J* 1983; 286:1609–1613.

Lavin G, Trabka S, Kahn M: Group therapy with aggressive, and delinquent adolescents, in Keith C (ed): *The Aggressive Adolescent*. New York, Free Press, 1984, pp 240–267.

Leton DA: Assessment of school phobia. *Ment Hygiene* 1962; 46:256–264.

LeVann LJ: Clinical comparison of haloperidol with chlorpromazine in mentally retarded children. *Am J Ment Defic* 1971; 75:719–723.

Levine MD, Karniski WM, Palfrey J, et al: A study of risk factor complexes in early adolescent delinquency. *Am J Dis Child* 1985; 139:50–56.

Lewis D, et al: Homicidally aggressive young children: Neuropsychiatric and experiential correlates. *Am J Psychiatry* 1983; 140:148–153.

Lewis D, Pincus J, Shauk S: Psychomotor epilepsy and violence in a group of incarcerated adolescent boys. *Am J Psychiatry* 1982; 139:882–887.

Lewis DO: *Vulnerabilities to Delinquency*. New York, SP Medical & Scientific Books, 1981, pp 39–56.

Lombroso C: *Crime, It's Causes, and Remedies* (Horton HP, trans). Boston, Little Brown, 1911.

Loomis SD: EEG abnormalities as a correlate of behavior in adolescent male delinquents. *Am J Psychiatry* 1965; 121:1003–1006.

Malamud N: Psychiatric disorders with intracranial tumors of the limbic system. *Arch Neurol* 1967; 17:113.

Masterson JF: *Treatment of the Borderline Adolescent: A Developmental Approach* New York, John Wiley & Sons, 1972.

McCracken J, Diamond R: Bipolar disorder in mentally retarded adolescents. *J Am Acad Child Adolesc Psychiatry* 1988; 27:494–499.

McElroy S, Keck P, Pope H: Sodium valproate: Its use in primary psychiatric disorders. *J Clin Psychopharmacol* 1987; 7:16–24.

McGlashan TH: Adolescent versus adult onset of mania. *Am J Psychiatry* 1988; 145:221–223.

McIntire M, Angle C, Schlict M: Suicide and self-poisoning in pediatrics. *Adv Pediatr* 1977; 244:291–309.

McManus M, Brickman A, Alessi N, et al: Neurological dysfunction in serious delinquents. *J Am Acad Child Psychiatry* 1985; 24:481–486.

Mendelson W, Johnson N, Stewart M: Hyperactive children as teenagers: A follow-up study. *J Nerv Ment Dis* 1971; 153:273–279.

Menkes D, Aghajanian G, McCall R: Chronic antidepressant treatment enhances alpha-adrenergic and serotonergic responses in the facial nucleus. *Life Sci* 1980; 27:45–55.

Minuchin S, Rosman B, Baker L: *Psychomatic Families*. Cambridge, Mass, Harvard University Press, 1978.

Mitchell J, Groat A: A placebo-controlled, double blind trial of amitriptyline in bulimia. *J Clin Psychopharmacol* 1984; 4:186–193.

Mitchell J, Laine D, Morley J, et al: Naloxone but not CCK-8 may alternate binge-eating behavior in patients with the bulimic syndrome. *Biol Psychiatry* 1986; 21:1399–1406.

Morgan HG, Purgold J, Wellbourne J: Management and outcome in anorexia nervosa: A standardized prognostic study. *Br J Psychiatry* 1983; 143:282–287.

Morgan HG, Russell GM: Value of family background and clinical features as predictors of long-term outcome in anorexia nervosa: Four-year follow-up study of 41 patients. *Psychol Med* 1975; 5:355–371.

National Institute of Mental Health: Admissions rate to state and county psychiatric hospitals by age, sex, and race. United States, 1975, statistical note 140, November 1977.

Normal D, Herzog D: A 3-year outcome study of normal-weight bulimia: Assessment of psychosocial functioning and eating attitudes. *Psychiatry Res* 1986; 19:199–205.

Noyes R: Beta adrenergic blocking drugs in anxiety and stress. *Psychiatr Clin North Am* 1985; 8:119–132.

Noyes R, Anderson D, Clancy J: Diazepam and propranolol in panic disorder and agoraphobia. *Arch Gen Psychiatry* 1984; 41:287–292.

Osterrieth P: Adolescence: Some psychological aspects, in Caplan G, Lebovici S (eds): *Adolescence*. New York, Basic Books Inc Publishers, 1969.

Oxley J, Roberts M, Danna-Haeri J: Evaluation of 24-hour 4 channel EEG taped recordings and serum prolactin estimations in the diagnosis of simulated and epileptic fits. Presented at the 12th Epilepsy International Symposium, Copenhagen, 6–10 Sept, 1980.

Patterson G: Interventions for boys with conduct problems: Multiple settings, treatments and criteria. *J Consult Clin Psychol* 1974; 42:471–481.

Patterson G, Fleischman M: Reciprocity and coercion: Two facets of social systems, in Neuringer C, Michael J (eds): *Behavior Modification in Clinical Psychology*. New York, Appleton-Century-Crofts, 1970.

Patterson G, Fleischman M: Intervention for families of aggressive boys: A replication study. *Behav Res Ther* 1973; 11:383–394.

Pearce J: Depressive disorder in childhood. *J Child Psychol Psychiatry* 1977; 18:79–82.

Peroutka S, Snyder S: Long-term antidepressant treatment decreases spiroperidol-labeled serotonin receptor binding. *Science* 1980; 210:88–90.

Platt JE, Campbell M, Green WH, et al: Cognitive effects of lithium carbonate and haloperidol in treatment-resistant aggressive children. *Arch Gen Psychiatry* 1984; 41:657–662.

Pool D, Bloom W, Mielke D, et al: A controlled evaluation of loxitane in 75 adolescent schizophrenic patients. *Curr Ther Res* 1976; 19:99–104.

Pope HG, Hudson J, Jonas J: Antidepressant treatment of bulimia: Preliminary experience and practical recommendations. *J Clin Psychopharmacol* 1983; 3:274–281.

Pope H, Hudson J, Jonas J, et al: Bulimia treated with imipramine: A placebo-controlled double-blind study. *Am J Psychiatry* 1983; 140:554–558.

Puig-Antich J: The use of RDC criteria for major depressive disorder in children and adolescents. *J Am Acad Child Psychiatry* 1983; 21:291–293.

Rabinowitz C: Therapy for underprivileged delinquent families, in Pollock O, Friedman A (eds): *Family Dynamics and Female Sexual Delinquency*. Palo Alto, Calif, Science and Behavior Books, 1969.

Rachman S, Hodgson R: *Obsessions and Compulsions*. Englewood Cliffs, NJ, Prentice-Hall International Inc, 1980.

Rado S: The problem of melancholia, in *Collected Papers,* vol 1. New York, Grune & Stratton, 1956 (original work published in 1927).

Rampling D: Aggression: A paradoxical response to tricyclic antidepressants. *Am J Psychiatry* 1978; 135:117–118.

Randall LO: The psychosedative properties of methaminodiazepoxide. *J Pharm Exp Ther* 1960; 129:163–171.

Reckless WC: *The Crime Problem.* New York, Appleton-Century-Crofts, 1967.

Reed JL: Hysteria, in Silverstone T, Barraclough B (eds): *Contemporary Psychiatry.* Kent, England, Headley Bros, 1975.

Reis DJ: The relationship between brain norepinephrine and aggressive behavior. *Assoc Res Nerv Ment Dis* 1972; 50:266–297.

Rexford E (ed): *A Developmental Approach to Problems of Acting Out:* A Symposium. New York, International Universities Press, 1966.

Richards DA, Woodings EP, Prichard BN: Circulatory and alpha-adrenoreceptor blocking effects of phentolamine. *Br J Clin Pharmacol* 1978; 5:507–513.

Rinsley DG: Theory and practice of intensive residential treatment of adolescents, in Feinstein SC, Giovacchini PL (eds): *Adolescent Psychiatry,* vol 1. New York, Basic Books Inc Publishers, 1971, pp 479–509.

Robin AA: Controlled evaluation of problem-solving communication training with parent-adolescent conflict. *Behav Ther* 1981; 12:593–609.

Robinowitz C: Therapy for underprivileged delinquent families, in Pollock O, Friedman A (eds): *Family Dynamics and Female Sexual Delinquency.* Palo Alto, Science and Behavior Books, 1969.

Rosen JC, Leitenberg H: Bulimia nervosa: Treatment with exposure and response prevention. *Behav Ther* 1982; 13:117–124.

Rotenberg M: Conceptual and methodological notes on affective and cognitive role-taking (sympathy & empathy): An illustrative experiment with delinquent boys. *J Gen Psychol* 1974; 125:177–185.

Rothner D: Diagnosis and management of headache in children and adolescents. *Neurol Clin* 1983; 1:511–526.

Rubin P, Poland R, Lesser I, et al: Neuroendocrine aspects of primary endogenous depression. *Arch Gen Psychiatry* 1987; 44:328.

Rubin RT, Poland RE, Lesser IM, et al: Neuroendocrine aspects of primary endogenous depression: III. Cortisol secretion in relation to diagnosis and symptom pattern. *Psychol Med* 1987; 17:609–619.

Rush A (ed): *Short-term Psychotherapies for Depression.* New York, Guilford Press, 1982.

Rutter M, Tizard J, Whitmore K (eds): *Education, Health and Behavior.* London, Longmans, 1970.

Ryan N, Meyer V, Dachille S, et al: Lithium antidepressant augmentation in TCA-refractory depression in adolescents. *J Am Acad Child Adolescent Psychiatry* 1988; 27:371–376.

Ryan N, Puig-Antich J, Cooper T, et al: Imipramine in adolescent major depression: Plasma levels and clinical response. *Acta Psychiatr Scand* 1986; 73:275–288.

Ryan N, Puig-Antich J, Cooper T, et al: Relative safety of single versus divided dose imipramine in adolescent major depression. *J Am Acad Child Adolesc Psychiatry* 1987; 26:400–406.

Satterfield J, Hoppe C, Schell A: A prospective study of delinquency in 110 adolescent boys with attention deficit disorder and 88 normal adolescent boys. *Am J Psychiatry* 1982; 139:795–798.

Satterfield J, Satterfield B, Schell A: Therapeutic interventions to prevent delinquency in hyperactive boys. *J Am Acad Child Adolesc Psychiatry* 1987; 26:56–64.

Schildkraut J: The catecholamine hypothesis of affective disorders: A review of supportive evidence. *Am J Psychiatry* 1965; 122:509–522.

Schlebusch L, Minnaar G: The management of parasuicide in adolescents. *South Afr Med J* 1980; 57:81–84.

Schneider S, Rice D: Neurological manifestations of childhood hysteria. *J Pediatr* 1979; 94:153–156.

Schneiderman G, Evans H: An approach to families of acting-out adolescents: A case study. *Adolescence* 1975; 10:495–498.

Schoenbach V, Kaplan B, Wagner E, et al: Prevalence of self-reported depressive symptoms in young adolescents. *Am J Public Health* 1983; 73:1281–1287.

Schwartz D, Thompson G: Do anorectic get well? Current research and future needs. *Am J Psychiatry* 1981; 138:319–323.

Sheehan DU: Reactive efficacy of phenalzine, imipramine, alprazolam, and placebo in treatment of panic disorder. Presented at the annual meeting of the American Psychiatric Association, Los Angeles, May 5–11, 1984.

Siever L, Cohen R, Murphy D: Antidepressants and alpha-2–adrenergic autoreceptor desensitization. *Am J Psychiatry* 1981; 138:681–682.

Sillanpaa M: Prevalence of migraine and other headaches during the first seven school years. *Headache* 1983; 23:15–19.

Spier SA, Tesar GE, Rosenbaum JF, et al: Treatment of panic disorder and agoraphobia with clonazepam. *J Clin Psychiatry* 1986; 47:238–242.

Spirito A, Stark L, Fristad M, et al: Adolescent suicide attemptors hospitalized on pediatric unit. *J Pediatr Psychol* 1987; 2:171–189.

Stanley J, Barter J: Adolescent suicidal behavior. *Am J Orthopsychiatry* 1970; 40:87–96.

Stanley M, Mann J, Gershon S: Serotonergic receptor alterations in the brains of suicide victims. Presented at the meeting of the Society for Biological Psychiatry, New York, May, 1983.

Strober M, Carlson G: Bipolar illness in adolescents with major depression. *Arch Gen Psychiatry* 1982; 39:549–555.

Swift W: The long-term outcome of early onset anorexia nervosa. *J Am Acad Child Psychiatry* 1982; 21:36–46.

Swift W, Ritholz M, Kalin N, et al: A follow-up study of early (?) hospitalized bulimics. *Psychosom Med* 1987; 49:45–55.

Talbot M: Panic in school phobia. *Am J Orthopsychiatry* 1957; 27:286–295.

Taylor E: Development of attention, in Rutter M (ed): *Developmental Psychiatry.* Baltimore, University Park Press, 1981, pp 185–197.

Thomas A, Chess S: *Temperament and Development.* New York, Brunner/Mazel, 1977.

Toner B, Garfinkel P, Garner D: Long-term follow-up of anorexia nervosa. *Psychosom Med* 1986; 48:520–529.

Toner B, Garfinkel P, Garner D: Long-term follow-up of anorexia nervosa. *Psychosom Med* 1986; 48:520–529.

Topol P, Reznikoff M: Perceived peer and family relationship, hopelessness and locus of control as factors in adolescent suicide attempts. *Suicide Life Threat Behav* 1982; 12:141–150.

Wallach M, Headley L: The effects of antihistamines in a modified behavioral despair test. *Communications Psychopharmacol* 1979; 3:35–39.

Walsh B, Roose S, Glassman A, et al: Bulimia and depression. *Psychosomatic Med* 1985; 47:123–131.

Warien W: Acute neurotic breakdown in children with refusal to go to school. *Arch Dis Child* 1948; 23:266–272.

Weathers L, Liberman RP: Contingency contracting with families of delinquent adolescents. *Behav Ther* 1975; 6:356–366.

Widom CS: Towards an understanding of female criminality. *Prog Exp Pers Res* 1978; 8:245–308.

Wold P: Trazodone in the treatment of bulimia, (letter). *J Clin Psychiatry* 1983; 44:275–276.

Wolff P, Waber D, Bauermeister M, et al: Neuropsychological status of adolescent delinquent boys. *J Child Psychol Psychiatry* 1982; 23:267–279.

Wurtman JJ, Moses PL, Wurtman RJ: Prior carbohydrate consumption affects the amount of carbohydrate that rats choose to eat. *J Nutr* 1983; 113:70–88.

6

Planning for Aftercare

Aftercare planning involves (1) planning for discharge, (2) anticipating the right type of placement after discharge, (3) knowledge of community resources, and (4) knowledge of the mental health code and the laws relating to the rights of adolescent patients.

The majority of hospitalized adolescents require further psychiatric treatment after discharge from the hospital. In fact, it is a rare adolescent who leaves the hospital without a recommendation for further treatment. Hospitalization is frequently a result of long-standing problems that reach crisis level before hospitalization occurs. It is necessary to begin discharge planning from the very onset of hospital treatment. In the majority of cases, outpatient psychiatric treatment is prescribed, and the adolescent is referred to a community mental health center, outpatient psychiatric clinic, or a private therapist. It is desirable in most cases, however, to make a recommendation for a specific type of therapy such as family counseling, marital counseling for parents, group therapy, or individual supportive or analytic therapy. The inpatient staff should be knowledgeable about the resources and the availability of various services in the community. It is necessary for aftercare planners to know the details of the services offered by each of the mental health facilities in the community in order to make an appropriate referral. The following facilities are generally present in most urban communities:

1. Outpatient facilities.
2. Day treatment programs.
3. Community support groups.
4. Foster homes.
5. Group homes.
6. Residential treatment centers.
7. General and special hospital psychiatric services.
8. Outpatient treatment for substance abuse problems.
9. Inpatient treatment programs for substance abuse.
10. Independent living facilities supervised and funded by private or state resources.

The staff of the hospital should also be aware of the jurisdictions of various mental health, law enforcement, and child and family agencies. A knowledge of the laws relating to parental rights and neglect, abuse, and abandonment is very helpful in dealing with complicated cases.

Kadushin (1974) has conceptualized community services for children and adolescents under three main categories:

1. Supportive.
2. Supplemental.
3. Substitutive.

These categories are by no means exclusive, and there is a great deal of overlapping among them.

Supportive services are generally recommended when an adolescent can be sustained in his family with the help of special educational, recreational, and mental health services available in the community. For example, an adolescent with academic and/or behavior problems may require special education services such as learning disability classrooms, a resource room, or a self-contained classroom for behavior disorders. Mental health services such as individual, group, or family therapy or counseling for substance abuse are generally available in most midsized communities. Recreational planning is frequently neglected in aftercare plans. Adolescents, in general, have a great deal of free time on their hands and have great difficulty in using their time efficiently. Adolescent patients frequently need help in planning their leisure activities. They should be helped to explore community resources to find some interesting activities that they can participate in.

Supplemental services include financial, homemaking, and other social services that are provided to a family in order to improve the social, psychological, and financial status of the family, thus benefitting the patient. The problems of adolescent patients in social relationships with peers are compounded by their poor hygiene, disheveled looks, and torn and dirty clothes. Although some of their problems may be self-imposed by the adolescents themselves, they may also have a genuine basis in their poor financial resources and poor home planning. Such a family can benefit from financial and/or homemaking services to help improve their home situation, thus helping adolescents with their hygiene, self-esteem, and peer relationships. Similarly, many families are not able or lack the knowledge to obtain proper health care services for their children. The condition of their house and lack of sufficient space for privacy may be a source of difficulty and embarrassment for an adolescent. Some parents may not avail themselves of local community and mental health services because of the lack of transportation, long working hours, and the unavailability of baby-sitting services for other children.

Substitutive services may be required when supportive and supplemental services do not fulfill their intended goal—to help the adolescent patient stay in his family while undergoing therapy. However, there are families that are completely unable to provide the necessary care and supervision needed by the adolescent patient. On the other hand, the problem of the adolescent may be so intense that all the supportive and supplemental services combined will not be sufficient to sustain him in his family.

Such cases require partial or complete removal of the adolescent from the home. It is possible that therapeutic day-care programs for half a day or a full day may be sufficient, thus allowing such adolescents to return home at night. In other cases, a foster home, group home, or a residential treatment center may be necessary.

OUTPATIENT MENTAL HEALTH SERVICES

These services are provided by community mental health centers, psychiatric clinics run by various not-for-profit organizations, and private clinics. Outpatient therapy is provided by mental health workers of various disciplines such as psychiatry, psychology, and social work. Many of these facilities offer individual, group, and family therapies; marital counseling; and counseling for substance abuse. However, the clinics rarely advertise their basic orientation and philosophy of treatment. The therapist's training, background, and discipline do not necessarily indicate the type of therapeutic technique employed by them. It is possible that a psychiatrist may practice behavior therapy while a psychologist may be using psychoanalytic techniques. It is frequently necessary to know a therapist and his type of therapy before referring a specific patient to him. However, in most cases a referral is made to a clinic or to a therapist without knowledge of the type of therapy that will be provided to the patient. Many community clinics are very busy and utilize therapists from various disciplines, some of whom lack adequate training and experience. Supervision of these therapists by senior staff may also be minimal. Some private therapists advertise their special brand of therapy. For example, some therapists call themselves eclectic, meaning that they are flexible and may utilize various therapeutic techniques to obtain maximum results. Behavior therapists generally identify the problem behavior and apply various behavioral techniques to resolve them. They frequently set up a contract between the adolescent patient and his parents. A system of reward and punishment is used to make the patient abide by the agreed-upon contract. Psychoanalytic psychotherapists focus on resolving underlying emotional conflicts, while rogerian therapists try to achieve a cure through a supportive relationship.

Outcome Studies

Earlier studies of outpatient treatment evaluated the overall efficacy of all the modalities of treatment provided in outpatient clinics. Shepherd et al. (1971), for example, compared a mixed group of children and adolescents receiving treatment in child guidance clinics with a normal control group from the community. Two years after the initial assessment, the two groups did not differ in outcome. The authors concluded that the improvement of the guidance clinic group was unrelated to the treatment. This study, however, was criticized for including a noncomparable control group and not taking into consideration the type of treatment provided in the clinics. A better controlled study was carried out by Kolvin et al. (1981). In this study, children with emotional and behavior problems were identified through an epidemiologic approach and were then assigned randomly to various treatment and control groups.

The children were assessed with a battery of measures at the conclusion of treatment and again at 18 months and 3 years after treatment. The results indicated that the children in the group therapy program showed much greater improvement than did the children in the control groups.

Most outcome studies in the past decade have tended to evaluate the efficacy of a specific modality of treatment rather than combining the effects of all treatment modalities carried out in outpatient clinics. Thus, the efficacies of various therapies such as group, family, marital counseling, individual counseling, and crisis intervention have been tested. Since the techniques of various therapies differ according to their theoretical basis, it is reasonable to expect differences in the outcome. Current research takes into account not only the type of theoretical background but also the type of patient treated. It has become evident that a therapist has to match specific patients with a specific modality of treatment based on a specific type of theoretical orientation in order to achieve the best therapeutic results. However, some studies (Kolvin et al., 1981) continue to find no consistent evidence that particular types of disorders respond better to a specific treatment modality. This finding may be explained on the basis of observation of several researchers that there are clear similarities among various types of therapies based on different theoretical orientations. For example, Wollersheim (1980) found some clear similarities between cognitive behavioral treatments for depression and psychodynamic approaches to the treatment of depression.

Among the various theoretical orientations, behavior therapy appears to have generated the largest number of controlled studies. Werry and Wollersheim (1989) presented a 20-year overview of behavior therapy with children and adolescents. They concluded that behavior therapy has made great progress and has a proven record of application in child and adolescent disorders. They also pointed out that the comparative efficacy and the complementarity of behavior therapy to other forms of psychotherapy and other forms of treatment remain to be demonstrated.

Referral to outpatient treatment is generally not well accepted by adolescent patients. They rarely believe that they have any problems of their own and tend to blame their families, schools, and community for their problems. Preparing an adolescent for outpatient treatment should be one of the goals of inpatient treatment. Unfortunately, most adolescents drop out of outpatient therapy after a few sessions. Family counseling is frequently helpful in sustaining an adolescent in outpatient therapy for longer periods.

DAY TREATMENT

Day treatment services are designed to keep an adolescent out of an institution. This type of care is provided in community facilities and may range from a few hours a day to an all-day program. The whole-day treatment programs usually include a combined program of education, recreation, and mental health counseling. The adolescents referred to these programs are frequently those who have problems at home, in the school, and in the community. However, their problems are not severe enough to warrant institutionalization. Many of those adolescents are institutionalized when partial-care services are not available in the community. The school problems may include a lack of motivation and behavior problems that have not been helped by such special education resources as a classroom for behavioral disordered children or special schools for behavior problems. Many of these adolescents are either suspended from school or are at the verge of being excluded from their schools. The problems in the relationship with the family include constant arguments, fighting, aggressive behavior toward various family members, and not abiding by the house rules.

Day treatment programs may comprise only a few hours of therapeutic and recreational programs for adolescents who may be doing fairly well in school but usually have problems at home and in the community after school hours. Some of these adolescents may be in special schools where highly structured educational programs can maintain them in the school without too much difficulty.

There are no clear-cut guidelines for choosing adolescent patients for day-care programs. It is not uncommon that many adolescent patients end up in these programs via a process of exclusion. They usually go through special educational and mental health counseling programs for some period of time until it is determined that they cannot be sustained in the school and in the community without more intensive help. It is apparent that acutely psychotic adolescents who are not stabilized by medication are inappropriate candidates for day treatment. Similarly, severely depressed adolescents with suicidal ideation are not appropriate for this type of treatment. The adolescents included in day treatment programs are mostly those with severe conduct problems. The associated problems include attention-deficit disorders, learning disabilities, and/or substance abuse. Herz et al. (1971) suggested that adolescent patients with the following problems be excluded from day treatment:

1. Those who are dangerous to themselves or to others.
2. Those who can best be treated in an outpatient setting without requiring all-day contact with mental health workers.
3. Those whose family or caretakers are seriously disturbed and abusive. Returning home in the evening would put these adolescents in danger.
4. Those with serious medical problems requiring round-the-clock care.

Day treatment programs were started in the early 1940s, but there was a very slow development of such facilities until the 1960s when this treatment modality became widely accepted. There were about 90 such programs in the country in 1972 and 353 in 1981 (Directory for Exceptional Children, 1981). The impetus for the proliferation of these programs was provided by the high cost of inpatient treatment. These therapeutic programs should be differentiated from other day treatment programs that provide substitutive care for children and adolescents during the time when their parents are working outside the home. Recreational and educational activities in such day treatment programs is provided by non–mental health staff who may have a consultative relationship with mental health professionals.

Lahey and Kupfer (1979) enumerated the following advantages of day treatment programs:

1. Part-time institutional treatment is more economical than full-time residential care.
2. Part-time programs provide needed relief to families.
3. In contrast to full-time institutionalization, part-time treatment allows the family to remain intact.
4. Part-time treatment programs can partially remove the child from maladaptive family environments.
5. The part-time treatment modality provides an excellent opportunity for families to learn new ways of acting toward their exceptional child.
6. Part-time treatment will not necessarily disrupt a child's education.
7. Part-time treatment will not necessarily disrupt a young person's social life.
8. Part-time treatment programs can be used to avoid some of the iatrogenic effects of institutionalization.
9. Part-time treatment is preferable for parents of exceptional children.
10. Part-time programs can be used to avoid the stress of separating the child and the family.
11. Part-time programs can be used to ease the transition between outpatient care and full institutionalization.
12. Part-time institutional programs can provide the opportunity for extended assessment.
13. Part-time programs can be used as the basis for the treatment of the whole family.

Day treatment programs may be situated in a hospital setting, in association with a community mental health center, or in outpatient psychiatric clinics. Each facility offers a unique combination of services and help from various professionals in carrying out these treatment programs.

A variety of psychotherapeutic interventions are provided in day treatment programs such as individual, group, and family therapy. The adolescent patient may spend a portion of his day treatment time with a therapist who focuses on day-to-day issues. The family therapy component is emphasized in most programs. Family therapy sessions, however, may take place at some other facility that may have trained family therapists.

Outcome Studies

There are few controlled studies of day treatment programs. However, several studies indicate that day treatment programs are frequently helpful in keeping adolescent patients out of institutions. One study (Valasquez and Lyle, 1985) evaluated 40 juvenile delinquents in a day program and compared them with a matched group that was placed in residential treatment centers. Post-treatment measures after a treatment of about 2 years indicated that the two groups were similar in their pattern of living in a family setting, in school attendance, and in post-treatment offenses. The two groups differed with regard to misdemeanors: the day group committed significantly more of these offenses following treatment than did the residential group. Probation officers and social workers reported a global assessment that 55% of the residential group and 44% of the day treatment group improved greatly or somewhat following treatment. For a substantial portion of delinquents in both groups, evaluators saw no beneficial change with treatment (38% of the residential group and 49% of the day treatment group). A small number of patients were considered to have become worse.

Simone (1986) reported some success in the day treatment of borderline adolescents. Most borderline adolescents are unwilling or unable to participate in the usual outpatient therapies. They often are uncooperative and act out their feelings destructively. Diagnostically, these adolescents were referred for psychiatric evaluation or hospitalization for a variety of symptoms including drug abuse, delinquent behavior, suicidal attempts, anorexia, withdrawal, and depression. The day treatment programs included a variety of group activities such as group therapy, psychodrama, work assignments, patient government, occupational therapy, social parties, field trips, and various projects planned by committees of patients and staff. The program was carried out between 8:30 A.M. and 3:00 P.M. on weekdays. Each patient received individual psychotherapy once or twice a week. The average length of stay was 6 months. Very few patients required hospitalization during the time they attended day treatment. Daily staff meetings were devoted to discussing individual patient problems and planning consistent approaches. Clear treatment goals were focused on the following issues:

1. Improving the range of affect through recognition and verbalization of feelings of anxiety, anger, and depression.
2. Fear of closeness and trusting others.
3. Problems of identity.
4. Depressive loneliness (which was decreased by participation in the program).
5. Integration of the personality (which was facilitated by focusing on projections, magical thinking, and splitting mechanisms).

Families were helped to understand patient problems. The author felt that this program was helpful to these patients primarily by facilitating further outpatient therapy and by reducing their frequency of hospitalization.

FOSTER HOME PLACEMENT

Recommendations to place a hospitalized adolescent patient into a foster home are usually made under the following circumstances:

1. Parents abandon or refuse to take an adolescent home.
2. The adolescent refuses to return home.

3. The therapy staff perceives very inadequate parental care and feels that the parents are not able to provide proper care to the adolescent because of their own severe problems.
4. There is a history of severe abuse and neglect or evidence of future potential for such acts.

Some parents have reached the end of their rope with their adolescent. Such conduct problems of the adolescent as aggressive and destructive behavior may be so severe that his parents fear for their safety. They have lost all control over the behavior of the adolescent. The adolescent may be constantly running away or staying out with friends overnight without the knowledge and permission of his parents. Such an adolescent has to improve his attitude and behavior before he can be placed in a foster home; otherwise, the same behavior is repeated in the foster home and leads to a series of unsuccessful placements or return to a hospital, group home, or residential treatment center.

Hospitalized adolescents frequently express angry and negative feelings toward their families. Some of them do not want to return home. They usually have severe conflicts with their natural or stepparent. Their conflicts usually revolve around their desire to have more privileges and to be more independent. Most parents are able to grant their adolescent new privileges. However, conflicts arise when the adolescent becomes slack in his normal responsibilities such as schoolwork, grades, chores, and substance abuse. Most adolescents do not recognize their contribution to the conflict and tend to blame their parents for being overly strict and unreasonable. They do not want to go home because they cannot get what they want. There are, however, some adolescents who fear severe sexual or physical abuse from their parents. The abuse may have been reported and investigated but not excessive enough to be "founded."

Occasionally, there are some adolescents who falsely acuse their parents of physical and sexual abuse in order to be placed away from home in the hope that they will have more privileges and independence in foster homes. Many of these adolescents threaten to run away if they are sent home. Such adolescents require intensive family therapy before they can return. However, the persistence of conflict with the family may require the adolescent to be placed in a foster home.

The most frequent reasons for foster home placement are physical and sexual abuse, parental neglect due to their own emotional problems, and lack of supervision on the part of the parents.

Protective services are required when an adolescent is severely neglected, abused, or exploited. Neglect usually occurs when the social, emotional, educational, and physical needs of an adolescent are not provided by his parents or guardians. However, these criteria may be difficult to apply in the teenage years since many adolescents are unmindful of their hygiene, wear dirty and torn clothes, eat junk food, experiment with drugs, and stay out after curfew hours. Many parents try to correct the behavior and appearance of their adolescent but give up after exhausting all methods of reward and punishment. There are, however, some parents who consider all adolescent behavior as an expression of normal adolescent rebellion. They may truly be neglecting their teenager when they refuse to seek help for extensive substance abuse, suicide attempts, or severe conduct problems.

Similarly, physical abuse during the adolescent years is a controversial issue. Many teenagers are physically larger and stronger than their parents. Sometimes physical abuse occurs in reverse—children threatening or actually beating their parents. We have found that many adolescents initially hit their parents in anger or in frustration. But once they discover that they can get away with hitting their parents, the physical abuse of the parents by the adolescent occurs more frequently, usually when parents try to control or set some limits on their behavior. Many single parents, usually mothers, have been frightened by physical abuse by their teenage sons or daughters and have allowed them to do what they pleased. Fistfights, slapping, and throwing objects between the parents and teenagers are not uncommon. At times the bruises on the adolescent's face may mirror the bruises on the parent's body. Parents generally do not bring charges against their adolescent, but the adolescent frequently relates his story of abuse in great detail, depicts his parents as villains, and accepts no responsibility for his own actions. Physical abuse in young teenagers who are physically small should be investigated carefully because these youngsters may not be able to defend themselves well.

Outcome Studies

The American Public Welfare Associations voluntary cooperative information system (1984) reported that during the fiscal year 1981 to 1982 a total of 434,000 children were in placement. A total of 161,000 entered placement during the year, and 172,000 were discharged. Several studies indicate that a high percentage of children stay in foster care for 2 or more years. Faushel and Shinn (1978) found that almost 42% of the children in their study had one placement and 30% experienced two placements. Lawder et al. (1986) reported that the majority of children who entered foster care returned to their families within a short period of time. Only a small group of children, because of the severity of their problems or those of their parents, needed extended care. Six of the variables in this study were significantly related to the length of stay in the foster home. For example, the frequency of visitation by members of the biological family was a strong predictor of whether the child returned to the biological family or remained in foster care. Similarly severe behavior problems, teenage parents, family crisis before placement, the presence of mental health problems in the parents, and neglect contributed heavily toward a continuing stay in the foster home.

Several other studies of the foster care system have examined the involvement of natural parents in foster care. These studies indicate that a large number of children in foster care are not visited by their natural parents. Columbia University studies of foster care placement in New York City observed that "at the end of five years, 57% of the children still in foster care were not being visited by their natural parents" (Faushel et al., 1978). The study found that greater frequency of parental visiting was significantly correlated with early discharge from foster care. Mech (1985) also reported similar findings indicating that the length of time children spent in foster care was related to the frequency of parental visiting. The association between parental visiting and time spent in foster care was significant for black families in which multiple parental contacts were observed. However, the results with respect to parental visiting as a factor associated with time and placement appeared consistent regardless of socioeconomic categories or geographic regions.

Several studies emphasize the extreme importance of the biological parents for the development of normal identity during the teenage years. Littner (1976) points out the traumatic effect of separation and placement. He indicated that foster children experienced anger toward their own parents for rejecting them. However, persistent angry feelings toward one's own parents become unacceptable after a while guilt is aroused in the child for having such feelings. To alleviate their guilt these children often behave in a manner that results in punishment. Also, loving foster parents may imply disloyalty toward the biological parents. A foster child may remain aloof in order to avoid further rejection by the foster parents. Many workers in this field (Tiddy, 1986) suggest involvement of the biological parents through visitation, joint therapy sessions, correspondence, and telephone calls. Such contacts should be initiated after careful planning with the foster and biological families while keeping the child's welfare at the forefront. Visitation should be carried out in an atmosphere of cooperation rather than mistrust among the families. Loyalty conflicts in the child can be reduced by family sessions involving the child and both families. Resolution of love and hate conflicts toward the biological parents requires family sessions with the biological parents.

Multiple Foster Placements

Adolescents who have stayed in several foster homes pose special placement problems.They do not have sufficient time to develop a relationship with adults and begin to depend on themselves, their impulses, and their frequently poor judgment. They rarely internalize adult values and often run away or behave badly when appropriate limits are set by foster parents. These behaviors frequently lead to shifting to other foster homes or placements in more restricted environments such as residential treatment centers. These adolescents consume a major portion of the service resources.

Several studies indicate that placement disruptions only partly result from the child's behavior problems. A great deal of variance is attributed to the service system and the manner in which children are placed in foster homes (Faushel and Shinn, 1978). Taber and Proch (1987) reported findings of the Chicago Service Project on the placement of youth who have had several placement disruptions. The typical youth in the study was 15 years old, had been in placement for 5 years, had lived in nine different substitutive care situations of increasing restriction, and had manifested various delinquent behaviors. The project staff focused on a series of specific steps and activities that resulted in the reduction of placement disruptions. The most important feature of this project was the involvement of the youth in the placement process. Each youth was interviewed by the staff within 5 days of his acceptance. In addition to the usual social, psychological, and psychiatric assessments, specific information was gathered on the youth's daily routine and the way in which the youth responded to stress, disappointment, and authority. The developmental needs of each youth were considered for specific placement. A planning team was formed for each youth accepted for the service. The team included the youth, the youth's significant others (family members, close friends), the clinician overseeing the assessment, the caseworker, and the project staff member. The planning team met a minimum of three times. The first meeting was focused on preparing the service description, including the type of services necessary for the placement. The second meeting was held to explain the nature of the placement to the youth and his significant others and have the placement agreement signed. The third meeting was held at the time of closing the case. Each case was kept open for 90 days after the placement of the youth. The project staff routinely contacted the foster family after placement and provided necessary help to reduce conflict in the family. The findings of the project indicated a strongly positive outcome. The frequency of placement was reduced by 60%, and placements after this service were in less restrictive settings.

Specialized Foster Homes

These may include therapeutic foster homes and foster homes for the medically handicapped, seriously disturbed, and pregnant teenagers. This decade has seen a variety of foster homes suited for the special needs of different adolescents. Some of these specialized foster homes have been developed in conjunction with group homes and residential treatment centers to serve their own adolescents who may be discharged to a less restrictive foster home situation. The foster parents of these homes may themselves be trained professionals or may have had a great deal of experience in working with adolescents in various mental health settings. These facilities allow greater flexibility so that an adolescent placed in a specialized foster home from a residential treatment center may return to the center if unable to adjust in the foster home. Consultation with the professional staff is provided to the foster parents on a regular basis. Therapeutic foster homes have been designed to avoid residential care for those adolescents who have not been able to stay in a regular foster home but may function well with the extra structure, supervision, and therapy provided in a specialized foster home.

There are few outcome studies of the success of these specialized foster homes. Sisto (1985) reported her findings on specialized foster homes for teenage mothers. Many of these teenagers suffered from severe social, economic, and emotional difficulties as a consequence of early pregnancy. Eight out of ten girls who gave birth between 15 and 17 years of age never finished high school. Social agencies around the country have provided group homes as well as specialized foster homes for these pregnant teenagers. Many of these teen homes provide a comfortable home environment both for the mother and the child. The mothers are encouraged to finish school and acquire additional training in some job skills. The baby's care is supervised by houseparents when the mother is at school or at job training. However, the mother herself is primarily responsible for providing care to her baby. Sisto found that many teenage mothers were quite immature. They resisted assuming their responsibilities as independent citizens. They also resented caring for the baby and the structure that the foster homes imposed on them.

GROUP HOMES

Historically, group homes came into existence to house those children and youths who could not be placed in foster homes and did not require institutionalization. The development of such homes was spurred by the movement of deinstitutionalization and the closing of a large number of residential facilities for children and youth. In addition, the continuing deterioration of the nuclear family has produced a large number of adolescents who cannot live with either of their parents and who require group homes or foster home settings.

The size of a group home may range from as few as 7 youths to over 100. The residents of such homes are usually divided into small structural living groups of 8 to 12. These programs are community based, and the residents of group homes utilize most of the community facilities such as public schools and recreational facilities. Staff supervision varies depending upon the degree of psychological and behavioral disturbance of the residents. Each structural unit or cottage is supervised by houseparents 24 hours a day. The houseparents usually have little or no training in mental health work. They are generally given training by the professional staff, which may be composed of social workers and therapists with bachelor or master levels of training. Some group homes may have psychiatrists as consultants providing direction to the professional staff in the management of the more severely disturbed children.

The quality of the programs varies among group homes. All homes provide basic needs such as shelter, food, clothing, health care, education, and recreation. However, the time and attention given to each child varies depending upon the number of staff available for such work. In a California study, Cohen (1986) classified the objectives of the treatment programs of group homes into three categories:

1. Resocialization and rehabilitation.
2. General developmental growth.
3. Mixture of the above.

Some group homes have focused their activities on improving the general developmental growth of their residents, whereas others have emphasized resocialization and rehabilitation. However, the majority of group homes appear to have the mixed objectives of treatment focusing on both developmental growth and resocialization. Similarly, the treatment modalities utilized by the different group homes also varied. Behavior modification and eclectic, psychodynamic, and social living approaches are commonly used to achieve treatment objectives. In this study, the behavior modification approach was defined as focusing on daily living behavior that is observable and accessible to intervention, the psychodynamic approach emphasized treating intrapsychic emotional conflict, and social living and peer pressure were the principal mechanism to bring about changes in behavior.

Curtis et al. (1985) studied 17 group homes in Kansas. None of these homes admitted residents with a history of severe violence. The group homes were divided into two groups:

1. Teaching family homes.—Each of these homes was directed by a live-in mar-

ried couple called teaching parents. Each teaching parent was extensively instructed and supervised in the application of specific skills such as teaching, self-government, motivation, relation development, and youth advocacy procedures.

2. Nonteaching family homes.—These were staffed by at least one full-time live-in staff member. Various staff members rotated the nighttime duties. Each of the homes had an outside director responsible for several homes.

During much of the 1970s the emphasis was on the development of community-based programs for juvenile delinquents who committed offenses such as school truancy, running away, and other nonviolent crimes. These programs included run-away shelters, alternate school programs, and small open group homes as an alternative to institutions. Juvenile delinquents were placed in these community facilities, mostly on the basis of the type of offense committed. However, many adolescents were placed in these facilities without regard to the emotional and developmental needs of each individual. Several studies have indicated that these programs have not been as successful as was initially expected. Simone (1985) studied the failures of placement in three group homes located in northeast Ohio. The term *failure* implied a youth who was terminated from the program prior to a satisfactory completion of the rehabilitation. Running away and/or chronic disruptive behavior were the most frequent reasons for termination. Many of these homes were not paid for the days that an adolescent was absent, which resulted in a substantial loss of revenue for the group homes. The homes were inclined to terminate runaways after a few days of absence. The author noted that most of these adolescents, when brought to court, received a more secure placement such as a residential facility. The author felt that institutionalization could have been avoided in some cases if the homes had been paid to keep the beds open until the adolescent returned.

Krueger and Hansen (1984) found that positive changes in self-esteem and self-concept are important predictors of successful outcome of group home treatment. The authors noted that the status offender youth in group homes frequently had low self-esteem that was often related to their anxiety, poor school performance, acting-out behavior, and substance abuse. They studied 46 youths (both male and female) between the ages of 12 and 16 years who resided in a group home for 12 months. The authors compared the scores on self-concept scales (Tennessee Self-concept Scale) at the time of arrival at the group home and 12 months later. The program of the group home included time spent in public schools, support, and role modeling by houseparents as well as family counseling. A tutor coordinated the schoolwork and homework and saw that the assignments were completed and returned. The families of these adolescents received counseling from family service workers. The primary goal of family counseling was improving parenting and communication skills. Youths needing individual counseling were provided the services in the community. A youth who showed improvement in behavior also showed improvement in self-esteem. The adolescents who continued to act out and ran away did not show much improvement in their self-esteem.

RESIDENTIAL TREATMENT CENTERS

In the early part of this century, residential centers for children and adolescents included group homes, orphanages, custodial institutions for the mentally retarded, training schools, and reform schools. Most of these institutions were geared to provide the basic necessities of daily life and possibly rehabilitate delinquent youths with harsh and punitive training methods. It was not until the 1930s and 1940s that attention was focused on the problems of the children themselves and that therapeutic elements were introduced in the treatment of children in residential centers. These trends were inspired and promoted by several well-known leaders in child psychiatry such as Aichhorn (1935), Redl and Wineman (1957), and Bettleheim (1974). Although these therapists differed in their treatment approaches, the common goal of residential treatment was identified as providing a comprehensive, therapeutic environment in which a child could grow, learn, and be rehabilitated. Residential treatment centers vary widely in their organizational structure, staff patterns, and treatment modalities. These variations depend upon the availability of resources and the training of the personnel. Most residential treatment centers provide a highly organized milieu; education programs; recreational facilities; individual, group, and family therapy; and medical services. Comprehensive vocational training programs are also available in some centers.

Milieu staff forms the backbone of the program. They are on the front line taking care of the children and helping them with day-to-day problems every day of the week, 24 hours a day. The milieu staff may be trained child-care workers or lay individuals with little or no experience in the mental health field. The professional staff of the center is expected to provide guidance to the milieu staff as well as work directly with the children and their families. The educational program forms a major component of the daily activities of the children. However, many of the children have learning and/or behavioral problems that reduce their capacity to function in a regular classroom. Most teachers at these centers are thus trained in special education techniques. Tutoring is provided in small classroom settings. After a period of treatment some children are able to attend regular or special classrooms in community schools. Most centers utilize the vocational facilities of the community for the training of their residents. However, some centers have developed extensive in-house facilities to train motivated residents in common trades.

The duration of stay in residential treatment centers varies greatly, depending upon the severity of the psychopathology, funding sources, and the ability of the staff to work with the resident. Most centers have an initial evaluation period of a few weeks to determine the suitability of a specific child for a particular treatment facility. The child may stay in the center for a few months to several years. Many residential treatment centers are associated with community facilities for a transition from center to community living. Many adolescents, especially those in their late teenage years, do not have a home to return to and need a place of transition such as a half-way house, foster family, or a group foster home in order to learn and adjust to semi-independent and consequently independent living.

There has been a strong trend against placing adolescents in residential treatment centers for various reasons such as cost, separation of the adolescent from his family, and the overly controlled environment of the institution. However, there are many adolescents who continue to be disturbed in spite of extensive outpatient treatment in mental health clinics, day treatment programs, and short-term hospitalization. It is generally difficult to identify adolescents who need residental treatment centers without first exposing them to outpatient or day treatment. Stone (1979) has suggested the following criteria indications for residential treatment center placements:

1. Severe individual intrapsychic disorder (mental, emotional, and behavioral).
2. Serious developmental disturbances, including a failure to achieve psychomotor development and mastery of psychobiological functioning, or pronounced fixations or regressions in various aspects of development.
3. Significant disturbances in environmental relationships such as in the family, community, and schools.

The most common types of adolescents referred to residential treatment centers include the following:

1. Adolescents with severe depression who have not responded to short-term hospitalization and continue to be suicidal and potentially harmful to themselves.
2. Schizophrenics who have not responded to short-term hospital treatment.
3. Adolescents with severe conduct disorders who have not been able to get along with their families and are a constant problem in the community and/or schools.
4. Abused children who have been taken away from their families and have significant psychopathology such as chronic depression, anxiety, and conduct disorders.

However, most of the adolescents placed in residential treatment centers have multiple problems (emotional, familial, and developmental).

Outcome Studies

There are very few follow-up studies of the effectiveness of residential treatment centers. This may be due to the fact that there are a large number of variables in the outcome of such treatment. In addition to the wide variability of organization, staff qualifications, and therapeutic interventions, the psychopathology of the adolescent patient varies greatly. The success of treatment may also depend upon parental participation, family therapy, vocational training, and the availability and readiness of the natural family to receive the adolescent after discharge.

Davids and Salvatore (1976) carried out a follow-up study through questionnaires of a number of residents who were discharged from a residential treatment center in Rhode Island. The follow-up questionnaires focused primarily on assessing the patient's outcome through responses to questions about other hospitalizations, school adjustments, problems with authorities, work history, overall emotional adjustments, and current symptoms of psychopathology. Seventy-one of the questionnaires returned were composed of the following diagnostic categories: passive/aggressive personality (41 subjects), psychoneurosis (7), schizoid personality (12), and child schizophrenia (11). The sample was subdivided into three groups on the basis of overall adjustment, including areas of aggressive behavior, obedience to parents, work history, school failure, truancy, and running away. The three groups were as follows: well-adjusted (29 subjects), fair (22 subjects), and poor adjustment (20 subjects). These groups were then compared on a variety of measures indicating problems they presented at the time of admission. The good-adjustment category included children who were fearful and withdrawn and had difficulty concentrating at the time of admission. The poor-adjustment group included children who manifested troublesome behavior such as lying, stealing, and peculiar behavior. No significant differences in age, length of stay, parental participation, or casework were noted. In comparing their adjustment at the time of follow-up with that at the time of discharge, 88% of those who were making a good adjustment were judged to be better than when discharged. However, of those individuals in the poor-adjustment group, 54% were judged to now be worse than when discharged. Eighty-eight percent of the parents of those patients who were making good to fair adjustments felt very positive about residential treatment centers.

Levy (1969) reported that in residential treatment centers psychotic children had a poor prognosis, particularly if the psychosis was associated with lower intelligence. Similarly, Barker (1974) reported a poor outcome for psychotic, organic, or conduct disorder children but a good prognosis for neurotic children in residential treatment centers. Garber (1972) reviewed follow-up studies of hospitalized adolescents and found a poor outcome for schizophrenia and organic disorders, while affective disorders and psychoneurosis showed a good outcome.

Lewis et al. (1980) followed up 51 children who were discharged within a 6-year period. They had received approximately 2 years of inpatient treatment. The follow-up information was obtained from case records, telephone reports, relatives, and outside agencies. Information was obtained on the number of placements prior to entering residential treatment centers, the number and kinds of subsequent placements, evidence of serious maternal or paternal psychopathology, and evidence of maternal or paternal legal difficulties. The criteria for poor outcome were three or more placements since discharge, difficulties with the law, and placement in a psychiatric hospital. If none of the above conditions existed, the outcome was rated as good.

The results indicated that of the 51 children sufficient information was available on 43 children for independent raters to decide on the outcome. Twenty-nine (67.4%) showed poor outcome, whereas 14 (32.6%) had a good outcome. Postresidential treatment adjustment was frequently characterized by serious psychiatric and antisocial problems.

Pearson (1987) followed 140 selected adolescents for at least 2 years after discharge from an adolescent service of a state hospital. The group included the following diagnostic categories:

1. Borderline personality disorders, 32 subjects.

2. Nuclear schizophrenia, 25 subjects.
3. Major affective disorders, 24 subjects.
4. Behavior and family problems, 22 subjects.
5. Conduct disorders, 17 subjects.
6. Developmental disabilities, 15 subjects.
7. Others, 5 subjects.

The outcome was divided into five categories on the basis of two major parameters:

1. The degree of phase-appropriate independence.
2. The presence of symptoms in the context of level of independence.

The five categories were as follows:

1. Independent/adaptive, 31 subjects.
2. Independent/symptomatic, 27 subjects.
3. Dependent/functional, 25 subjects.
4. Dependent/impaired, 30 subjects.
5. Institutionalized, 23 subjects.

About two thirds of the adolescents with borderline personality disorders showed good outcomes, while three fourths of the adolescents with major affective disorders had favorable outcomes. The author pointed out the need of seriously disturbed adolescents for a stable, long-term relationship with a therapist. Good outcomes were frequently associated with such a relationship.

There are few studies evaluating program outcomes for adolescent boys in residential treatment facilities. Gilliland-Marlo and Judd (1986) have reported on the effectiveness of residential care facilities for 101 males between the ages of 11 and 17 years. The residential facility was located in rural Colorado and was organized into four program components: diagnostic programs, a 30-day evaluation; treatment programs providing individual and group therapy and educational and recreational activities; the World of Work Program for boys over the age of 16 years, which was designed to develop independent living skills; and on-ground group homes for individuals who needed a supportive, transitional environment before going home or into other facilities. This program focused on finding and sustaining work and promoting living skills and personal growth.

Data were collected on demographic information, social history (prior history of aggressive behavior, court involvement, police contacts, runaway behavior, drug abuse, learning problems, and medical problems), and program involvement (length of stay, family counseling, and other components of the program in which the residents participated).

Program outcome was divided into successful or unsuccessful. A successful outcome included placement into the homes of parents, a significant other, foster care, a group home, or some other residential facility. An unsuccessful outcome included placement into a detention facility or termination for running away from the facility. The results included the following: age was not related to outcome; race had significant effects (70.2% of the white boys had a successful outcome as opposed to 47.1% of the nonwhites); boys with no history of substance abuse had a better outcome than did those with a positive history; and boys on probation before or upon entering the facility had a 53.8% successful outcome, while those with no probation had an 80% successful outcome. There was a very significant effect of running-away behavior in the outcome of those who ran from the facility: 47.5% were ultimately able to achieve successful outcomes as compared with the nonrunners, 88.2% of whom had successful outcomes.

Overall, 59 (62.1%) of the boys had a successful outcome: 43 (45.3%) went home; 6 (6.3%) went into foster homes; 6 (6.3%) went into another residential facility; and 4 (4.2%) went into a group home. Thirty-six (37.9%) had an unsuccessful outcome (7 went into a detention facility, while 29 were terminated because they were constantly running away from the facility).

Although the overall results of residential treatment are not very convincing, this modality of treatment is definitely needed for those adolescents who do not benefit from any of the other mental health services provided in a community. Unfortunately, third-party payers have withdrawn their financial support from these institutions, so they are now run primarily with the support of state and private funds. There are many adolescents who can be identified during their first short-term hospitalization as requiring residential treatment, but the unavailability of funds keeps them in the community. They continue to suffer and create problems for their families and communities and are hospitalized repeatedly until financial support becomes available from the state or private sources to pay for their residential treatment.

COMMUNITY SUPPORT GROUPS

A large number of community support groups have been developed for various health- and mental health–related problems. Such groups exist both for the parents as well as for the adolescent patient. The groups for the parents focus on helping them understand the mental health problems of their children and/or sharing techniques of dealing with their problem children. For example, parents who are overprotective of their children and are easily manipulated by them can benefit from attending community groups called "Tough Love." There are other groups of parents whose children suffer from schizophrenia, autism, and Tourette's syndrome. If a community does not have a certain type of group, parents may write to the national headquarters of a specific group and receive information with regard to their specific problems.

Adolescent patients themselves may join self-help groups relating to their specific problems such as obesity, bulimia, anorexia, schizophrenia (National Schizophrenia Fellowship), children of alcoholic parents (Alateens), alcoholism (Alcoholics Anonymous), substance abuse, and past sexual abuse. These groups frequently include both adult and adolescent patients. There are few controlled studies evaluating the effectiveness of these groups. A few studies of groups involved in weight control were mentioned in Chapter 5. Marc Galanter (1988) studied Recovery Incorporated, a self-help program for people with psychiatric problems. The organization was established in 1937 by Dr. Abraham Low. It has more than 900 local groups spread around the country with an attendance of about 10,000 members in weekly meetings. Each 2-hour meeting follows the same format: an initial reading or listening to an audio tape by Dr. Low followed by member presentation and then open exchange. The group does not discuss psychiatric therapies or medications. The speaker describes an incident from his life that was upsetting and points out how an untoward attitude led to distress. Other members help the speaker by pointing out other attitudes in the situation that may have contributed to the distress.

In Galanter's study 201 leaders (one from each group), 155 new members, and 195 control subjects filled out questionnaires. The questionnaire contained 216 multiple choice questions relating to general well-being, neurotic distress, social cohesiveness, ideological commitment to recovery, and psychiatric treatment. The results indicated a decline in both symptoms and psychiatric treatment after the subjects had joined the group. Scores for neurotic distress were considerably lower than those reported for the period before joining. The author concluded that support groups were a helpful adjunct to the psychiatric treatment of mental patients.

PLACEMENT INTO JUVENILE JUSTICE OR THE MENTAL HEALTH SYSTEM?

A small number of adolescents with severe conduct problems are placed in the mental health system for treatment. A great deal of ambiguity exists in the society with regard to the management of adolescents with severe conduct problems. In some communities, all adolescents with severe conduct problems are first brought to mental health facilities unless they have committed a felony. On the other hand, in some communities the department of corrections handles the majority of cases of adolescents with severe conduct problems. Since neither of the two systems (the mental health system and the juvenile correction system) claims major success in dealing with these adolescents, the selection of one or the other system seems to depend on certain parameters. Several studies in the past have indicated that race, ethnicity, and social class differences frequently account for the placement of adolescents in the juvenile justice or mental health system (Hatke, 1978; Stewart, 1976). Westendorp et al. (1986) compared 221 adolescents who were admitted to six mental health programs with 55 adolescents who were presented for correction placement by juvenile courts. The authors collected data on four broad areas: demographic variables (ethnicity, race, social class, gender, parental/marital status), personality/psychopathology variables, academic variables, and social adjustment. Personality, academic, and social adjustment variables were assessed by the following measures: the Minnesota Multiphasic Personality Inventory (MMPI), the Peabody Individual Achievement Test, and the Child and Adolescent Adjustment Profile.

The results indicated that demographic variables (race or ethnicity, gender, and the marital status of the parents) were the primary determinants of which system (mental health or juvenile justice) the adolescent was placed in. The psychological measures used in this study were of little significance in differentiating the two groups with the exception of the MMPI depression subscale. Adolescents funneled to the juvenile justice system were usually minority males with a history of drug abuse and no previous mental health history whose parents were single, divorced, or remarried. There was no significant difference with regard to the level of academic achievement. On the five adjustment variables (peer relationship, dependency, hostility, productivity, and withdrawal), the juvenile justice group was somewhat better adjusted than the mental health group in expression of hostility and productivity.

Three psychopathology variables (depression, hysteria, and schizophrenia) were statistically more prevalent in the mental health groups than in the juvenile justice group. The authors emphasized the need for further research and the necessity of redefining mental illness and its associated legal statutes in order to eliminate barriers to quality cases and to protect the rights of all those involved.

REFERENCES

Aichhorn A: *Wayward Youth.* New York, Viking Press, 1935.

Barker P: History, in Barker P (ed): *The Residential Psychiatric Treatment of Children.* New York, 1974, pp 1–26.

Bettelheim B: *A Home for the Heart.* New York, Alfred A Knopf Inc, 1974.

Child Welfare Planning Notes: Characteristics of children in substitutive and adoptive care. Washington, DC, Hecht Institute: A division of Child Welfare League in America. 1984, pp 2–3.

Cohen N: Quality of care of youths in group homes. *Child Welfare* 1986; 65:481–494.

Curtis J, Bedlington M, Belden B, et al: Effects of community-based group-home treatment programs on male juvenile offenders' use of drugs and alcohol. *Am J Drug Alcohol Abuse* 1985; 11:249–279.

Davids A, Salvatore P: Residential treatment of disturbed children and adequacy of their subsequent adjustment: A follow-up study. *Am J Orthopsychiatry* 1976; 46:62–73.

Directory For Exceptional Children, 1980–1981. Boston, Porter-Sargent Publishers, 1981.

Faushel D, Shinn E: *Children in Foster Care: A Longitudinal Analysis.* New York, Columbia University Press, 1978.

Galanter M: Zealous self-help groups as adjustments to psychiatric treatment: A study of Recovery, Inc. *Am J Psychiatry* 1988; 145:1248–1253.

Garber B: *Follow-up Study of Hospitalized Adolescents.* New York, Brunner/Mazel, 1972.

Gilliland-Marlo D, Judd P: The effectiveness of residential care facilities for adolescent boys. *Adolescence* 1986; 21:311–321.

Hatke WF: *A Critique and Test of Labeling Theory—A Social Psychological Account of Deviance.* Ann Arbor, Mich, University Microfilms International, 1978.

Herz MI, Endicott J, Spitzer R, et al: Day versus inpatient hospitalization: A controlled study. *Am J Psychiatry* 1971; 127:1371–1382.

Kaduskin A: *Child Welfare Services.* New York, Macmillian Publishing Co Inc, 1974.

Kolvin I, Garside R, Nicol A, et al: *Help Starts Here: The Maladjusted Children in the Ordinary School.* London, Tavistock, 1981.

Krueger R, Hansen J: Self-concept changes during youth-home placement of adolescents. *Child Care Q* 1984; 13:126–141.

Lahey B, Kupfer D: Partial hospitalization programs for children and adolescents, in Luber R (ed): *Partial Hospitalization.* New York, Plenum Publishing Corp, 1979, pp 73–90.

Lawder E, Poulin J, Andrew R: A study of 185 foster children five years after placement. *Child Welfare* 1986; 65:241–251.

Lewis D, Shanok S, et al: The undoing of residential treatment, a follow-up study of 51 adolescents. *J Am Acad Child Psychiatry* 1980; 19:160–171.

Levy EZ: Long-term of follow-up of former inpatients at the children's hospital of the Menninger Clinic. *Am J Psychiatry* 1969; 125:1633–1639.

Littner N: *Some Traumatic Affects of Separation and Placement.* New York, Child Welfare League of America, 1976.

Mech E: Parental visiting and foster placement. *Child Welfare* 1985; 64:67–72.

Pearson GT: Long-term treatment needs of hospitalized adolescents, in Feinstein SC (ed): *Adolescent Psychiatry,* vol 14. Chicago, University of Chicago Press, 1987.

Redl F, Wineman D: *The Aggressive Child.* New York, Free Press, 1957.

Shepherd M, Oppenheim B, Mitchell S: *Childhood Behavior and Mental Health.* London, University of London Press, 1971.

Simone M: Group home failures in juvenile justice: The next step. *Child Welfare* 1985; 65:357–366.

Simone J: Day hospital treatment for borderline adolescents. *Adolescence* 1986; 21:561–572.

Sisto G: Therapeutic foster homes for teenage mothers and their babies. *Child Welfare* 1985; 64:157–163.

Stewart PL: *Deviance, theory, black youth and mental health professionals.* Presented at the National Conference on the Black Family in America: Black Youth, Louisville, Ky, 1976.

Stone LA: Residential Treatment, in Noshpitz ID (ed): *Basic Handbook of Child Psychiatry,* vol 3. New York, Basic Books Inc Publishers, 1979, pp 231–262.

Taber M, Prech K: Placement stability for adolescents in foster care: Findings from a program experiment. *Child Welfare* 1987; 66:433–445.

Tiddy S: Creative cooperation involving biological parents in long-term foster care. *Child Welfare* 1986; 65:53–62.

Valasquez J, Lyle CG: Day versus residential treatment for juvenile offenders: The impact of program evaluation. *Child Welfare* 1985; 64:145–156.

Werry J, Wollersheim J: Behavior therapy with children and adolescents: A twenty year overview. *J Am Acad Child Adolesc Psychiatry* 1989; 28:1–18.

Westendorp F, Brink K, Robertson M, et al: Variables which differentiate placement of adolescents into juvenile justice or mental health systems. *Adolescence* 1986; 21:23–37.

Wollersheim J: Direct Cognitive Therapies, in Wilson HF (chairman): *Direct Cognitive Therapies: Psychological and Philosophical Foundations and Implications.* Presented at the convention of the Rocky Mountain Psychological Association, Las Vegas, 1980.

7 | Adolescent Medicine

Adolescent patients hospitalized for psychiatric reasons tend to have many acute and chronic health problems. Although some of the physical symptoms such as headaches, stomachaches, and sleeping difficulties may apparently be related to stress, other acute and chronic problems may be more ambiguous and require further investigations. It is not uncommon for the staff of a psychiatric unit to question the genuineness of physical complaints before responding. This caution is frequently justified since the majority of the physical complaints may have a basis in heightened tension and desire for extra attention. However, all physical complaints should be investigated and appropriate interventions provided. If the primary cause of a physical symptom is found to be an emotional stress, this should be communicated to the patient. It is often of the utmost value for an adolescent to know the relationship between stress and physical symptoms and learn some techniques to decrease stress in order to relieve symptoms.

Most of the health problems of adolescents may be divided into three categories:

1. Health problems related to the developmental stage of adolescence, i.e., growth, nutrition, obesity, dermatologic problems, orthopedic problems.
2. Exacerbation of chronic medical problems during adolescence, i.e., diabetes, asthma, epilepsy, hemophilia.
3. Acute medical and surgical problems more common to adolescent years, i.e., sexually transmitted diseases, physical injuries.

GROWTH AND DEVELOPMENT

All adolescents have some concern about their height, weight, and sexual maturity. These concerns are rarely expressed directly or spontaneously to physicians. Only after careful questioning do these concerns become apparent. The use of height and weight charts is helpful in explaining the normal pattern of growth. Until girls enter their adolescent growth surge, there is little difference in height between the two

175

sexes. The mean age for the peak of the growth spurts for girls is 12.14 ± 0.14 (SD = 0.88) years; the mean age for the peak of the growth spurt for boys is 14.06 ± 0.14 (SD = 0.92) years. Girls tend to become taller than the boys in their early teens, but boys catch up in height and surpass girls by the mid and late teens. This difference in height is explained on the basis of the different rate of bone growth in the two sexes. Ossification centers appear earlier in the long bones of girls, and there is an earlier cessation of bone growth in girls that results in the lesser average height of adult women.

Short Stature

Height is genetically determined, and the short stature of an adolescent should be compared with that of his parents. Normal lower limits for height are set at the 3rd percentile and the height below the 3rd percentile should be investigated carefully. There are multiple causes of short stature including genetic and familial, constitutional, endocrinological, and chromosomal, as well as from chronic diseases.

Genetic or familial short stature is suggested by the presence of short stature of parents, a growth curve that is within the 3rd percentile for height, bone age consistent with chronological age, and a normal history and physical examination findings.

Endocrinological causes of short stature are uncommon and relate to hyperthyroidism, a deficiency of growth hormones, and an excess of adrenal cortical hormones. Hyperthyroidism and hyperactivity of the adrenal cortex are associated with other physical systems and can be detected easily. However, an isolated deficiency of growth hormone may be difficult to detect, especially in adolescents with a constitutional delay in puberty.

Chronic diseases of the kidney, intestine, heart, and lung frequently cause nutritional and metabolic changes resulting in short stature. Similarly, skeletal dysplasias relating to the abnormal growth of the bone and cartilage reduce physical height.

Chromosomal abnormalities such as Turner's syndrome cause short stature in girls. In addition, several other congenital syndromes are frequently associated with short stature such as Prader-Labhart-Willi syndrome, Laurence-Moon-Biedl syndrome, Rosewater syndrome, Down syndrome, etc.

Tall Stature

Excessively tall stature is at times a matter of concern, especially in girls during early adolescent years. Normal causes of excessive tallness are familial and early onset of puberty. Other causes include excessive growth hormone, an excess of anabolic steroids (from an adrenal tumor, gonadal tumors, etc.), hyperthyroidism, Marfan Syndrome, etc.

SEX MATURATION

Physiology

The sex of an individual is determined at the time of fertilization of the ovum by a sperm. However, the process of sexual differentiation may be broken down into three stages:

1. Establishment of genetic sex.
2. Establishment of gonadal (genital) sex.
3. Establishment of phenotypic sex (body sex).

Genetic sex is determined at the time of fertilization and depends upon whether an X or the Y chromosome is present in the fertilizing sperm. It appears that the Y chromosome is essential for the development of maleness, more specifically, the development of testes. No matter how many X chromosomes are present, if a Y chromosome is also present, testes will develop. In the absence of a Y chromosome, a female develops.

The establishment of gonadal sex, that is, the development of testes or ovaries, occurs by about the 10th or 12th week of gestation. A group of cells in the developing gut becomes separated fairly early from the rest of the rapidly somatic cells in the embryo and can be recognized as germ cells by approximately the 22nd day of gestation. Shortly thereafter, the germ cells leave the gut and migrate toward the future site of gonadal development (called the gonadal ridge). This migration seems to be caused by some substances (chemotactic) produced by the prospective gonadal region. During the migration, the germ cells increase steadily in number by mitotic division. Beginning about the sixth week of gestation the germ cells (or the primitive testes) in the human male embryo undergo rapid development to form tiny tubules (seminiferous tubules) and then other cells. In the female, potential ovaries grow in size but undergo little differentiation during this period. Later in development the germ cells in the ovaries become grouped and then divide by meiosis. Still later, they become surrounded by follicular cells, and eventually a definite ovary with follicles and supporting structure (stroma) develop by the third month of gestation.

The establishment of phenotypic sex relates to the development of internal and external genital organs. Each human fetus develops a dual system of structures— wolffian and müllerian duct systems—that gives rise to internal genital organs other than the gonads. The male genital structures (epididymis, vas deferens, and seminal vesicles) are derived from the wolffian ducts; the female genital structures (the fallopian tubes, the uterus, and the upper part of the vagina) are derived from the müllerian ducts. If the fetus is to develop into a male, the müllerian ducts regress while the wolffian ducts develop into male genital structures. In the female, the wolffian ducts regress while the müllerian ducts give rise to female genital structures.

The internal genital organs of the two sexes develop from different sets of structures, whereas the external genitalia in both sexes develop from a common set of structures. It is through the action of the gonads that phenotypic sex develops. Between the sixth and eighth weeks of gestation the ovaries begin to synthesize estrogens while the testes synthesize testosterone. The two hormones from the fetal testes are responsible for the differentiation of male internal and external genitalia: testosterone and the müllerian regression factor. Testosterone, secreted by the Leydig cells of the testes, is also converted into another potent hormone, dihydrotestosterone

(DHT). Testosterone and DHT are responsible for the development of the wolffian duct system into the male internal organs. DHT is also responsible for the differentiation of the external genitalia of the male. At the seventh week of gestation the external genitalia of the two sexes look identical. At about the eighth week of gestation testosterone and DHT induce formation of the penis and the scrotum.

The establishment of sexual differentiation of body structures involves a complicated series of developmental events, and each step presents a potential disaster for normal outcome. For example, deficiency of an enzyme (5α-reductase) that converts testosterone into DHT would result in a person whose internal genital organs are male (including testes, vas deferens, and seminal vesicles) but whose external genitalia are predominantly female. The defects may also occur in the responsiveness of the fetal tissue that are acted upon by the sex hormones to differentiate them. In the testicular feminization syndrome, a person is born with testes and produces normal testosterone levels, but there is an absence of internal genital tract development, the presence of female external genitalia, feminization of body contours, and breast development at puberty.

The hypothalamus and the pituitary gland regulate the synthesis of sex hormones from the ovaries, the testes, and the adrenal cortex. The regulation is carried out through the influence of gonadotropic hormones secreted by the pituitary, primarily, follicle-stimulating hormones (FSH) and luteinizing hormone (LH). The initial synthesis of testosterone by the testes and the sexual differentiation in the fetus are not dependent upon gonadotropic hormones. However, the gonadotropic hormones are essential for further development of the ovaries and the testes. By the eighth week of gestation, the hypothalamus begins to secrete a factor (gonadotropin-releasing hormone) that induces the pituitary to begin to secrete gonadotropic hormones by the 10th to 13th week of gestation, and by the 20th week these hormones reach their peak concentration. At the end of the first week after birth, pituitary gonadotropins rise in concentration and exhibit wide fluctuations for several months until about 6 months to 1 year of age when these hormones settle at their low level, which continues in boys until the onset of puberty. In girls FSH shows a greater and more prolonged rise in concentration that gradually declines to its prepubertal level at about 2 years of age.

During early and late childhood, gonadal hormones are present in small concentrations and probably exert only a minor influence in the sexual differentiation of boys and girls. At the beginning of puberty, however, gonadal hormones increase in concentration, and they are essential in bringing about further development of external genitalia and other sex characteristics. Plasma testosterone levels show only a very slight rise during the prepubertal years in both sexes. However, during early puberty there is a very steep rise in boys and only a slight rise in girls. Estrogen levels rise steadily throughout puberty in girls, and its plasma concentration varies with the menstrual cycles.

Gender Identification

Gender identification is generally divided into three underlying processes:

1. Gender assignments.
2. Gender identity.
3. Gender role.

Gender assignment is certainly determined by the sex chromosomes and intra-uterine environment. Gender identity refers to an individual's self-awareness of his maleness or femaleness. The gender role is the outward expression of gender identity. In the majority of the cases, all three of these aspects go hand in hand, that is, a child born with male genitalia recognizes himself as a male and expresses his sexuality as a male. Specific problems arise when all three of these processes do not go along together. In the cases of failure of clear differentiation of external genitalia (such as in hermaphrodites), an ambiguity of gender assignment occurs that, if continued without correction for any length of time, creates severe problems in gender iden-tification and gender role.

The influence of the environment in the acquisition of gender identity and gender role is greatly emphasized. Differences in the play of male and female infants can be detected during the first year of life. These differences may result from differences in parental expectation and attitude toward the girls and boys. In cases of herma-phroditic babies whose sex is reassigned at around 12 to 18 months of age through operative procedures, the mothers and fathers of these children become aware of the changes in their own behavior toward these children. For example, a father reported that he found himself no longer encouraging his child, newly assigned at the age of 16 months as a daughter, to roughhouse with her brother, a year older. A few cases have been described where operative corrections at the age of 5 years or later required a great deal of preparation and psychotherapy of the children and the parents before changing the sexual genitalia.

Sex identity is part of the general process of maturation called self-identity. The self-identity is acquired in childhood through an influence of various factors such as parental teachings and reward and punishment for certain attributes of the personality and identification. Identification plays a major role in the acquisition of self-identity after the first 2 years of life. Identification is an unconscious process that leads the child to think, feel, and behave after another person (called "model"), usually a parent in the case of a child. Two conditions appear to facilitate the development of iden-tification with a model: (1) a child must want to possess some of the model's attributes, and (2) he must have some basis for believing that he and the model are similar in some ways. The identification is facilitated if the model is a desirable person. The identification, however, is not an "all-or-none" phenomena. Each child identifies to some degree with both parents and, as his social contacts become wider, with adults and peers outside the family.

Acquisition of sex roles is an even more complex process. Every culture and different classes of society in each culture characterize certain attributes for males and females. By the age of 3 years most children can properly label themselves as "boy" or "girl." By the age of 4 years they are able to label both themselves and others correctly. However, even by 5 years of age most children are not certain of the consistency of their sex identity. In one study 4- to 8-year-old children were asked whether a girl could become a boy if she wanted to, if she played boys' games, or if she wore a boy's haircut or clothes. Most 4-year-olds said that she could be. By the age of 6 or 7 years most children were certain that a girl could not become a boy regardless of appearance or behavior.

A great many difficulties in sexual behavior seem to arise primarily from problems in the acquisition of gender roles; this leads to homosexuality, transexualism, transvestism, and fetishism.

Sexual Maturity Rating

Adolescents vary in the timing at which pubertal events occur, but the sequence in which they occur are the same for all adolescents. Tanner's chart on stages of sexual maturation (1962) is very helpful in identifying the maturational stage of an adolescent. Two separate ratings are used for boys and girls. In girls, patterns of pubic hair growth and configuration of breasts are rated on a scale of 1 to 5, whereas size of the testicles and penis and patterns of pubic hair growth are rated in a similar manner. Menarche usually occurs in stage 4 but may start in stage 3. The average age of menarche for American girls is about 12 years and 4 months, and normal variation is 9 to 17 years. It usually takes about 18 months to 2 years to establish regularity of menstrual periods. For the first 1 to 2 years menstrual cycles are usually anovular.

Delayed Puberty

It is suggested that a male may be considered to have delayed puberty if genital stage 1 persists beyond the age of 13.7 years or pubic hair stage 1 persists beyond 15.1 years. Similarly, a female is considered to have delayed puberty if breast stage 1 persists beyond the age of 13.4 years or pubic hair stage 1 persists beyond 14.1 years.

Causes of delayed puberty are multiple. However, common causes include constitutional delay, gonadotropin deficiency, congenital gonadal disorders, and chronic diseases. The vast majority of the adolescents (90% to 95%) with delayed puberty are constitutional and have a positive family history of constitutional delay of puberty. A deficiency of gonadotropin hormones may occur in isolation or in association with a deficiency of other pituitary hormones. Hypothalamic and/or pituitary lesions from a neoplasm may result in delayed physical and sexual development. Functional hypogonadism may result from chronic systemic diseases such as chronic renal disease and inflammatory bowel disorder. Congenital disorders of the gonads include Klinefelter's syndrome, Turner's syndrome, Prader-Lebhart-Willi syndrome, and Laurence-Moon-Biedl syndrome.

An investigation of an adolescent with delayed puberty should include a family history; physical examination; laboratory tests to rule out systemic diseases, find chromosomal abnormalities, and determine gonadotropin levels; x-ray films of bone for age; skull x-ray films; thyroid function studies; and a determination of testosterone or estradiol levels.

ADOLESCENT SEXUALITY

Premarital sexual activity among U.S. teenagers has increased significantly over the past three decades. Zelnik and Kantner (1980) reported estimates of the proportion of teenagers who had ever experienced premarital sexual intercourse. The data were collected in three national surveys of young women (NSYW) in 1971, 1976, and 1979. These studies indicated that in all teenagers between the ages of 15 and 19 years the percentage reporting sexual activity rose from 30.4% in 1971 to 43.4% in 1976 and 49.8% in 1979. The trend for white teenagers was similar to that of all teenagers combined, but the trend for black teenagers was different: it rose from 53.7% in 1971 to 66.3% in 1976 and was 66.2% in 1979.

In another survey, the National Survey of Family Growth (NSFG) in 1982, teenagers were asked the age at which their first sexual experience occurred. These data are combined in Table 7–1 with other data from three NSYW studies (Hofferth et al., 1987). Table 7–1 indicates some decline in the percentage of sexually active teenagers

TABLE 7–1

Percentage of U.S. Metropolitan Teenage Women Who Had Ever Had Premarital Sexual Intercourse by Race and Age: 1971, 1975, and 1979 National Surveys of Young Women and 1982 National Survey of Family Growth*

Race and Age	Survey Year			
	1971	1975	1979	1982
Total	N = 2,739	N = 1,452	N = 1,717	N = 1,157
15–19	30.4	43.4	49.8	44.9
15	14.8	18.9	22.8	17.0
16	21.8	30.0	39.5	29.0
17	28.2	46.0	50.1	41.0
18	42.6	56.7	63.0	58.6
19	48.2	64.1	71.4	72.0
White	N = 1,758	N = 881	N = 1,034	N = 767
15–19	26.4	38.3	46.6	43.3
15	11.8	14.2	18.5	15.4
16	17.8	25.2	37.4	27.3
17	23.2	40.0	45.8	39.4
18	38.8	52.1	60.3	56.3
19	43.8	59.2	68.0	70.4
Black	N = 981	N = 571	N = 683	N = 390
15–19	53.7	66.3	66.2	53.6
15	31.2	38.9	41.7	24.8
16	46.4	55.1	50.9	37.6
17	58.4	71.9	74.6	49.4
18	62.4	78.4	77.0	73.6
19	76.2	85.3	88.7	81.4

* From *Family Planning Perspectives*, 1987;19:47. Used with permission.

between 1979 and 1982. However, the difference is slight and statistically nonsignificant.

Several studies (Sorenson, 1973) have indicated that teenagers are very versatile in finding a place to carry out sexual activities. In spite of parental strict watch over their intimate activities most teenagers have their first intercourse in a home. The availability of their own or a friend's home has especially become much more common in this decade because an increasing number of both parents have been working outside the home. Sorenson also found that sexual activity was mutually consented to in 60% to 80% of the cases. Thirteen percent to 28% of the girls indicated that they went along with their boyfriends, whereas 5% to 12% indicated that they could not say no or were afraid that the boyfriend would leave for another girl (2% to 6%).

Hass (1979) noted that only 42% of the sexually active teenage females reported to have experienced orgasm during coitus, whereas 25% did not experience orgasm and 33% were unsure.

Contraception

The use of contraception by teenagers is a very complex problem. It is influenced by knowledge, attitude, availability, and socioeconomic status of the teenager. Zelnik and Kantner (1980) found that, in 1979, 27% of 15- to 19-year-old females had never used a contraceptive during coitus and 39% used it only inconsistently. Bachrach in 1982 found that 31% of never-married, sexually active 15- to 19-year-old females were not using any contraceptive.

Kalmuss (1986) evaluated the effects of pregnancy on the subsequent use of contraceptives in teenagers. Four hundred twenty-five sexually active, unmarried teenage women who had access to contraceptives were interviewed. The findings indicated that ever-pregnant youths were less likely to have used contraceptives at their last intercourse than their never-pregnant teens. The negative effect of pregnancy on the subsequent use of contraceptives appeared to be related to a more positive attitude of the ever-pregnant teenagers toward pregnancy than their never-pregnant peers.

Lowe and Radius (1987) studied 283 unmarried college students between the ages of 18 and 22 years. Each student filled out an anonymous questionnaire containing questions regarding personal background, relationship with the opposite sex, health beliefs, self-esteem, attitude toward sex and contraception, knowledge about reproduction and contraception, and the use of contraception at last coitus, and 68.2% of the students described themselves as having experienced coitus. Among this sexually active group, 76.9% reported the use of effective contraceptive methods at the last coitus. These methods included the following:

1. Condoms, 24.4%.
2. Diaphram, 21.1%.
3. Birth control pills, 26.0%.
4. Intrauterine device (IUD), 4.2%.
5. Other, 1.2%.

Among their ineffective contraceptive use the most common method was withdrawal during sexual intercourse. Other ineffective methods included foam, jelly, cream, douching, and rhythm.

Several misconceptions were noted during evaluation of the knowledge items. More than one third of the students did not recognize the fact that abstaining from coitus at midcycle was necessary for the effectiveness of the rhythm contraceptive method. Miscalculations of the probability of pregnancy was also frequent. Approximately 43% agreed that "pregnancy just is not something that would happen to me or a sexual partner." Emans et al. (1987) investigated compliance with the use of oral contraceptives in 209 unmarried adolescents initiating the use of oral contraceptives in three different locations: an inner-city adolescent clinic, a birth control clinic, and a suburban private practice group. At the third month follow-up visit, 66% of the adolescents (134) were compliant. Only 11 patients had reported having read the instruction sheet. The mean age of the compliant group was higher than that of the noncompliant one. The private practice group had the highest compliance rate (84%), and the adolescent clinic group had the lowest compliance rate (48%). Forty-nine percent of the black and 70% of the white teenagers were compliant. Older age and prior experience with contraception increased compliance.

On long-term follow-up, 34% of the adolescent clinic patients and 55% of the private practice patients were compliant at a mean duration of 13 months after the initial prescription. Ten pregnancies occurred during the long-term follow-up. All of the pregnancies occurred among the noncompliant adolescent population.

Frequent reasons cited by the nonusers of contraceptives included the following:

1. They did not expect to have intercourse.
2. They thought they could not become pregnant at the time they had the intercourse.
3. Contraceptive was not available.
4. The sexual partner objected to its use.
5. There was a belief in the harmful effects of contraceptives.

ADOLESCENT GYNECOLOGY

Pelvic Examination

Pelvic examination is not carried out routinely during a physical examination for the psychiatric admission of adolescents. The exact age at which a pelvic examination is indicated without a history of gynecologic problems is controversial. Some gynecologists believe that it should be carried out within 1 year after menarche. Others believe that it is not necessary until later teen years. However, most adolescents do not present themselves for pelvic examinations unless they suffer from some symptoms relating to gynecologic problems. The clear indications for pelvic examinations include menstrual disorders, vaginal or uterine infections, the use of birth control pills, and lower abdominal pain.

Most gynecologists emphasize careful preparation of an adolescent for the first pelvic examination. The purpose of the examination should be stated clearly. Questions should be answered with regard to the method of examination, possible pain during the examination, losing virginity, and unexpected findings from the examination.

Disorders of Menstruation

About 50% of the adolescent females suffer menstrual dysfunctions including dysmenorrhea, abnormal vaginal bleeding, and amenorrhea.

Dysmenorrhea

Dysmenorrhea refers to pain associated with menstrual flow. At least one out of every three adolescent females experience intolerable and incapaciting abdominal discomfort and pain during menstrual flow. Some adolescents also suffer from premenstrual tension characterized by headaches, weight gain, breast congestation, depression, irritability, and aggression. These symptoms are relieved with the onset of the menstrual flow. Dysmenorrhea is considered primary when no organic pathology is found in the reproductive system. Secondary dysmenorrhea is associated with organic diseases such as ovarian cysts, pelvic adhesions such as following a ruptured appendix, pelvic inflammatory disease, etc. Pain in secondary dysmenorrhea is usually spasmodic and is felt the strongest in the lower part of the abdomen with radiation to the back and to the interior aspect of the thighs.

Therapy involves reassurance that the problem is a physiological one and the use of pain-relieving medications such as ibuprofen or acetaminophen. Oral contraceptives may be prescribed because they will provide both contraception and relief of primary dysmenorrhea by supression of ovulation and lack of progesterone production.

Abnormal Vaginal Bleeding

This may occur in the form of excessive and prolonged bleeding during menstrual flow, in the form of polymenorrhea (uterine bleeding at regular intervals of less than 21 days), and metrorrhagia (uterine bleeding occurring at irregular intervals). The abnormal bleeding may be caused by an anovulatory cycle, miscarriage, infection, polyps or tumors of the uterus, cervix, or vaginal cavities, systemic diseases such as blood dyscrasias and endocrine disorders, and ovarian dysfunctions. In 90% of the cases abnormal vaginal bleeding in adolescents is caused by an anovulatory menstrual cycle in which secretory endometrium does not develop due to a lack of progesterone (which is produced by the corpus luteum). The lack of progesterone and consequent low levels of local uterine prostaglandins result in less than normal myometrial and vascular contractions and cause heavy and prolonged menstrual flow. Estrogen breakthrough bleeding occurs when the estrogen level falls to a low level so that it cannot support the maintenance of a thick proliferative endometrium. This can happen at irregular intervals.

Management of abnormal vaginal bleeding involves a careful menstrual history and thorough physical and pelvic examination to rule out other causes of bleeding. Frequent bleeding from an anovulatory cycle is usually treated with hormone therapy.

Amenorrhea

Primary amenorrhea is diagnosed in an adolescent by lack of a menstrual period by the end of her 17th birthday. Secondary amenorrhea occurs when an adolescent has had previous menstrual flow but has missed three such cycles in a row.

The investigation of primary amenorrhea requires extensive evaluation of the pituitary-ovarian-uterine axis as well as all the systemic causes including disorders of thyroid, adrenal, and nutritional status; chronic diseases; etc. The most common cause of second amenorrhea is pregnancy. However, other causes include emotional problems, pituitary and ovarian dysfunctions, thyroid and adrenal disturbances, and systemic diseases.

Polycystic Ovarian Disease

This should be suspected in cases of secondary amenorrhea or oligomenorrhea in late teens with a tendency toward obesity and hirsutism. The ovaries are covered with a thick capsule and contain numerous small follicular cysts. This is a disorder of the hypothalamic-pituitary-ovarian system that gives rise to temporary or persistent anovulation. The ovarian dysfunction is caused by aberrations of gonadotropin secretion. LH levels are persistently elevated, and FSH is usually in the low normal or normal range. This causes a lack of normal secretion of estrogen and progesterone and the production of excessive androstenedione and testosterone. The diagnosis should be verified through laparoscopy, culdoscopy, or exploratory operations.

Vaginal Infections

The vagina is normally protected by a low acid pH of 4 to 5 and a protective thick epithelium lining supported by estrogen secretion. Various factors predispose adolescent girls for vaginal infection such as multiple sex partners, the use of broad-spectrum antibiotics, tight clothing, and low estrogen levels. *Candida albicans, Trichomonas vaginalis,* and *Haemophilus vaginalis* cause 90% of the nongonococcal vaginal infections.

Clinical manifestations frequently include a vaginal discharge, pruritus, and sometimes associated symptoms of dysuria. Infection with *Candida albicans* is diagnosed by finding yeast cells in a KOH preparation and Gram staining of a vaginal smear. Similarly, *Trichomonas vaginalis* infection is diagnosed by demonstrating flagellating protozoa in a wet mount of vaginal discharge.

Breast Disorders

Common disorders of the breast in females include a symetrical benign hypertrophy, tumors, and galactorrhea. Sometimes one breast may develop faster than the other, but they usually equalize after puberty. Surgical treatment may be required to correct a significant asymmetry for cosmetic reasons if it persists in adulthood. Breast hypertrophy may result in the development of very heavy and pendulous breasts. Some adolescents feel very self-conscious with large breasts and may require surgical correction.

The occurrence of cancerous tumors is very low during adolescent years. However, various types of benign tumors do occur in adolescence, including fibroadenoma, lipoma, cystic mastitis, etc. Management of these tumors requires surgical removal. However, adolescent patients should not be approached with urgency or alarm and should be assured that only minimal scarring occurs after such surgeries.

Galactorrhea is a milky or watery discharge from one or both breasts that occurs either spontaneously or from manual expression in a nonpuerperal breast. Etiologic factors frequently include neuroleptic drugs, hypothalamic-pituitary lesions, chronic renal disease, and thyroid dysfunction.

Gynecomastia

Gynecomastia is a benign increase in glandular and stromal tissue that leads to the enlargement of breasts in adolescent males. It is frequently a source of great concern for boys who may shy away from changing clothes for gym activities and taking showers with other boys. Breast enlargement may be unilateral or bilateral. The hypertrophy is usually in the form of small discoid, subareolar growth that is discrete and movable and has varying degrees of tenderness. There usually is no major imbalance of endocrine functions, and it may not require any endocrine work-up if the general physical examination is normal. Gynecomastia does occur in association with various disorders such as drug intake (phenothiazine, reserpine, tricyclic antidepressants, cimetidine, amphetamines, etc.), chronic hemodialysis hyperthyroidism, hypothyroidism, chronic liver diseases, and testicular, pituitary, and adrenal tumors. These conditions may be ruled out fairly easily in most adolescents through careful examination.

Pubertal gynecomastia usually resolves in 12 to 18 months. In a small number of cases it may last longer and may persist into adulthood. In addition to reassurance any therapy is rarely necessary. In cases of massive breast enlargement surgery may be considered.

Sexually Transmitted Diseases

Most hospitalized adolescents are reluctant to reveal symptoms relating to their genital problems. It is rare for an adolescent to make a spontaneous complaint about discharge, itching, or a rash in their genital area. Symptoms usually progress to moderate or severe degrees before they are revealed. The examining physician or psychiatrist must question adolescent patients about each of the symptoms relating to venereal diseases.

The history must include the age of onset of the menstrual period, the regularity of menstruation, menstrual cramps, sexual activities, the use of contraceptives, and any symptoms relating to genital organs such as discharge, itching, rash, ulcers, warts, growths, lower abdominal pain, etc. The onset of symptoms relating to sexual activity must be noted. Table 7–2 shows the frequency of gonorrhea and syphilis in adolescents.

Trichomonas vaginalis

Infection with *Trichomonas vaginalis* is one of the most common sexually transmitted infections. There are about 3 million reported cases in the United States. Adolescent cases account for about 28% of the total. The organism colonizes primarily in the vagina, urethra, and periurethral glands. It can survive on a wet towel for about 90 minutes and can possibly be transmitted through the common use of a towel and tub.

The infection may remain asymptomatic for some time. However, it is frequently associated with a vaginal discharge (usually grayish white or white tinged with green and malodorous), pruritus, dysuria, and lower abdominal pain.

Examination may reveal edema and excoration of the external genitalia, a discharge, inflammation of the vaginal walls and cervix, and occasionally abdominal tenderness.

A laboratory diagnosis is best made with a wet preparation of vaginal discharge. Mix a drop of discharge with a drop of saline on a glass slide, apply a coverslip, and observe under a microscope as soon as possible. *Trichomonas vaginalis* appears as a pear-shaped, motile organism about the size of a polymorphonuclear leukocyte with anterior flagellae. Staining smears is more time-consuming. Examination of urinary sediments is useful in diagnosing infection in males.

Both the female and her male contacts should be treated with metronidazole, 2 mg, in a single dose.

Chlamydia trachomatis Infection

This infection causes nongonococcal urethritis and vaginitis. In females symptoms frequently include a vaginal discharge (non–foul smelling), pruritus, and a urethral

TABLE 7–2

Morbidity and Rate per 100,000 Population for Gonorrhea and Syphilis* (Source: U.S. Department of Health and Human Services — Center for Disease Control 1987)

Age Groups (yr)	Calendar Year	Male Case	Female Cases	Total Cases	Male Rate	Female Rate	Total Rate
Syphilis							
10–14	1980	51	117	168	0.5	1.3	0.9
	1987	51	178	229	0.6	2.2	1.4
15–19	1980	2,014	1,560	3,574	19.2	15.1	17.2
	1987	1,826	2,505	4,331	19.7	27.7	23.7
Gonorrhea							
10–14	1980	2,199	6,674	8,873	23.6	74.8	48.7
	1987	1,775	5,267	7,041	21.0	65.6	42.7
15–19	1980	99,994	147,245	247,239	953.4	1,424.6	1,187.3
	1987	73,570	114,663	188,233	793.2	1,269.2	1,028.1

* From Centers for Disease Control, U.S.Department of Health and Human Services, 1987.

discharge; in males, pruritus and scanty to moderate urethral discharge are present. However, the discharge could occasionally be purulent. Dysuria is associated with urethral infection.

The symptoms usually start 8 to 14 days after sexual contact. However, many infected individuals may remain asymptomatic. A differential diagnosis should rule out gonococci and other organisms. The lack of intracellular gram-negative gonococci suggests a nongonococcal urethritis.

Treatment is usually carried out with tetracycline, 500 mg orally four times a day for 7 to 14 days. The sexual partner must also be diagnosed and treated.

Gonorrhea

Adolescents account for about 25% of 1 million reported cases in the United States. Females between the ages of 15 and 19 years report about 35% of all cases. The etiologic organism, *Neisseria gonorrhoeae,* is a gram-negative organism that is usually located within polymorphonuclear leukocytes.

Presenting symptoms include burning upon urination and a purulent penile discharge usually 3 to 6 days after contact. The majority of the infected females may remain asymptomatic. Symptomatic females may develop transient dysuria and a foul-smelling vaginal discharge. The infection may spread to the prostate, epididymis, and seminal vesicles in males and to the uterus, fallopian tubes, and upper part of the abdomen in females.

The diagnosis is generally made by microscopic detection of a urethral discharge containing gram-negative intracellular diplococci. Uncomplicated gonorrhea may be treated with penicillin, ampicillin, or tetracycline. Adolescents weighing 100 lb or more should receive the adult dosage. Adolescents weighing less than 100 lb are generally treated as follows: amoxicillin, 50 mg/kg with probenecid, 25 mg/kg body weight (maximum, 1 gm); or tetracycline, 40 mg/kg body weight per day orally in four divided doses for 5 days.

Syphilis

Since the mid-1960s there have been 20,000 to 25,000 cases of primary and secondary syphilis reported each year. The actual occurrence rate may be higher because private physicians report only a fraction of their cases. The etiologic organism *(Treponema pallidum)* enters the body through minute breaks in the skin and mucosa. The infection spreads via lymphatics and blood vessels and causes cellular infiltration and obliterative endarteritis. These pathological processes cause necrosis and ulceration. The ulcer or primary chancre appears at the site of inoculation, usually on the external genitalia after an incubation period of 9 to 90 days. It may, however, appear on the lips, face, mouth, arms, or cervix. The lesion has the appearance of a punched-out, shallow ulcer that is painless. Regional lymph nodes are enlarged, firm, and usually painless. The chancre usually heals in 4 to 6 weeks.

Manifestations of secondary syphilis appear between 6 and 8 weeks after the contact. The symptoms usually include flulike syndrome, general skin eruptions, and generalized lymphadenopathy. Laboratory diagnosis includes a demonstration of spirochetes in a darkfield microscopic examination and specific treponemal antibodies in serum. The antibodies are detected by the following tests:

1. Fluorescent treponemal antibody absorption test (FTA-ABS).
2. Microhemagglutination assay for *Trepomena pallidum* (MHA-TP), which has replaced the FTA-ABS test in many laboratories to confirm a positive VDRL test response.

Treatment of primary and secondary syphilis includes: benzathine penicillin G, 2.4 million units intramuscularly in a single session, or for patients allergic to penicillin, tetracycline, 500 mg four times daily for 15 days.

The treated patients should be followed with VDRL tests, usually done at 1, 3, 6, and 12 months after therapy. VDRL responses should become negative 3 to 12 months after the initial treatment.

Herpes Genitalis

Herpes genitalis is caused by herpes simplex virus (HSV). This is a virus with two serotypes: type 1 is generally recovered from oral lesions, but it also causes genital lesions in 10% to 20% of the cases, and type 2 is predominately involved in genital lesions. These viruses have the ability to become latent and then recur. Chuang et al. (1983) demonstrated that patients 15 to 20 years of age accounted for 47% of genital herpes infection. Transmission usually occurs through genital or oral-genital contact.

Typical burning of the skin is followed by the appearance of grouped vesicles. Rupture of the vesicles leaves multiple shallow ulcers that may coalesce to form one or more large ulcers. In women, the labia minora and majora and fourchette are commonly affected. In males, herpetic lesions usually affect the glans, prepuce, and shaft of the penis. Inguinal lymphadenopathy appears in about 50% of the cases. The virus can be cultured from the lesion. It is easier to recover virus from the vesicle fluid of early ulcers than late ulcers.

Primary infection heals within 10 to 14 days. Symptomatic relief is obtained with sitz baths, wet dressing with Burrow's Solution, and analgesics. Acyclovir ointment is used in the initial herpes genital infection in patients with normal immune systems. This drug seems to reduce the healing time from an average of 14.3 days to 10.9 days. Viral shedding is also decreased.

Acquired Immunodeficiency Syndrome

The acquired immunodeficiency virus (AIDS) is a disease caused by the human immunodeficiency virus (HIV). The AIDS virus may live in the human body for years before the actual symptoms appear. This virus compromises the immune system of the body and impairs the ability of an infected person to fight other diseases that usually do not cause fatality. This virus is transmitted in two main ways. First, a person may become infected during sexual contact—oral, anal, or genital—with someone who has already been infected with the AIDS virus. Second, a person may become infected by sharing drug needles and syringes with an infected person. The virus may also be transmitted from an infected mother to her baby, who becomes infected before or during birth. Also, some individuals who have received blood transfusions may become infected by receiving blood infected with HIV. Individuals with hemophilia are particularly prone to this infection because of their requirement for frequent blood transfusions.

The infected person usually has AIDS virus in semen or vaginal fluids. The virus can enter the body through the vagina, penis, rectum, or mouth. Rectal intercourse, especially in homosexuals, is particularly risky because the rectum is easily injured during anal intercourse, and this makes the entrance of the virus from an infected person easier. The AIDS virus is not transmitted through casual daily contact with the infected person. In fact, it has been shown that a person coming in contact with the saliva, sweat, tears, urine, or a bowel movement of an infected person will not contact AIDS. Although cases of AIDS in the adolescent age group have been proportionately fewer than in the adult population, this group is particularly at high risk because of their casual and frequent involvement in sexual contact with multiple partners.

DERMATOLOGIC PROBLEMS

Acne is the most common skin problem that concerns all adolescents. Although a majority of adolescents complain about the disfiguring aspect of facial acne, only a few actually seek professional help. Most of them try remedies suggested by their families and friends. Some adolescents with severe acne may become very self-conscious of the disfigurement of their faces and may withdraw from social contact. Psychiatrists dealing with such adolescents should assess the extent and severity of their facial acne and help them seek dermatologic help.

In addition to acne, hospitalized adolescents may manifest a whole range of dermatologic problems such as contact dermatitis, warts, and parasitic, bacterial, and fungal infections. Adolescents treated with psychotropic medications should also be watched for skin rashes.

Acne

Acne occurs in areas where sebaceous glands are in the highest concentrations such as the face, chest, and back. Sebaceous glands enlarge and produce sebum under the influence of androgenic hormones (gonadal and adrenal) to lubricate the skin. Increased production of sebum is associated with colonization of sebum by bacteria.

There are two common types of lesions in acne: noninflammatory and inflammatory. The noninflammatory lesions include comedones (blackheads) and closed comedones (whiteheads). The comedones represent a sebaceous follicle that has become filled with infection of keratinized material, sebum, and bacteria. The inflammatory lesions include papules and pustules. The inflammatory lesions result from the rupture of a sebaceous follicle, the content leaking into the adjacent dermis and causing an intense inflammatory response.

There are many therapies in vogue, some with proven and others without proven success. However, there are no specific therapies that are successful for all patients. Some patients may respond well to topical treatment, while others may require additional systemic therapy. Topical treatment with antibiotics such as tetracycline and erythromycin lotion are quite effective. Topical tetracycline preparations often leave a color residue on the skin, and its vehicle is at times irritating. Benzoyl peroxide is also an effective topical agent, but it may be irritating and cause an allergic reaction in some individuals.

Systemic therapy with antibiotics may be necessary in many cases of moderate to severe acne. Tetracycline, erythromycin, and minocycline are frequently used. Tetracycline may be started at 1 gm/day (500 mg twice daily [BID]) for 4 to 6 weeks. Then it is gradually reduced to find an optimum dose for each patient. Some patients may do well with as little as 250 mg or 500 mg tetracycline per day, whereas others may need a higher dosage for several months. Treatment is continued for a year or more. Common side effects to systematic antibiotics include gastrointestinal distress, phototoxicity, and vaginitis from yeast infection.

A large distressing papulopustular acne lesion may be treated with an injection of a diluted suspension of repository corticosteriod. Triamcinolone acetonide suspension is diluted to 2 to 3 mg/mL. A dose of 0.02 to 0.04 mL is injected at a depth of 4 to 5 mm with a 30-gauge needle.

Contact Dermatitis

Dermatitis is an inflammatory response of the skin to exposure to a causative agent. There are two varieties: (1) chemical agents that would cause inflammatory skin reactions in almost every person and (2) chemical agents that would cause inflammatory skin reaction only in some people, and it is mediated immunologically to produce an allergic reaction.

Contact dermatitis resulting from cosmetics and poison ivy are common in adolescents. Although the reported incidents from the use of cosmetics is only 1%, it may occur more often from excessive use.

Treatment involves a careful history to determine the offending agent and removing its further contact. Inflammation and pruritus can be helped with the use of calamine lotion three or four times daily. The use of local steroids may be necessary in more severe local lesions. The systemic use of steroids is limited in more widespread lesions. Antihistamines taken orally are helpful in reducing pruritus.

Warts (Verrucae)

Warts are caused by a DNA virus called papovavirus. It is more common in females, with a peak incidence between the ages of 12 and 16 years. It occurs in about 10% of the general population and is usually transmitted by direct contact with warts. The warts are frequently classified on the basis of their shape and location into four categories:

1. Verrucae vulgaris (common wart).
2. Verrucae plana juvenilis (flat wart).
3. Verrucae plantaris (plantar wart).
4. Verrucae acuminata (venereal wart).

Warts are easy to recognize. Sometimes plantar warts may be difficult to distinguish from corns. A differential diagnosis should also be made from molluscum contagiosum, which is a smooth papule with umbilication.

Warts can disappear spontaneously, but they may spread or persist for years. A number of therapeutic techniques have been utilized to treat warts. The goal of the treatment is not to destroy the underlying skin. It is usually an overzealous treatment that causes skin scarring and disfiguration. Treatment modalities frequently include cryotherapy, electrodessication, and acid treatment. Cryotherapy is generally carried out with liquid nitrogen. The wart is lightly frozen with a cotton applicator dipped in liquid nitrogen and applied to the wart long enough to turn it white. Avoid touching tissue surrounding the wart. Within 1 to 2 weeks the wart usually turns into a hemorrhagic blister that peels off later on. The procedure may need to be repeated. Acid treatment usually involves painting the wart with trichloroacetic acid, nitric acid, or phenol acid. The acid is worked into the wart by carefully pricking the wart with a needle or toothpick.

Fungal Infection

Common fungal infections during adolescent years include "athletes foot" and "jock's itch." Jock's itch refers to a fungal infection of the skin in the groin. The lesions are usually well demarcated with scaly patches. Microscopic demonstration of typical hyphae in the specimen from the edge of the lesion with the addition of 10% to 20% KOH clinches the diagnosis.

Unfortunately, lesions frequently recur after treatment and require further treatment. Common fungicides sold over the counter such as Tinactin are well tolerated. When dermatitis occurs along with fungal infection, it is treated with a combination of corticosteroids and antifungal topical applications.

Newer broad-spectrum fungicides include miconazole, haloprogin, and clotrimazole. These drugs are best used in the form of topical creams. The systematic use of fungicides such as griseofulvin is reserved for severe cases because it may cause many side affects.

Parasitic Infections

Infections with lice and scabies mites are not uncommon in adolescents. Scabies is frequently missed as a cause of pruritus. A differential diagnosis of these infections is made by finding the etiologic parasite. However, visualization of scabies mites is generally difficult. Generalized eruptions of scabies are usually due to a hypersensitivity reaction. The best chance of finding a mite is on the hand and wrist and on webs between the finger. Apply a drop of mineral oil to the burrow and then scrape the skin with a small blade. Examine the scrapings under a microscope.

Current treatment for scabies is usually one application of 1% gamma benzene hexachloride (Kwell) to the entire body from the neck downward. The medication is thoroughly rubbed into the skin. The patient bathes 24 hours later. Sometimes a second application may be applied if necessary 1 week later.

Kwell causes neurotoxicity, and some physicians prefer to use other drugs such as crotamiton (Eurax) cream. Kwell shampoo is also used for treating lice infections. The shampoo is worked into the hair and left there for 5 to 10 minutes before washing. A solution of vinegar with an equal amount of water may be used to wash the hair following Kwell application to dissolve the nits. Also a fine-toothed comb may be helpful in removing the nits.

INFECTIOUS MONONUCLEOSIS

Infectious mononucleosis is common among adolescents and young adults. Epstein-Barr virus (EBV) appears to be the etiologic agent. The lymphoreticular system including the lymph nodes, spleen, liver, and bone marrow are affected and infiltrated by mononuclear cells. EBV antibodies are present in most children and adolescents. About 50% to 85% of the children in lower socioeconomic groups show positive serology by the age of 4 years. However, in the middle and upper-middle class, only 14% of the students develop positive serology by college age. Although EBV infection is common in children, it is usually asymptomatic. However, infection during the adolescent years frequently results in clinical symptoms. EBV has a low communicability. It is probably transmitted through frequent personal contact and oropharyngeal excretions. Infected patients do not require quarantine. The incubation period ranges from 20 to 50 days.

Symptoms usually begin with general malaise, fatigue, and headaches. Fever, pharyngitis, and adenopathy are very common. Enlargement of the spleen and liver and a skin rash may occur in a small proportion of cases.

Laboratory tests show lymphocytosis, atypical monocytes, positive EBV antibodies titers, and positive heterophil antibodies. The monospot test utilizes horse erythrocyte agglutination in a rapid slide test and is highly sensitive (96% to 97%). Heterophil antibodies agglutinate or hemolyze erythrocytes from other species of animal such as sheep, horse, and oxen. These antibodies are present in normal individuals in low titer. Heterophil antibodies are maximal during the second and third week of sickness. Sheep and beef agglutination tests remain positive for 3 to 6 months, but horse agglutination tests remain positive up to 18 months. Liver function test values are generally elevated.

Acute symptoms of fever and sore throat usually disappear within 7 to 10 days. Fatigue and malaise may persist from 2 to 4 weeks. Ten percent to 20% of patients may not be able to resume normal activities for 2 to 3 months. There are a few who may continue to have a low-grade fever and fatigue for 6 to 12 months. The differential diagnosis is made from other viral infections. Fatigue and tiredness frequently resemble a lack of energy and depression.

Patients are advised to rest during the acute stage of illness and take the appropriate analgesics for sore throats and fever. Activities should be resumed as tolerated after the fever subsides. If the spleen is enlarged, sports activities in which a person might be hit in the spleen area are avoided. If throat infection with β-hemolytic streptococci is present, appropriate antibodies are used.

CARDIOVASCULAR SYSTEM

Many children with congenital heart diseases and cardiac infections are now surviving into their adolescent years because of the better management of these disorders in childhood. Rapid growth during adolescent years produces compensatory changes in the cardiovascular system and may at times result in clinical symptoms. These adolescents may require special counseling with regard to the common issues of adolescents such as birth control, pregnancy, smoking, exercise, proper nutrition, and the preventive aspects of heart disease.

Birth Control

Birth control pills generally are not appropriate for many heart patients and are contraindicated in some cardiac patients who have experienced complications such as pulmonary hypertension, cynosis, obstructive lesions, bacterial endocarditis, or thrombophlebitis. However, patients with cardiac problems such as left-to-right shunts and rheumatic heart disease without valvular damage may be prescribed oral contraceptives. A preferred method of contraception for many adolescents with cardiac problems may be a well-fitting diaphgram.

Pregnancy

Pregnancy in a cardiac patient carries a high risk, both for the mother and the baby. There is an increase in blood volume by about 40% during the pregnancy. The increase is rapid during the first trimester, but the volume continues to rise slowly until the termination of the pregnancy. The primary concern about pregnancy in a cardiac patient relates to the ability of her heart to tolerate this increase in volume. Intrauterine growth retardation, miscarriage, and prematurity are common complications for the fetus. Pregnancy in these patients frequently requires careful monitoring by a cardiologist.

Smoking

The percentage of those smoking in the 12- to 18-year-old age group is 10% to 12%. Smoking increases the risk of premature coronary heart disease and lung cancer. Effects of nicotine include an increase in heart rate, blood pressure, cardiac output, and oxygen consumption of the heart. A patient with cardiac illness who smokes would certainly be more at risk of serious complications of heart and lung diseases.

Exercise

Adolescents with cardiac disease need not limit their activities. They may be helped to find interesting hobbies, games, and sports that require less vigorous physical efforts such as golf, archery, swimming, etc. A careful evaluation of each patient would reveal the limit of physical activity and their ability to participate in certain sports. Various committees of the American Heart Association have prepared guidelines and specific recommendations for heart patients suffering from different types of cardiac malformations. These recommendations are very helpful for adolescents to find the type of activities that they may be interested in.

Hypertension

Blood pressure, both systolic and diastolic, increases with age. Many facilities use the 96th or 97th percentile for age as the high cutoff point for hypertension. A World Health Organization technical report recommended below 140/90 as the normal range and 160/95 and above as the abnormal range (hypertensive). Blood pressure levels vary widely among individuals and within the same individual on a given day. The prevalence of hypertension in adolescents is 1.4% to 8.9% (systolic) and 1.4% to 12.2% (diastolic). Most of the hypertension in children is secondary. The risk of primary hypertension increases with age.

Multiple factors contribute to the etiology of hypertension in adolescents such as renal, endocrine, vascular, and metabolic disorders. Many of the secondary causes of hypertension can be identified by history, physical examination, and laboratory tests. Common secondary causes of hypertension in adolescents may include the following:

1. Renovascular disease.
2. Unilateral renal parenchymal disease.
3. Coarctation of the aorta.
4. Cushing's syndrome.
5. Primary aldosteronism.
6. Pheochromocytoma.

Management of primary or essential hypertension in adolescents requires careful counseling with regard to diet, exercise, smoking, and other risk factors such as the use of birth control pills and abuse of drugs. Pharmacological treatment may include diuretics, β-blockers, and vasodilator agents.

Rheumatic Heart Disease

Rheumatic heart disease results from upper respiratory tract infection by β-hemolytic streptococci. Only 3% of the untreated individuals develop rheumatic fever. Factors contributing to susceptibility for rheumatic fever are not known. Acute rheumatic fever causes inflammatory disease involving the heart, joints, subcutaneous tissue, and the central nervous system. Jones' criteria (1967) for the diagnosis of rheumatic fever includes major and minor manifestations. The major manifestations include carditis, polyarthritis, chorea, erythema marginatum, and subcutaneous nodules. Minor manifestations include a history of previous rheumatic fever or rheumatic heart disease, arthralgia, fever, and the presence of a high sedimentation rate, C-reactive proteins, leukocytosis, and prolonged PR intervals.

Once the diagnosis of rheumatic fever is established, streptococcal infection is treated with a course of penicillin for 10 days. After the completion of 10-day therapy, penicillin is continued in small dosage (250 mg BID) as prophylaxis. Alternatively, 1.2 million units of long-acting bicillin may be given once a month. The length of the prophylactic treatment is variable. In the presence of heart disease, it has to be continued indefinitely. However, in the absence of heart disease, it may be continued until the age of 21 years when the incidence of recurrence of rheumatic fever drops significantly.

About 50% of the patients with rheumatic fever are left with residual heart disease, mostly involving heart valves—mitral insufficiency, mitral stenosis, aortic stenosis, and aortic insufficiency are the most common residual heart diseases. All patients with rheumatic heart disease should be informed of their susceptibility to recurrent attacks of rheumatic fever and bacterial endocarditis.

GASTROINTESTINAL DISORDERS

Gastrointestinal disorders in adolescents include irritable bowel syndrome, peptic disorders, and inflammatory bowel disease.

Irritable Stomach and Bowel Syndrome

Stomach upsets, nausea, abdominal discomfort, occasional diarrhea, or constipation are common symptoms in hospitalized adolescents. Irritable bowel syndrome is characterized by alternating cycles of diarrhea and constipation associated with abdominal pain. The abdominal pain may be generalized or localized to areas of the cecum and sigmoid colon, these two areas of the colon being more irritable.

Other causes of diarrhea and pain should be ruled out such as dysentery, lactose intolerance, and inflammatory bowel disease. Investigations may include an examination of stool for blood, bacteria, and parasites. Sigmoidoscopy may be necessary in some cases to rule out inflammatory bowel disease. A barium enema may be indicated when the symptoms are persistent.

Treatment frequently includes management of associated stress and anxiety. The constipation may be helped by an increased intake of foods and vegetables. Chemical laxatives and enemas are to be avoided. Diarrhea usually requires no special treatment.

Peptic Disorders

Common symptoms relating to the upper gastrointestinal tract include nausea, vomiting, distention, heartburn, and pain. These symptoms frequently occur from the irritation of esophageal, gastric, and duodenal mucosa. Continued peptic irritation of the mucosa may cause a break and formation of an ulcer in the stomach or duodenum. There are a number of mechanisms and factors that give rise to the formation of peptic ulcers:

1. Decreased physiological resistance of the mucosa.

2. High production of acid.
3. Gastrin oversecretion.
4. Influence of certain drugs such as steroids, aspirin, coffee, or alcohol.
5. Stress ulcers as in burns.
6. Anxiety-related ulcers.

The pain of peptic ulcers is typically characterized by an onset a few hours after meals and is relieved by antacids and food. Nocturnal pain, occurring 2 to 3 hours after retiring, is suggestive of peptic ulcers.

Inflammatory Bowel Disease

Inflammatory bowel disease usually includes two disease entities: ulcerative colitis and Crohn's disease.

Ulcerative colitis is a chronic inflammatory disease of the bowel that affects primarily the colon and rectum. There are many known causes of colitis including amebic colitis, shigellosis, and factitial colitis of homosexuals. However, the etiology of idiopathic ulcerative colitis is unknown. Multiple factors have been attributed to its etiology such as genetic, immunological, and psychological. Proctoscopic examination reveals red, friable, edematous mucosa covered with mucopus. Ulcerations are not present in the early stages but may become evident later on. These ulcers are superficial, usually mucosa deep. The lumen of the colon is of normal caliber, and haustration of the colon is absent. Radiologic examination of the colon with a barium enema may show an irregular surface, particularly in the rectosigmoid area. With extensive ulceration, a pseudopolypoid pattern may be present.

The clinical picture is characterized by acute episodes of variable duration with periods of remissions. During an acute attack the patient passes frequent unformed bloody stools and has abdominal pain and urgency. As many as 20 bowel movements may occur in 1 day. Additional symptoms include fatigue, diminished appetite, loss of weight, headaches, dizziness, and weakness. Patients may develop hypochromic microcytic anemia due to blood loss and diminished food intake.

Crohn's Disease

Crohn's disease is an inflammatory disease that involves the terminal ilium and segments of the duodenum, jejunum, and colon. The ulcerations are deep, well into the submucosa and muscular layer of the bowel wall. Healing of the ulcers causes extensive fibrosis and narrowing of the lumen and gives a hose pipe appearance. A barium enema may show minimal findings in the early stages, but later on it may show a characteristic appearance of diffused cobblestones. A small bowel series will show dilated loops of intestine with widening folds and localized strictures.

The onset of Crohn's disease is generally insidious with mild diarrhea, abdominal pain and cramping, loss of appetite, and fever. Gross rectal bleeding is minimal. Sometimes the initial course of the disease resembles that of ulcerative colitis. The course of Crohn's disease is variable with some remissions and excerbations.

Management of ulcerative colitis and Crohn's disease is at best difficult and protracted. In the absence of definitive treatment, multiple approaches have been utilized. Treatment is individualized to help each patient meet his nutritional, vocational, and psychological needs. Acute attacks are sometimes treated with steroids, which frequently suppress the acute symptoms. The use of immunosuppressive agents such as azathioprine has been found helpful in some cases.

Although the primary management of inflammatory bowel disease rests in the hands of surgeons, pediatricians, or internists, psychiatrists become involved in the treatment of a fairly large proportion of these patients. The role of psychotherapy in the treatment of inflammatory bowel disease is not well defined. The mortality and incidence of colectomy in psychiatrically treated patients have been about the same as in the control groups (O'Connor et al., 1964). Such studies, however, do not adequately answer the questions of whether outpatients with inflammatory bowel disease would benefit from psychotherapy or from other types of psychological interventions. Most patients have a great deal of difficulty in adjusting to the chronic, debilitating nature of their disease. Psychotherapy does not cure inflammatory bowel disease, but it should be considered an important part of the total management. Many adjustment problems created by the chronicity of the disease may alone warrant psychological intervention.

COMMON ORTHOPEDIC PROBLEMS

Common orthopedic problems of adolescents may be divided into three main categories:

1. Skeletal problems that are present from childhood but that become more apparent in adolescence, i.e., scoliosis and kyphosis.
2. Skeletal problems occurring during adolescence, i.e., knee problems (Osgood-Schlatter disease, subluxation, dislocated patellae, osteochondritis dessicans) and hip problems (slipped capital epiphysis), and back pain.
3. Skeletal problems resulting from sports injuries such as a concussion; injuries to the lumbar spine, knees, and ankles; muscle cramps; and shin splints.

Scoliosis

Lateral curvature of the spine occurs in 2% to 5% of the children in adolescence. It is more common in females. Structural deformity of the spine should be distinguished from a functional or nonstructural deformity. A nonstructural deformity may be postural scoliosis that disappears when lying down or compensatory scoliosis usually as a result of a discrepancy in the length of the two legs. Structural scoliosis may result from multiple causes including genetic, congenital abnormalities of the vertebrae, neuromuscular diseases such as poliomyelitis and cerebral palsy, myopathies such as muscular dystrophy, etc. However, 70% to 85% of the cases appear idiopathic. The deformity is usually asymptomatic and is diagnosed on physical examination. However, if the scoliosis is untreated, it progresses in severity and frequently leads to disabling pain. Scoliosis does not stop at skeletal maturity and may continue to deteriorate in 1% to 2% per year during adulthood.

The best screening test for determining spine curvature is the forward-bending test. The patient is asked to bend forward at the waist with the trunk parallel to the floor, legs straight, and arms dangling with fingers and palms together. The back should be examined while the patient is standing straight; look for level shoulders, tips of the scapulae deviating from the midline and trunk, and head alignment. Radiologic examination should include erect anteroposterior and lateral views of the spine from the occiput to the sacrum.

Exercise alone is of little benefit in structural scoliosis. However, exercises are helpful in conjunction with a brace. Various types of braces are used that may have to be worn for a year or more. Surgical intervention is required in many cases.

Kyphosis

Kyphosis is characterized by forward bending of the spine with a rounded back deformity, winging of the scapulae, forward displacement of the shoulders, the head and neck carried forward from their center of gravity, and a protuberant abdomen. The deformity usually begins in adolescents from avascular necrosis of the growth center surrounding the upper and lower margins of the vertebrae. This produces delayed growth and softening of the bone to the point of anterior wedging of the vertebrae, especially in the thoracic spine. In some cases lateral wedging may occur and produce scoliosis.

About 50% of the patients present with persistent back pain localized to the involved area, which may be tender on palpation. Pain is aggravated by flexion and extension of the spine, and it is not relieved by rest in all cases. Radiologic examination is necessary for a diagnosis and determination of the degree of curvature.

Mild cases may be treated with postural exercises, sleeping on a hard bed board without a pillow, and limited activity. Many of the patients may require a cast or braces to correct the deformity.

Osgood-Schlatter Disease

Osgood-Schlatter disease results from a painful enlargement of the tibial tubercle. Bone and muscle growth during adolescence produces considerable tension in the quadriceps and patellar tendons, which in turn produces stress on the tibial tubercle. As a consequence, an inflammatory process is induced in the tibial tubercle that causes pain, tenderness, and soft-tissue swelling over the tubercle. It is usually unilateral but may be bilateral in some cases. The diagnosis is made on the basis of the history and physical examination. Actually, an examination may be necessary to eliminate other structural abnormalities.

Treatment usually consists of rest and restrictive activities for 3 to 4 weeks, after which patients may return to normal activity in a gradual manner. Adolescent patients must understand the nature of their disease in order to improve their cooperation with the treatment. Severe cases may require a cylindrical cast to immobilize the knee joint for a few weeks. The prognosis is generally excellent, and the problem stops at the completion of growth, a permanent tubercle being left behind.

Subluxation and Dislocation of the Patella

Instability of the patellofemoral joint may allow the patella to dislocate laterally during contraction of the quadriceps muscles. In partial dislocation the patella snaps back into the joint, but in complete dislocation the patella is pulled laterally and can be seen out of the socket. Symptoms include pain, swelling, giving way of the knee, and a popping sensation. Reduction of the joint often occurs spontaneously. Gentle straightening of the knee by lifting up the foot may allow the patella to return to its place.

Treatment includes exercises to strengthen the quadriceps muscles, temporary restriction of activities, and elastic support of the knee. Immobilization of the knee in a cylinder cast for 3 weeks may be necessary in dislocation. Surgical intervention is occasionally required to realign the pull of the quadriceps muscles.

Chondromalacia Patella

This results from the degeneration and softening of the patellar cartilage, which possibly occurs as a result of direct and indirect trauma to the cartilage. It is more common in female adolescents than in males. Symptoms include pain in the peripatellar or retropatellar regions. The pain worsens with activity and improves with rest. The symptoms are bilateral in one third of the cases. Physical examination may reveal patellar malalignment, external tibial torsion, genu valgum, and tenderness of the articular surface of the patella. Acute symptoms of pain are helped by rest and restriction of activities, analgesics for a few weeks, and then gradual resumption of exercise to strengthen the muscles.

Osteochondritis Dessicans

This condition results from asceptic necrosis in a segment of subchondral bone in the weight-bearing areas of joints such as the head of the femur, the talus, and the capitulum but is more common in the lateral femoral condyle. Its exact cause is unknown, but trauma and ischemia appear to play a major role in the etiology. Symptoms include intermittent, nonspecific knee pain usually related to activity. Swelling of the knee and pain may be present for months before consultation is sought. X-ray films of the knee show a segment of subchondral bone separated from its bed.

The object of treatment is to revascularize the bone without restoration of the normal contour of the joint. This is achieved by rest, by restriction of activity, and possibly by a cast. Occasionally bone pegs and screws may be necessary to hold the fragments together. Healing usually occurs in 6 to 12 months.

Slipped Capital Epiphysis

In this condition there is a slipping of the femoral head posteriorly, inferiorly, and medially on the femoral metaphysis. The condition results largely from certain mechanical factors. The epiphyseal plate of the proximal part of the femur in children is situated horizontally in relation to the ground. As the child approaches adolescence, the neck-shaft angle increases to the adult average of 120 degrees. The epiphyseal plate in turn becomes more vertical. Newly formed bone is less able to withstand sheer stress, and this results in slipping inferiorly. This is more likely to occur in the overweight adolescent.

Characteristic physical signs are elicited by flexion of the involved hip. The motion is blocked at about 60 degrees, and further flexion is possible only if the hip is externally rotated and abducted. X-ray examination of the hip reveals the degree of slipping.

A failure to diagnose and treat this condition may result in irreparable damage and an early onset of arthritis. Treatment should be provided immediately with hospitalization and traction for the relief of pain. Further surgical treatment aims at establishing a firm bony union of the femoral head to the femoral neck.

Severe complications may include avascular necrosis of the femoral head, loss of hip motion and shortening of the limb, acute cartilagenous necrosis, and destruction of the joint.

Sports Injuries

Sports injuries can be largely avoided if proper conditioning, muscle strengthening, and flexibility training is provided before an adolescent participates in regular games. Conditioning primary improves the body's energy efficiency, while training includes both improvement of energy utilization and sport-specific skill development. Adequate warm-ups should be a prerequisite of each sport. The four most common sports injuries include the following:

1. Concussion.
2. Lumbar spine injuries.
3. Knee injuries.
4. Sprained ankles.

Rehabilitation of injured athletes is a gradual process with the aim of return to full function. The rehabilitation is usually carried out in phases. For example, in phase 1 the injured area is protected, rested, and relieved of pain while uninjured body parts are exercised. In phase 2, the injured part is subjected to gradual exercise until its functions catch up with the rest of the body. In phase 3, reconditioning, muscle strengthening, and flexibility exercises are carried out before returning to active sports. Ligaments and tendons normally heal in about 6 weeks. It may take several more months before they regain their full strength. A fracture may heal in 4 to 12 weeks, depending upon various factors.

TABLE 7–3
Prevalence of Chronic Conditions*

Diseases	Rate per Thousand
Asthma	18.3
Epilepsy	9.3
Rheumatic heart disease	5.7
Congenital heart disease	2.0
Severe retardation	3.6
Deafness	2.0
Cerebral palsy	1.8
Mongolism	1.2
Legg-Perthes disease	1.2
Diabetes mellitus	0.8
Cystic fibrosis	0.4
Blindness	0.2

* From National Center For Health Statistics. Hyattsville, Md, 1983.

CHRONIC DISEASES IN ADOLESCENTS

Approximately 7% to 10% of all adolescents are afflicted with chronic illness of primary physical origin (Table 7–3). The number of visits made by chronically ill adolescents to an outpatient department or to a pediatrician's office far outnumber the visits made by adolescents with acute illnesses. A fair proportion of the pediatrician's time is spent not only treating the chronic disease process but also managing acute crises and counseling the adolescent and his parents on developmental issues, achievement problems, social relationships, and vocational choices.

Emotional problems frequently result from difficulties in adjusting to chronic illnesses, and these in turn affect the course of chronic illnesses. The influence of emotional problems upon a chronic disease may be quite apparent in some illnesses but completely obscure in others. For example, emotional problems are clearly present when a diabetic adolescent is hospitalized with severe acidosis and it is discovered that he has not followed his diet or insulin injection schedule for several days. Similarly, difficulties in the acceptance of his disease are apparent in a hemophiliac who joins in the practice of the neighborhood football game without consideration to injuries. However, the influence of emotional problems may be not as apparent as in other cases of chronic illnesses such as an exacerbation of epilepsy or an increased frequency of acute asthmatic attacks.

By the beginning of puberty most children usually understand the major causes of their chronic illnesses. However, these emotional reactions become more complex during adolescent years. They begin to ask questions such as "Why me?" They may feel sorry for themselves and brood about their illness for days. Many parents try to answer such questions by telling them how much better off they are when compared with other children suffering from worse types of illnesses. Also, various philosophic and religious explanations are given to help them make the best of their handicap:

"Life is not a matter of holding good cards, but playing a poor hand well," or "God gives hardship to those who can bear it."

While normal adolescents struggle to find an identity for themselves, handicapped adolescents have a much more difficult time in this regard. Feelings of inadequacy and of not being a complete or satisfactory human being dominate their thoughts. Their self-esteem, which is governed greatly by peer reinforcement, also suffers some loss. Some of these adolescents, plagued by low self-esteem and confused identity, begin to deny their illness and begin to behave in an irrational manner, for example, a diabetic adolescent joining his peers in an all-night drinking and eating party or a hemophiliac picking a fight with his peers.

The chronic illnesses that begin during adolescence cause various degrees of regression in behavior, motivation, and achievement. Such an adolescent may become more dependent upon his family or become more demanding of his peers and friends. In some cases withdrawal and a sad mood may prevail for months.

Factors Influencing Adjustment to Chronic Illness

The conditions necessary for a better adjustment to chronic illness are a realistic role definition and parental acceptance. Optimal adjustment requires the child's role to be clearly and realistically defined by the important authorities in his life (parents, teachers, and peers) and that his parents value him even when he is not playing his expected role with consistency. The difficulties encountered by handicapped adolescents lie in the fact that they are confronted with more severe and more frequent adjustment problems due to the varying course of chronic illness than are normal adolescents. Adjustment problems are also exaggerated for handicapped children because their parents and other role definers often cannot furnish them with appropriate and unambiguous behavior standards for their new role and because cultural norms (from which few parents are immune) define any handicap as a loss of value or work. The adolescent with a handicap is thus in a limbo between two social worlds—the world of the healthy (with which his parents and other authorities are more familiar) and the world of the handicapped (which is poorly defined and devalued). In fact, the handicapped adolescent does indeed tend to see his role as somewhere between that of the healthy adolescent and that of the sick adolescent.

The following generalizations are helpful in understanding the adjustment of adolescents to chronic illnesses (Zachmeister, 1970):

1. The greater the amount of physical discomfort associated with a chronic illness, the poorer will be the adjustment. For example, regular injections of medication will be more upsetting to the child than regular oral medication will.

2. The greater the limitation of physical activity, the poorer will be the adjustment. A paraplegic child who is taught to use braces and crutches is likely to be better adjusted than is the child skilled in the use of a wheelchair.

3. The greater the visibility of the handicapping condition, the less well adjusted the child will be. Cosmetic surgery done at an earlier age will lead to better adjustment (even if it must be repeated later) than will cosmetic surgery done at a later age.

4. The greater the loss of sensory abilities (sight, hearing), the poorer will be the child's adjustment. A partially sighted child will have a better chance at adjusting to his disability than the totally blind child will.

5. The later the age at which a chronic condition is diagnosed (or occurs), the poorer will be the child's adjustment. A congenital handicap will be adjusted to more easily than will an acquired handicap of the same kind and severity.

6. The greater the amount of parental rejection, overindulgence, or disinterest, the poorer will be the child's adjustment. Genetically transmitted illnesses produce greater guilt (and rejection or overprotection) in parents and, therefore, lead to poorer adjustment by the child. Increased support of the parents of a handicapped child by the physician will increase the parents acceptance of that child and thus improve the child's adjustment.

7. The larger the number of siblings younger than the chronically ill child, the poorer will be the adjustment. The parents of chronically ill children tend to have smaller families than do parents without chronically ill children. Siblings younger than the handicapped child are likely to suffer more adjustment problems than siblings older than the handicapped child.

8. The severity of the handicap interacts with the family socioeconomic status: from middle- and upper middle-class families, the milder the degree of handicap, the poorer will be the child's adjustment, while for lower-class families the milder the degree of the handicap, the better the child's adjustment.

Parents of middle-class status are more likely to set unrealistically high goals for a mildly handicapped child than for a severely handicapped child, which results in poorer adjustment for the mildly handicapped child. Lower-class parents tend to seek less medical attention for their handicapped children than do middle-class parents, and this results in poorer adjustment for handicapped children of lower-class parents, especially those with a severe handicap.

9. The less intelligent the child, the poorer is the adjustment to a chronic illness. A child must have a minimum level of intelligence to adjust to a loss of sensory ability, a handicap, or a chronic illness. The more intelligent child is better able to understand his handicapped condition and, as a result, to have a more realistic self-image.

REFERENCES

Chuang TY, Su WP, Perry HO, et al: Incidence and trends of herpes progenitalis: A 15-year population study. *Mayo Clin Proc* 1983; 58:436–441.

Emans ST, et al: Adolescents compliance with the use of oral contraceptives. *JAMA* 1987; 257:3377–3381.

Hass A: *Teenage Sexuality—a Survey of Teenage Sexual Behavior.* Los Angeles, Pinnacle Books, 1979.

Hofferth S, Kahn J, Baldwin W: Premarital sexual activity among U.S. teenage women over the past three decades. *Fam Plann Perspect* 1987; 19:46–53.

Jones Criteria (revised). Chicago, American Heart Association, 1967.

Kalmuss D: Contraceptive use: A comparison between ever and never pregnant adolescents. *J Adolesc Health Care* 1986; 7:332–337.

Lowe C, Radius S: Young adult's contraception practices: An investigation of influences. *Adolescence* 1987; 22:291–304.

O'Connor JF, Daniels G, Karush A, et al: The effects of psychotherapy on the course of ulcerative colitis. *Am J Psychiatry* 1964; 120:738–742.

Sorenson RC: *Adolescent Sexuality in Contemporary America.* New York, World Publishing, 1973.

Tanner JM: *Growth at Adolescence; With a General Consideration of the Effects of Heredity and Environmental Factors Upon Growth and Maturation From Birth to Maturity,* ed 2. Oxford, Blackwell Scientific Publications, 1962.

Zachmeister C: *Services for Chronically Ill Children* (unpublished paper). Chicago, Children's Memorial Hospital, 1970.

Zelnik M, Kantner F: Sexual activity, contraceptive use and pregnancy among metropolitan area teenagers 1971–1979. *Fam Plann Perspect* 1980; 12:230.

8

Theoretical Models for Short-Term Treatment

Psychiatric care for children and adolescents was provided primarily in long-term residential centers until the 1950s and 1960s when a large number of these centers were closed, primarily for a lack of financial support. Adolescents with acute psychosis, depression, and suicidal tendencies began to be hospitalized in the adult psychiatric services of general hospitals. The population of adolescents gradually increased in the adult units even though they did not fit into the general adult milieu. The needs of adolescents for structure, discipline, activity, recreation, education, and peer contact cannot be met in the adult units. Also, adolescent patients tend to disrupt the serenity of the adult milieu with frequent episodes of aggressive acting-out behavior. Staff members often spend more time dealing with a handful of adolescents than with the rest of the adult patients. It is generally difficult to organize a separate milieu just for a small group of adolescents within the large adult units.

The aforementioned considerations led to the development of separate adolescent units in general hospitals. Most of the adolescent units tended to hospitalize adolescents for much longer periods of time than they did adult patients in similar settings. This was justified on the basis of the extra time spent in dealing with the developmental needs of the adolescent patients in addition to treating their psychiatric problems. However, the length of hospital stay for adult patients continued to decrease. In 1980, the median length of stay for adult patients in state and county mental hospitals was 23 days (Rosenstein et al., 1986). This drastic decrease in the length of hospital stay was brought about gradually by a number of events that occurred during the 1970s and 1980s including the following:

1. Escalating medical costs.
2. Resistance of third-party payers to reimbursement of high costs.
3. Development of prepaid health maintenance organizations (HMOs).
4. Pressure from regulatory agencies for documentation of the need for hospitalization.
5. Establishment of diagnosis-related groups (DRGs).
6. Changes in the philosophy of treatment and in the right of treatment.

Proposals to establish prospective payment for treatment based on DRGs caused the most stir in the psychiatric community. Although psychiatry is still exempt from such systems, pressure has continued to mount from other sources such as insurance companies, regulatory agencies, and the general public to reduce the length of psychiatric hospitalization. Several studies have tried to correlate psychiatric diagnoses with the length of hospitalization. The results have been inconsistent and inconclusive. For example, Heinman and Shanfield (1980) noted that psychiatric diagnoses were very helpful in determining the length of hospitalization. However, Doherty (1975) found a much less stronger relationship between diagnosis and length of hospitalization. Canton and Gralnick (1987) reviewed several studies related to the factors surrounding the length of psychiatric hospitalization. They divided these factors into two broad categories:

1. Patient characteristics.
2. Environmental characteristics.

The patient characteristics included the psychiatric diagnosis and the severity of the illness. The environmental characteristics included the stability of the family situation and the availability of community resources for aftercare. It was found that the predictive value of the psychiatric diagnosis improved when the severity of the illness and the environmental characteristics were also taken into consideration.

Mezzich and Coffman (1985) surveyed a panel of mental health professionals (psychiatrists, psychologists, social workers, and administrators) about the factors that most frequently influenced the length of hospitalization. The respondents considered the patient's symptomatology (including the severity of the illness), the level of adaptive functioning, and social support to be more important predictors than the specific psychiatric diagnosis.

Financial pressures have been placed on hospitals to reduce the length of hospital stays. Rupp et al. (1984) examined the difference between two forms of prospective hospital payment systems: per-case vs. per-service payments. The study utilized a 20% sample of 58,000 mental disorder discharges from 21 per-case– and 24 per-service–reimbursed hospitals. The results indicated that the per-case payment method provided more incentive for hospitals to reduce the length of hospital stay.

Unfortunately, changes in the philosophy of treatment for acute care have lagged behind the financial pressures. Although a number of studies (Herz et al., 1979; Endicott et al., 1979; and Rosen et al., 1976) have shown that brief hospitalization for the acutely ill is as beneficial as long-term hospitalization, especially when a discharged patient is provided appropriate aftercare services in the community, debate over the usefulness of short-term hospitalization continues. The issue is particularly important in adolescent psychiatry. Munoz-Millan (1986), in an editorial comment, pointed out the vulnerability of adolescent egos to reactivation of infantile conflicts, increased intensity of drives, identity issues, and conflict with authority figures. It is the presence of these developmental issues, he emphasized, that makes it impossible for adolescents to benefit from short-term hospitalization focused only on the control of overt symptoms. The majority of adolescent patients feel forced to accept hospital treatment because the hospital admissions are generally initiated and requested by the parents or other guardians and not by the adolescent patients themselves. This creates intense opposition and negative feelings that take from several days to a couple of weeks to subside before treatment is accepted. There are a few adolescent patients who do not benefit from short-term hospital treatment because they continue to be intensely negative and oppositional to any effort on the part of the staff to help them. Programs designed to improve cooperation and the motivation of adolescent patients to work on their problems would certainly reduce the length of hospitalization. A well-planned hospital admission in which adolescent patients in outpatient treatment are prepared by therapists for hospitalization will enhance cooperation and facilitate early discharge.

One of the objectives of hospital treatment is to modify the environment of the patient including the home, the school, and the community so that the patient has a better chance to adjust after discharge from the hospital. Working with families, schools, and community agencies and planning cooperatively for aftercare are extremely essential to achieve treatment goals and to reduce the length of hospitalization.

Selection of the right type of patients for brief hospitalization is also important. There are few studies to guide clinicians in making such a selection. A large number of patients in general hospitals are admitted through emergency rooms, and clinicians have little opportunity to weed out long-term patients. Most psychiatrists avoid admitting adolescents with conduct problems and borderline personality disorders for brief hospital treatment. In our experience, the following categories of patients do fairly well during brief hospitalization:

1. Complex cases requiring diagnostic evaluation through close observation in the hospital setting.
2. Patients requiring a safe and protective environment, i.e., suicidal patients and runaways.
3. Aggressive and homicidal patients who are severely emotionally disturbed.
4. Patients who are uncooperative in outpatient treatment and who require brief hospitalization to initiate treatment, i.e., patients with anorexia nervosa or a chronically ill child who refuses medical treatment.
5. Adolescents with substance abuse problems.
6. Acute psychiatric problems such as psychosis, obsessive compulsive disorder, major depression, agitation, and anxiety disorders.

THEORETICAL MODELS

Several theoretical models have been proposed to work with hospitalized adolescents. Most of these models emphasize the clear identification of the reasons for hospitalization. The goals of hospital treatment are frequently limited to resolving a crisis or stabilizing the patient before discharge. Aftercare plans are structured to provide continuity of care in a less restrictive setting.

Problem-Oriented Approach

Larry Weed (1968) introduced a system of medical record keeping called the "Problem-Oriented Medical Record." It contains four sequential sections:

1. Database.
2. Problem List.
3. Plans.
4. Follow-up.

This system has now been used in medicine for many years. Its application in psychiatry is described in detail by Ryback and associates (1974, 1981). The components of the database include the usual initial history comprising identifying data, chief complaints, the history of the present illness, developmental history and family history, past history, and mental status examination.

The second portion of the record, labeled the "Problem List," includes the following sections:

1. Diagnosis.
2. Physiological Findings.
3. Physical Symptoms.
4. Abnormal Laboratory Findings.

It is suggested that the problem list should include everything that is known or observed about the patient. The problems should be stated in words that can be understood easily by all levels of staff. The problems may be listed in various formats and divided into various workable or meaningful categories such as physiological, social, behavioral, and familial.

A plan of treatment is carried out for each problem identified. The authors suggest that the initial treatment plan be described in the following manner:

Problem 1

Title of problem:	Depression.
Problem description:	Feeling sad.
Problem assessment:	Patient appears sad from affect, low-energy level, and lack of interest in activities.
Diagnostics:	Dexamethazone suppression test.
Treatment:	Antidepressants.
Education:	Mental health education with regard to dealing with a depressed mood and stress.

The problem description is usually obtained from the patient's own version of the problem, and assessment is based on observation and evaluation of the patient's version of the problem. However, these two aspects of the problem are frequently continuous and should not be artificially separated. The treatment plan may require further diagnostics, collection of additional information, or prescription of certain types of therapy and patient education.

Follow-up of each problem is extremely essential in determining the outcome of the treatment. The follow-up is carried out through systematic progress notes.

This system has been criticized for various reasons. For example, the problem list frequently accumulates descriptions of behavioral trivia that do not require hospitalization for their management. Differences among mental health workers frequently arise with regard to the importance of a particular problem. Some staff, because of their special biases, continue to spend their time working on simple problems that can easily be worked through in outpatient therapy. The problem-oriented record rarely describes the primary reason for hospitalization in dynamic terms. Most of the staff rarely acquire an overall understanding of the reasons for hospitalization and continue to work on minor problems in the absence of such understanding.

Goal-Directed Treatment Planning

Setting goals and objectives in psychiatric treatment has become much more acceptable in recent years. In the past, setting specific goals frequently implied an imposition of the therapist's preconceived notions on his patient, thus restricting the patient's ability to fully explore himself. Cautious optimism about goal orientation, however, emerged with the necessity and popularity of short-term psychotherapy. A fair number of studies (refer Chapter 3) now show that it is clearly possible to carryout goal-directed individual and group therapy for certain types of patients. Similar principles are being applied in the short-term treatment of hospitalized patients.

Nurcombe (1989) viewed the primary purpose of hospitalization as stabilization of the patient in the hospital so that he can safely be treated outside the hospital. Stabilization is achieved through understanding the patient's problems through diagnostic evaluation and setting the goals of the treatment to eliminate the behaviors that precipitated the hospitalization (such as suicidal attempts or ideations).

In summary, a patient is evaluated through a comprehensive history, mental status determination, physical examination, and laboratory and psychological tests. From this database, an extensive list of problems is prepared. Then each problem is assessed objectively for its severity and relevance to presenting problems. The treatment plan is then outlined for each of the problems identified. Each symptom should be followed with a specific treatment to determine the outcome of treatment.

In addition, treatment goals include preparation of the family and the community to receive the adolescent patient for further therapy.

In this model of treatment the clinician collects the initial data in a standardized manner with a comprehensive history, mental status check, physical examination, and laboratory tests. The diagnostic formulation is based on a biopsychosocial concept of mental illness. Pivotal problems are extracted from the formulation and are rephrased to represent the goals of treatment. For example, in a case of separation anxiety disorder with school refusal, the pivotal problems include not going to school, spending a great deal of time at home, and not socializing outside the home. The goals of hospital treatment include (1) going to school from the hospital for several days before discharge and (2) leaving home to visit and socialize with friends. This goal may be achieved by the use of a pass to go home after a couple of weeks of treatment and socialization in the hospital. Other treatment goals include family therapy, medication to relieve anxiety, and other interventions based on a dynamic understanding of each case.

Eliminating the reasons for hospitalization such as suicidal thoughts, aggressive impulses, and uncooperation with medical treatment requires understanding the relationship of the adolescent patient with his family and peers and the underlying motivation for his behavior. Goal-directed treatment may at times be similar to problem-oriented treatment in dealing with superficialities and the trivialities of behavioral expression.

Focal Inpatient Planning

Harper (1989) have popularized the concept of focal inpatient treatment planning. Their form of treatment planning forces the clinical team to choose one focal problem from a myriad of problems presented by most patients at the time of hospitalization. The clinical team progresses quickly in a systematic manner to the following steps toward the primary goals of treatment, that is, to get the patient out of the hospital:

1. Choosing a focal problem.
2. Developing a list of all the factors contributing to the focal problem.
3. Developing a short list (working list) of the contributing factors.
4. Devising treatment to diminish or eliminate the contributing factors.
5. Planning for discharge.

The focal problem is the primary reason for the patient's hospitalization. It may be only one of the many problems that the patient complained of at the time of admission. Defining a focal problem requires a thorough evaluation and investigation of all areas of adolescent functioning, including biological, developmental, familial, social, and peer relationships. All the factors in the various areas of adolescent functioning are identified with regard to their current contribution to the focal problem. Developmental, familial, and other areas may have provided only a background context for the focal problem and may not have contributed actively toward development of the focal problem.

Not all the identified factors contributing to the focal problem need to be worked on in the hospital. Those factors (or problems) that can be ameliorated during hospital treatment should be identified and worked on while arranging therapy for other problems to be carried out outside the hospital. Treatment must also focus on those problems whose diminution or amelioration will facilitate discharge from the hospital.

The process of arriving at the focal problem may be quite difficult, and not all members of the clinical team may agree on one specific focal problem. Similarly, differences also arise with regard to the list of factors that may be currently contributing to the focal problem. Differences in the clinical sophistication, experience, and biases of the members of the treatment team contribute heavily to the differences in their opinion about the focal problem. It is extremely important to carry out these treatment planning exercises in an atmosphere of cooperation and openness.

The theoretical background of this approach resides in various concepts advanced in the psychotherapy literature by several authors. For example, Balint et al. (1972) advocated the concept of focal psychotherapy. They emphasized the need for determining a focal conflict in patients and directing therapy toward the resolution of that conflict. The term *focal conflict* was used to imply the link between the patient's character structure and the presenting symptoms. Similarly, several other authors (Mann, 1973; Malan, 1979) have suggested focusing therapy aims on a "focal concept" or "focal theme." Also, the similarities between this model and the previously described models such as the problem-oriented approach and the goal-directed approach are clearly apparent.

Transactional Risk Model

This model emphasizes the transactional nature of a child's psychopathology and advocates a very close involvement of family and school during inpatient treatment. The term *transactional* refers to a continual and progressive interplay between the child and his environment.This view contrasts with the linear model of causality in understanding children's problems. Although this model is more suited to younger children, it can be applied with some modification to adolescents. Woolston (1989) suggests the following steps for parental involvement in the planning of inpatient treatment in order "to change the fitness of the child/environmental transactions so that positive development occurs":

1. The first step for parents is to observe and understand the strengths and weaknesses of their child, his perception of himself and his environment, and the relationship of his perception to his interpersonal behavior.
2. The second step for parents is to implement a new strategy to reduce the child's anxiety, impulsivity, and other developmental problems.
3. The third step for parents is to generalize their newly acquired strategies in their interaction with the child after discharge.

In this model, parents serve as a special member of the treatment team and participate in all aspects of the child's hospitalization. After the initial orientation, parents help in evaluation, treatment, and discharge planning. The parents are assigned tasks to carry out some of the treatment goals. These treatment assignments frequently pertain to modification of interaction between themselves and their child. They may be required to give the child a time-out period or to put him in seclusion. Most parents need the help and support of the staff in carrying out such disciplinary techniques since they are afraid their child will reject them.

Various behavioral protocols are developed for parents to practice the treatment goals on the inpatient unit. The staff acts as a consultant to the parents during such periods of practice. The protocols are discussed frequently and revised if they appear to be unrealistic for the parents to carry out. After a protocol is mastered by the parents and the child, they are given longer and longer passes to go outside or to go home to try them out.

The major source of failure in this type of program is the parents' own characterological problems that prevent them from working in the treatment program. Many parents refuse to work with the staff in the hospital. Others, deciding that their own needs and lifestyle do not allow them to invest enough time and energy in dealing with the child, request longer-term hospitalization for the child.

The Behavioral Model

Many aspects of inpatient programs are designed on behavioral principles. For example, most programs have a level system to reinforce acceptable behavior. An adolescent with acceptable behavior progresses to higher levels that have more rewards and privileges. Similarly, progress in other aspects of the treatment program are based on a system of token economy. For example, an acceptable amount of academic work and good behavior in the classroom may earn a patient some points that he can trade for other items such as food and candy. Specific behavior programs can be designed for different patients to help them progress in their specific problem areas such as peer relationships, adult relationships, self-care, hygiene, and family relationships.

A behavior therapist deals with the specifics of behavior and analyzes each behavior with regard to its reinforcement pattern. Moss and Mann (1978) conceptualized various patterns of behavior in the following manner:

1. Behavior against the community, or crime.
2. Behavior against one's self, or drug abuse and suicide.
3. Withdrawal from the community, in schizoid and schizophrenic disorders.

The placement of an adolescent with behavior problems in the hospital removes the adolescent from the sources of reinforcement for his problem behavior. The structured environment of the hospital helps the adolescent to experience consistency in his daily life, which prior to hospitalization may have been very chaotic and inconsistent. Initially, all adolescents behave in their habitual pattern. However, the reinforcement system of the hospital unit helps them learn more acceptable behaviors. It is generally expected that learning in the hospital environment will generalize to the home and to community situations after discharge from the hospital.

The behavior model of therapy seems to work well in facilities for medium- and long-term hospitalization. Short-term hospitalization, however, cannot depend heavily on behavior modification techniques. Three or 4 weeks are not enough time to make substantial changes in a disturbed behavior pattern, especially in behaviors against society or withdrawal from the community. Sometimes, some adolescents go along with the staff and hospital rules for a period of 3 to 4 weeks but return to their original patterns of behavior after discharge.

Crisis Intervention Model

The crisis intervention model of psychopathology assumes that most individuals function in a homeostatic way during complex interactions among biopsychosocial factors. A crisis is produced by a disturbance of homeostasis that results from problems in one or more areas of the biopsychosocial sphere. If a person is unable to deal with his disturbed homeostasis by himself or with the help of his family or community resources, he needs psychiatric help and should be removed to a treatment facility or a hospital. The goal of hospital treatment then becomes to restore the person to the original or a new level of homeostasis and return him to the community.

A crisis is a state of temporary disequilibrium precipitated by unavoidable life events. A person in crisis feels overwhelmed and helpless and is temporarily unable to resolve his problems by himself. In addition to anxiety, there are manifestations of cognitive uncertainty, emotional distress, psychophysiological symptoms, and disruption of social relationships.

Crisis, by definition, is a temporary state lasting for a limited period of time. The life events that precipitate the crisis may be a part of normal development or external events beyond the control of the individual. These events may be obvious and easily identifiable, or they may be quite elusive. Some crisis situations are universal, such as death and fatal illness, while other situations are experienced as a crisis only by certain individuals. People differ vastly in their capacity to cope with crisis. Persons who are less vulnerable seem to possess better coping skills than do individuals who are highly vulnerable. Low-vulnerable individuals are better able to reorient themselves rapidly and are able to take decisive steps in response to change and emergency situations. Highly vulnerable people, on the other hand, fall apart easily in similar situations.

Phases of Crisis

Studies of individuals, families, and groups in crisis reveal that crisis is a regular process and that people in crisis undergo a fairly predictable sequence of emotional events. There are various classifications of the phases of crisis (Tyhurst, 1957; Lindemann, 1944; Hirschowitz, 1973), but most authors tend to differentiate a beginning, middle, and final phase of a crisis. Caplan (1964) described the following four phases of a crisis:

1. There is an initial rise of tension that calls forth habitual problem-solving responses to achieve equilibrium.

2. If these problem-solving responses are unsuccessful in resolving the crisis, there is a further rise of tension.

3. The individual then mobilizes his emergency problem-solving mechanisms. He may try new problem-solving methods and may define the problem in a new way so that it becomes similar to previous experiences. He may compromise and give up certain aspects of the goal as being unattainable. Trial-and-error behavior continues until all avenues are explored and the problem is resolved.

4. Tension mounts to a dangerous level if the problem remains unresolved.

Manifestations of severe emotional disturbance and personality disorganization may then appear.

Healthy and Unhealthy Crisis Coping

Individuals in crisis utilize a habitual mode of problem solving that they have used successfully in the past. Crises are often novel situations and may not be amenable to old problem-solving methods but may require new problem-solving techniques.

Hirschowitz (1973) identifies the following behaviors as characteristic of people who cope well with crisis.

1. Such a person is able to deal simultaneously with both the affective dimensions of his experience and the tasks that confront him. He is aware of his painful emotions and gives them appropriate expression but does not engage in interminable catharsis or ventilation. As he expresses his pain, he frees energy for mastery of his environmental changes. Crisis mastery proceeds by the conversion of uncertainty into manageable risk. This process of situational mastery is crucial. When life change is anticipated, this intelligent worry work can begin in advance, with significant diminution of the intensity of the crisis. Programs of anticipatory guidance or emotional prophylaxis incorporate these principles of anticipatory planning and action rehearsal.

2. He has the ability to acknowledge his increased dependency needs and to seek, receive, and use assistance.

3. He values the active mastery of environmental challenges and recognizes their value in promoting increased understanding and personal growth.

4. In coping with anxiety, he uses defenses (such as substitution) and modes of tension relief that do not have destructive consequences.

The person who copes badly with crisis has some or all of the following traits:

1. He exhibits excessive denial, withdrawal, retreat, or avoidance with fantasy replacing or merging with reality.

2. His behavior is often impulsive, and he ventilates his rage on vulnerable, relatively powerless family members who lend themselves to being scapegoats.

3. He meets his dependency needs by excessive clinging or counterdependent avoidance of assistance. These patterns, described by Bowlby (1952) as protest, despair, and detachment, resemble the behavior of separated infants. These actions are either annoying or indicate to others that the individual neither wants nor needs help; thus they do not usually evoke ministration responses from others.

4. He denies and overcontrols his emotions with eventual eruption of his feelings.

5. His malcoping may assume the form of hopelessness, helplessness, or the "giving-up syndrome" described by Engel (1954).

6. He may resort to hyperritualistic behavior, which serves little or no purpose.

7. His rest/work cycle is poorly regulated due to the fatigue of the crisis state.

8. He may rely on pain-reducing substances such as drugs or alcohol or adopt an addictive pattern of compulsive food intake.

9. He cannot ask for help and cannot use it when it is offered.

Crisis as Opportunity

The stimulation of personal growth by exposure to small doses of stress and challenge has long been successfully used by educators and scout leaders. Thomas (quoted by Volkhart, 1951) perceives crisis as a catalyst that disrupts old habits, evokes new responses, and becomes a major factor in the creation of new actions. Crisis illicits new coping mechanisms, thus strengthening the individual's adaptive capacity and thereby generally raising the level of mental health.

Crisis often gives a person a second chance to correct overly relied upon but faulty problem-solving techniques or to develop new problem-solving strategies more appropriate to the new situation.

Hospitalization of an adolescent is a crisis not only for the adolescent but for his whole family. Working with the family and helping them deal with the problems of the adolescent by developing new responses provides the opportunity for growth in parental skills.

Crisis Intervention

An accurate assessment of the reasons for hospitalization is essential for effective crisis intervention. The intervener usually deals with the factors that are directly related to the crisis. Morley and associates (1967) have outlined the following steps in crisis intervention:

1. The first phase of crisis intervention involves an assessment of the individual and his problem. Persons with severe suicidal or homicidal potential are referred for individual evaluation and possible hospitalization. Of critical importance in crisis intervention is the accurate assessment of the precipitating factors and the resulting crisis that brought the individual to treatment.

2. Next, the nature of the therapeutic intervention depends upon several factors such as the amount of time elapsed since the onset of the crisis, the coping skills of the individual, the degree of support offered by the family, the ego strength of the adolescent prior to the onset of the crisis, and the degree to which the adolescent's life has been disrupted.

3. The therapist may utilize various techniques with which he is familiar as long as he keeps in mind the basic philosophy and goal of crisis intervention. Morley et al. have found the following techniques useful:

- Help the individual gain a cognitive understanding of his crisis. Many individuals may have no idea that a connection exists between some life events and their state of crisis.
- Help the person to talk about his present situation and his feelings associated with the crisis. People in crisis frequently express feelings of anger, hate, aggression, and guilt. The therapist should be uncritical and accepting of such feelings.
- Explore the behaviors and techniques the person is using to deal with the crisis. Also, explore the coping behaviors and techniques the person utilized in similar past situations. The therapist should point out the ineffectiveness of the present coping behaviors and techniques and should suggest alternate methods.

• The final step is the resolution of crisis and anticipatory planning. As anxiety and depression subside and the person begins to readjust his daily life, the therapist should reinforce the change and help the individual realize the gains he has made. Help is also given in making realistic plans for the future.

Clinical Applications

Substance abuse, sexual forays, delinquent activities, and other conduct problems frequently emerge with the onset of adolescence. The crisis model views these problems as resulting from a disturbed homeostasis at the outset of puberty. Biological changes at puberty increase the adolescent's desire for association with peers and enhances the individual's drive for independence. However, these urges and drives may come into direct conflict with parental desire to maintain control over the adolescent's activities. The adolescent's constant struggle with his family may lead to alienation from the family, greater dependency on peers, emotional turmoil, and at times, severe conduct problems. The crisis created by the adolescent's turmoil is experienced by both the adolescent and his family. Crisis resolution is achieved by focusing the treatment efforts on the conflict between the adolescent and his family. Once the conflict is resolved, both the adolescent and the family will acquire a new level of homeostasis.

Many other events in the life of an adolescent (parental separation, divorce, sickness and death in the family, breaking up with a girlfriend or a boyfriend, and school failures) may create a crisis with symptoms of anxiety, depression, and behavior problems. Focusing treatment goals on helping adolescents to adjust to new life events will help resolve the symptoms associated with the crisis.

However, not all problems during adolescence begin with the onset of puberty. Many problems begin in childhood and become worse during adolescence. These adolescents may never have received any help in childhood and come to the attention of the mental health system during adolescence because of the fact that their problems have become unmanageable by their parents and the community. Such families are frequently disorganized and ignore the presence of problems in their child in the early years. Treatment strategies based on the crisis model do little to rectify the problems. The family continues to experience a perpetual state of crisis with frequent hospitalizations of the adolescent. Some of these adolescents may require long-term facilities where they can grow within a structured environment and develop sufficient ego and superego to function as independent persons.

In summary, all models share the same basic principles. All models recognize that the hospital environment is necessary only to stabilize acute psychopathology or to resolve an acute crisis and that the patient must be returned to his natural environment as soon as possible to continue treatment under the less-restrictive setting of the community. The need to modify the family, school, and community situations through early aftercare planning or transactional interventions is also recognized by all models.

Acute-care models provide clinicians with better directions for planning and clear goals for hospitalized patients. These models do not exclude goals and objectives based on psychodynamic or behavioral understanding of the patient's problems. The goals, however, must be attainable by the efforts of the clinical team during the short period of hospitalization.

REFERENCES

Balint M, Ornstein P, Balint E: *Focal Psychotherapy.* London, Tavistock Publications, 1972.

Bowlby J: *Maternal Care and Mental Health.* Geneva, World Health Organization, 1952.

Canton C, Gralnick A: A review of issues surrounding length of psychiatric hospitalization. *Hosp Community Psychiatry* 1987; 38:858–863.

Caplan G: *Principles of Preventive Psychiatry.* New York, Basic Books Inc Publishers, 1964.

Doherty EG: Length of hospitalization in a short-term therapeutic community. *Arch Gen Psychiatry* 1975; 33:87–92.

Endicott J, Cohen J, Nee J, et al: Brief vs. standard hospitalization. *Arch Gen Psychiatry* 1979; 36:706–712.

Engel GL: Studies of ulcerative colitis. I. Clinical data hearing on the nature of the somatic process. *Psychosom Med* 1954; 16:496.

Harper G: Focal inpatient treatment planning. *J Am Acad Child Adolesc Psychiatry* 1989; 28:31–37.

Heinman E, Shanfield S: Length of stay for patients in one city's hospitals with psychiatric units. *Hosp Community Psychiatry* 1980; 31:632–634.

Herz M, Endicott J, Gibbon M: Brief hospitalization: Two-year follow-up. *Arch Gen Psychiatry* 1979; 36:701–705.

Hirschowitz RG: Crisis theory: A formulation. *Psychiatry Ann* 1973; 3:33.

Lindemann E: Symptomatology and management of acute grief. *Am J Psychiatry* 1944; 101:141.

Malan DH: *Individual Psychotherapy and the Science of Psychodynamics.* London, Butterworth Publishers, 1979.

Mann J: *Time-limited Psychotherapy.* Cambridge, Mass, Harvard University Press, 1973.

Mezzick J, Coffman G: Factors influencing length of hospital stay. *Hosp Community Psychiatry* 1985; 36:1262–1260.

Morley W, Messick J, Aguilera D: Crisis: Paradigms of intervention. *J Psychiatry Nurs* 1967; 5:531.

Moss GR, Mann RA: A behavioral approach to the hospital treatment of adolescents. *Psychiatr Clin North Am* 1978; 1:263–275.

Munoz-Milan R: The optimal length of hospitalization of adolescents. *Hosp Community Psychiatry* 1986; 37:545.

Nurcombe B: Goal-directed treatment planning and the principles of brief hospitalization. *J Am Acad Child Adolesc Psychiatry* 1989; 28:26–30.

Rosen B, Katzoff A, Carrillo C, et al: Clinical effectiveness of 'short' vs. 'long' psychiatric hospitalization. *Arch Gen Psychiatry* 1976; 33:1316–1322.

Rosenstein M, Steadman H, Milazzosayre L, et al: Characteristics of admissions to the inpatient service of state and county mental health hospitals, United States, 1980. Mental Health Statistical Note, 1977. Rockville, Md, NIMH, 1986.

Rupp A, Steinwach D, Salkever D: The effects of hospital payment methods on the pattern and cost of mental health care. *Hosp Community Psychiatry* 1984; 35:456–459.

Ryback R, Longabaugh R, Fowler D: *The Problems Oriented Record in Psychiatry and Mental Health Care.* New York, Grune & Stratton, 1981.

Ryback R: *The Problem Oriented Record in Psychiatry and Mental Health Care.* New York, Grune & Stratton, 1974.

Tyhurst J: The role of transition states including disasters in mental illness, in *Symposium on Preventive and Social Psychiatry.* Washington, DC, Walter Reed Army Institute of Research, 1957.

Volkhart E (ed): *Social Behavior and Personality Contributions of W.I. Thomas to Theory and Social Research.* New York, Social Science Research Council, 1951.

Weed L: *Medical Records, Medical Evaluation, and Patient Care.* Cleveland, Case Western Reserve University Press, 1969.

Woolston JL: Transactional risk model for short and intermediate term psychiatric inpatient treatment of children. *J Am Acad Child Adolesc Psychiatry* 1989; 28:38–41.

9

Follow-up Studies

There are few follow-up studies of adolescents treated in short-term psychiatric hospitals. Most of the follow-up studies have been carried out on adolescent patients discharged from medium-term (less than 6 months) and long-term inpatient treatment facilities. Short-term psychiatric treatment is defined not only in terms of duration of treatment (less than 6 weeks) but also in terms of philosophy of treatment relating to the achievement of short-term goals—stabilization of the patient and crisis resolution. Similarly, medium-term psychiatric hospitalization is based on a treatment philosophy that tries to accomplish the same goal as short-term hospitalization for a population of adolescents who cannot be stabilized in short-term programs. The primary aim of hospital treatment (short-term or medium-term) is to stabilize the patient enough to return him to his community to continue psychiatric treatment in a less restrictive and more natural environment.

Major differences in the philosophy of treatment make it difficult to compare the outcome studies of the 1950s and the 1960s with the studies of the last two decades. The leisurely pace of diagnosis and treatment in the older studies cannot be compared with the intensive and rapid pace of diagnosis and treatment of present-day short-term treatment. The older treatment philosophy of character building and character change has been replaced by a focus on conflict resolution and crisis orientation. These trends are apparent in the selection of parameters that the long-term studies have utilized in their investigation. These studies have monitored changes in the severity of psychopathology, family dysfunction, adaptation to the society, academic and vocational achievements, and changes in personality. Several authors (Avison and Speechley, 1987; Canfield et al., 1988; Durkin and Durkin, 1975) have pointed out other deficiencies of such outcome studies, such as the use of small and heterogeneous samples, omission of preadmission variables, and a failure to examine the interactions among the patient, his environment, and the treatment. Pfeiffer (1989) reviewed 32 outcome studies of inpatient treatment of children and adolescents. He compared these studies on a 22-item list grouped into three broad categories: description of the patient population; description of treatment; and design, instrumentation, and methodological considerations. He noticed that most of the studies did not provide information on preadmission background. Diagnostic labels were broad, such as personality disorder or psychosis, and lacked specificity. The description of treatment was scanty and failed to mention the type and the frequency of psychotherapy.

The outcome of short- and medium-term hospitalization cannot be evaluated on the same principles as the outcome studies of long-term treatment. An evaluation of the outcome of short-term treatment should include the type of disposition at discharge, compliance with treatment in community facilities, and the frequency of readmissions. Changes in adjustment and coping capacity may show some improvement with hospital treatment but may not progress beyond their precrisis level. Further improvement in coping capacity and adjustment will depend upon the aftercare variables such as compliance with aftercare recommendations and the availability of community resources to meet the mental health, educational, and recreational needs of the adolescent and his family.

SOUTHERN ILLINOIS UNIVERSITY OUTCOME STUDY OF SHORT-TERM HOSPITALIZATION

This study has taken some of the hospital variables into consideration such as philosophy of treatment, adjustment of patients to the hospital milieu, family intervention, disposition at discharge, and readmissions. We studied 800 adolescents admitted between 1985 and 1988. These adolescents were hospitalized in a 23-bed adolescent psychiatric unit situated in a community hospital. The unit is a teaching facility of Southern Illinois University Medical School for medical students and residents from general psychiatry, child psychiatry, and pediatrics. The unit is a controlled access facility. It is staffed by round-the-clock nursing personnel and mental health technicians, one recreational therapist, three social workers, one psychologist, one unit administrator, a medical director (child psychiatrist), and three part-time teachers. In addition, medical students, general psychiatry trainees, and child psychiatry trainees spent variable amounts of time in the care of the patients. The patients were hospitalized primarily by three child psychiatrists who supervised the management of their patients. The components of the treatment program included the following:

1. Group psychotherapy—1 hour daily.
2. Individual psychotherapy—20 to 30 minutes daily.
3. Special purpose focused group (i.e., adoption group, group for sexually abused girls)—one to two times a week.
4. Mental health education groups for patients (personal growth and developmental groups)—1 hour daily.
5. Family therapy—once a week.
6. Mental health education groups for parents—once a week.
7. Family process groups—one to two times a week.
8. Special nursing activities—daily.
9. Formal education—daily.
10. Medical lectures—once a week.
11. Recreational therapy—daily.

TABLE 9–1.
Age and Sex Distribution of 800 Patients

Sex	Total Number	Age (yr)					
		12	13	14	15	16	17
Males	374	34	47	73	81	83	56
Females	426	18	58	88	111	88	63

The program required all patients to participate in all activities. Each patient is assigned a therapeutic focus for a week or more, depending on his specific problem. The therapeutic focus is spelled out in practical and simple terms such as increasing peer interaction, expressing anger in an acceptable manner, participating more in group discussions, and relating appropriately to boys or girls. A level system (based on the principles of reinforcement) is utilized for monitoring behavior adjustment to the treatment program. After an initial evaluation involving a detailed history from the adolescent, his family, and the referring sources, a mental status examination, and laboratory investigation and psychological testing if indicated, a formulation of the problem is arrived at within the first 5 days. Treatment goals and aftercare plans are discussed in a multidisciplinary staff conference. The rest of the time in the hospital is spent in accomplishing the treatment goals and setting up aftercare plans.

Patient Population Characteristics

Age and Sex Distribution

The study included 374 boys (47%) and 426 girls (53%). The age distribution of both sexes is represented in Table 9–1.

There was no significant difference between the number of male and female patients at the ages of 13, 14, 16, and 17 years. However, at 12 years of age a significantly greater number of boys composed the group, whereas at the age of 15 years a significantly greater number of girls composed the group. Table 9–1 also indicates that the number of both boys and girls increases in each age category until 15 and 16 years of age, after which there is a sharp drop in the number of admissions at the age of 17 years.

Sources of Referral and Funding

The hospital is surrounded by the rural counties of central Illinois and receives patients living within an area of about a 50- to 80-mile radius whose total population is 500,000 to 800,000. Psychiatric services in the community are provided by community mental health centers, grant-in-aid agencies, and private practitioners. Although the sources of referral to the hospital vary at different times of the year, the overall sources of referral are as follows:

- Physicians—30%.
- Hospital emergency room—20%.
- Social service agencies and private therapists—20%.

- Self-referral—10%.
- School-initiated referral—8%.
- Other hospitals—4%.
- Others—8%.

Admissions through the emergency room of the hospital are mostly self-referred. Parents bring their suicide-attempting and aggressive adolescents to the emergency room because they perceive the urgency of the problem and the necessity for hospitalization. Some parents may call the adolescent unit directly and ask for an evaluation of their adolescent for a possible psychiatric admission.

The economy of the area is based on agriculture and some small industries. A fairly large proportion of the patients are covered by health insurance. The approximate distribution of mental health coverage was estimated to be as follows:

- Commercial insurance—60%.
- State of Illinois—3.3%.
- Health maintenance organizations (HMOs)—9.5%.
- Medicaid—18.5%.
- Private payment—8.7%.

Length of Hospital Stay

This is an important measure in brief psychiatric hospitalization. The average length of stay for all patients was 27.33 (SD = 13.6) days. The total patient population was divided into three subgroups for further analysis.

Group I consisted of 127 adolescents who stayed less than 2 weeks. The average length of hospital stay for this group was 7.59 days (SD = 4.48). Group II stayed for 14 to 42 days and consisted of 583 patients with an average length of hospital stay of 27.77 days (SD = 8.98). Group III remained in the hospital for more than 42 days and consisted of 90 adolescents with an average length of stay of 52.4 days (SD = 12.65). The rationale for distinguishing between these three groups is the assumption that a minimum of 2 weeks is required for an adolescent patient to benefit from the program. A period of less than 2 weeks does not provide sufficient time for diagnosis, trial of treatment, family intervention, and aftercare planning. Thus, patients who leave within the first 2 weeks after admission are unlikely to have benefited much from the program. Similarly, patients who stay longer than 42 days present special types of problems requiring extended stays in the hospital. Further analysis of these groups is discussed at the end of this study.

Psychiatric Diagnoses

The diagnosis at discharge was considered the final diagnosis. However, a diagnostic work-up was generally completed by the end of the first 5 days. Diagnostic labels were discussed once a week during a multidisciplinary staff meeting, and changes were made based on new observations and information. The diagnoses were based on the criteria of DSM III and DSM III-R. These criteria were reviewed frequently in teaching rounds with psychiatric residents and students. A variety of structured interviews and inventories such as Beck's Inventory, Hamilton's Scale for Depression, KIDDIE Schedule for Affective Disorders and Schizophrenia (K-SADS), and Hamilton's Anxiety Scale were used in relation to ongoing clinical research in the unit.

Table 9–2 shows the proportion of adolescents under various diagnostic categories. Mood disorders appear to be the most frequent diagnoses (45%) given to the hospitalized adolescents. The second most common diagnosis is conduct disorder (27%).

Table 9–3 shows common primary diagnoses by age and sex distribution. This table shows that a significantly higher number of female adolescents suffered from mood disorders at all ages. There were more boys with diagnoses of conduct disorder than there were girls, but the difference was not significant.

The most common secondary diagnoses under axis I included the following:

1. Psychoactive substance abuse disorder (mostly alcohol and marijuana abuse).
2. Attention-deficit disorder with hyperactivity.
3. Specific developmental disorders such as reading, arithmetic, and language disorders.
4. Dysthymic disorder.
5. Parent/child problem.

Substance abuse is very common among adolescents. In our area the substances

TABLE 9–2.

Primary Diagnoses of Hospitalized Adolescents (Southern Illinois University Study)

Primary Diagnosis	Diagnosis by Age (yr)						Percentage of Total
	12	13	14	15	16	17	
Dysthymic disorder	10	18	37	41	32	28	20.75
Major depression	8	17	23	56	45	33	22.75
Bipolar mood disorder	—	2	2	—	1	3	1.00
Adjustment disorder	6	15	13	21	20	19	11.75
Oppositional disorder	10	12	10	12	5	4	6.30
Conduct disorder	9	25	56	50	55	21	27.00
Substance abuse disorder	—	—	3	7	3	—	1.60
Schizophrenia	—	3	2	—	3	1	1.00
Schizoid disorder	—	1	2	2	4	3	1.50
Attention-deficit disorder	7	6	5	2	2	1	2.90
Organic brain syndrome	—	1	1	—	—	—	0.25
Borderline	—	1	1	—	—	3	0.62
Impulse control disorder	—	1	1	—	—	—	0.25
Overanxious disorder	—	1	2	1	—	2	0.75
Separation anxiety disorder	2	2	1	—	—	—	0.62
Somatization disorder	—	—	—	—	1	—	0.125
Anorexia nervosa	—	—	1	—	—	1	0.25
Bulimia	—	—	1	—	—	—	0.125

TABLE 9–3.
Primary Diagnoses of Hospitalized Adolescents: Age and Sex Distribution
(Southern Illinois University Study)

Primary Diagnosis	Sex	Diagnosis by Age (yr)						Percentage of Total
		12	13	14	15	16	17	
Mood disorder	M	12	12	15	36	30	27	16.50
	F	6	25	47	61	48	37	28.00
Conduct disorder	M	3	13	34	27	33	13	15.30
	F	6	12	22	23	22	8	11.60
Oppositional disorder	M	8	2	5	5	2	2	3.00
	F	2	10	5	7	3	2	3.60
Adjustment disorder	M	4	6	6	5	7	7	4.30
	F	2	9	7	16	13	12	7.30

abused were mostly alcohol and marijuana. Although substance dependency was suspected in many cases, it was actually present in only a few cases. Parent/child conflict was present in almost all cases. The secondary diagnoses of substance abuse and attention-deficit disorder were most frequently associated with a principal diagnosis of conduct disorder. There were very few diagnoses on axis III. They included bronchial asthma, diabetes, ulcerative colitis, and Osgood-Schlatter disease.

Treatment Outcome

The components of the treatment program are listed in the description of the program. All adolescents were required to participate in all aspects of the program. However, acceptance of the program varied from complete acceptance to complete opposition. Usually, by the end of the first week of hospitalization, most patients had accepted the program and were willing to work on their problems. It was usually in the beginning of the second week of hospitalization that some predictions could be made with regard to the benefit of the program to a particular patient. It was easy to pick out those patients who had maintained a negative attitude toward the program. The majority of those patients carried the diagnoses of conduct disorder or oppositional disorder. However, not all patients who started out with a negative attitude remained negative. In fact, the majority of them accepted help but to varying degrees. Those who remained negative at the end of the second week did not change their attitude to any great extent throughout the remainder of the period of hospitalization.

There was yet a third group of about 10% to 15% of the patients at any one time who tended to slide through the program without much emotional investment. They were not vocal about their opposition and had secretly decided to go through the "sentence" without any protest. This group was frequently difficult to spot because of their apparent compliance with the program. They participated in all aspects of the program but did not reveal themselves and avoided discussing their problems.

Behavior in the program was monitored by the level system that is described in Chapter 4. The attainment of certain levels in the program was indicative of the degree of compliance with the rules of the program but did not reflect personal attitudes toward acceptance of help or willingness to work on personal problems.

Based on these broad clinical assessments, it was concluded that about 50% of the adolescents participated in the program with a positive attitude and benefited to the fullest extent possible. The remaining 50% included about 20% of those who benefited to varying degrees, 15% who slid through quietly without much benefit, and 15% who remained overtly oppositional throughout their stay in the hospital. The adolescents who benefited the most tended to have a positive attitude toward receiving help, talked about their problems, were more self-confident, and admitted contributing to the problems in their family and in peer relationships.

We believe that certain changes in the program can maximize the benefits of the program, especially for those groups who remain negative or slide through the program quietly. A careful and early assessment of the attitude of the patient and the degree of his participation in the program may lead to more effective interventions. The overall outcome of the treatment program does not depend solely on the treatment provided in the hospital. Other variables such as the strength of the family and availability of resources in the community contribute heavily to the overall outcome. It should be emphasized that a short-term inpatient treatment program cannot function well without adequate community resources to maintain the small gains acquired in the hospital and to continue further progress.

Disposition

Early discharge planning is an important aspect of brief hospitalization. This planning is carried out during the first week of hospitalization. Community resources are found to meet the needs of the patient and his family after his discharge. Early aftercare planning is especially critical in cases requiring substitutive care such as a foster home, group home, or placement in medium- or long-term facilities.

The type of disposition is frequently based on the severity of psychopathology, the strength of the family, and the availability of appropriate community resources. The following dispositions were made in our study:

1. Discharged to family home—706 patients.
2. Discharged to foster care—23 patients.
3. Discharged to group homes or residential treatment centers—27 patients.
4. Discharged to a medium-term state psychiatric facility—17 patients.
5. Transferred to another psychiatric hospital primarily for substance abuse disorder—5 patients.
6. Discharged against medical advice—19 patients.
7. Transferred to other acute hospitals—3 patients.

Recommendations for counseling in the community mental health facilities were made in all cases of returning to home and discharge to foster care. The compliance rate with these recommendations was only about 62% for the first 12 weeks after discharge. Many families did not follow the aftercare plan because they felt that the patient had improved enough not to require further therapy. Financial and other difficulties prevented some families from seeking further help. A few families had very negative experiences with mental health professionals during the hospitalization, and this prevented them from seeking further help.

Further Analysis of the Subgroups

The study population was divided into three subgroups, primarily on the basis of the length of the hospital stay. Group I included 127 patients (15.8%) who stayed in the hospital for less than 14 days (mean, 7.59 days; SD = 4.48). Group II included 583 patients (72.9%) who stayed in the hospital for 14 to 42 days (mean, 27.77 days; SD = 8.98). Group III included 90 patients (11.3%) who stayed in the hospital for longer than 42 days (mean, 52.39; SD = 12.65).

With the exception of the length of stay, the three groups were similar with regard to the age and sex distribution, diagnoses, and disposition. These findings were surprising, but further analysis revealed some of the factors that contributed to earlier or later discharge. The patients who were discharged before the end of 2 weeks were inclined to be great manipulators of their family system. They tended to deny their problems and appealed to their families to take them out of the hospital. They complained about the treatment program, hospital staff, and other patients. The hospital staff was not successful in providing enough support to these patients and their families to keep them in the hospital. Although the discharge in most cases was considered against medical advice, it was not stated in the actual discharge notes in order to avoid difficulties with the third-party payers. A few cases of early discharges included adolescents whose parents were divorced and were in disagreement with regard to the necessity of hospital treatment for their child.

The patients in the third group of longer hospitalization manifested characteristics that were quite different from those of the other two groups. The majority of these adolescents stayed longer in the hospital because they had no appropriate place to return to. About half of these adolescents were wards of the state. They had lived in foster homes or group homes before the hospital admissions. The Department of Children and Family Services had to make appropriate arrangements in a new foster home, group home, or residential treatment facility before these children could be discharged. These arrangements frequently required extra time before an appropriate place was found. Other factors contributing to delayed discharges included child abuse by parents, refusal by patients to return to their parents' homes, and abandonment of patients by parents. All these patients required appropriate homes for placement. There were only 12 adolescents in this group who stayed longer in the hospital due to medical necessity: they continued to be depressed and suicidal.

Readmissions

Fifty-eight adolescents were readmitted within the 3-year period of this study. Five of the adolescents had three admissions during this period. Table 9–4 shows that the readmissions included more depressed girls than boys. The readmissions were primarily the result of recurrence of the disorders for which they were hospitalized initially. Twenty-nine of the patients did not follow the recommended treatment after the first discharge. Only 13% of this group were discharged after fewer than 14 days of the first hospitalization. Ten percent had stayed longer than 42 days

TABLE 9–4.
Patient Characteristics of Readmissions (58 Patients)

Mean Age (yr)	Sex/No.	Diagnoses (No. of Cases)						
		Major Depression	Dysthymic Disorder	Bipolar Mood Disorder	Oppositional Disorder	Conduct Disorder	Anxiety Disorder	Schizophrenia
15.6	Female/36	14	7	2	4	8	—	1
15.2	Male/22	1	4	—	5	9	2	1

during the first hospitalization. These data indicated that more than half of the readmissions were the result of recurrences of episodes of mood disorders. Lack of cooperation with the aftercare planning and early discharge contributed to the readmissions of the rest of the patients.

REVIEW OF FOLLOW-UP STUDIES

A brief review of long-term psychiatric treatment in residential treatment centers was provided in Chapter 6. The following discussion is limited to a review of selected follow-up studies of short- and medium-term psychiatric treatment for adolescents.

Most follow-up studies have tried to determine the effects of hospital treatment on recovery from primary psychopathology, stability of the initial diagnosis, and psychosocial adjustment. Typically, a follow-up study is carried out several years after discharge via a telephone interview with the patient, a personal interview, a questionnaire sent by mail, and psychological tests administered at the time of follow-up.

The length of stay in medium-term psychiatric facilities for the adolescent ranges from 2 to 6 months. The median length of stay has gradually decreased but still centers around 3 months. Some of the old studies emphasized the necessity of at least 3 months of hospitalization for optimal benefit. In fact, patients leaving earlier than 3 months were considered by many psychiatrists to be discharged against medical advice.

Treatment programs in most hospital units included group therapy, individual psychotherapy, recreational programs, formal education, casework with families, a strong therapeutic milieu, and occasional pharmacotherapy. The units, however, differed with regard to the frequency of various types of therapies and the amount of casework carried out with families. Although few studies described their exact philosophy of treatment, most tended to assume that recovery from psychiatric symptomatology and character building through therapy were the primary aims of hospital treatment.

Patients admitted by different hospitals have varied with regard to the nature and severity of their psychopathology. Urban hospitals tend to treat a greater number of patients with character problems (conduct disorders), whereas suburban hospitals treat more neurotic patients. Similarly, differences exist between closed and open units with regard to the severity of psychiatric problems. Open units tend to exclude more severely affected patients because of difficulties in managing them within the open unit. It is difficult to compare the follow-up studies of the 1970s and 1980s with earlier studies because of major differences in their diagnostic criteria and philosophy of treatment. Most psychiatrists in the 1950s and 1960s were less meticulous in selecting a diagnostic label, especially for children and adolescents. Psychodynamic and behavioral terminologies were frequently used to describe the problems of hospitalized adolescents. The five studies summarized in Table 9–5 are fairly representative of the follow-up studies of the 1950s and 1960s. Some later studies are listed in Table 9–6.

TABLE 9–5.
Follow-up Studies of Hospitalized Adolescents

Study Parameters	Masterson, 1958	Annesley, 1961	Hartmann et al., 1968	Beavers & Blumberg, 1968	King & Pittman, 1969
No. of patients	158	78	30	47	55
Follow-up period (yr)	5–19	2–5	5–19	2–4	6
Schizophrenic disorder (%)	52	22	46	55	2
Affective disorder (%)	5	4	0	0	38
Psychoneuroses (%)	22	19	9	11	15
Psychopathic personality (%)	13	0	0	0	16
Personality disorders (%)	0	0	11	0	0
Transient situation disorder (%)	0	0	14	0	0
Organic syndromes (%)	5	0	0	13	22
Behavior disorders (%)	0	55	0	28	0
Significantly improved at discharge (%)	52	76	52–75	79	0
Significantly improved at follow-up (%)	33	42	33–94	62	79

TABLE 9–6
Follow-up Studies of Hospitalized Adolescents

Study Parameters	Frank, 1980	Kivowitz et al., 1974	Garber, 1972	Welner et al., 1979
Number of patients	23	61	100	77
Follow-up period (yr)	2–4	2–9	1–10	8–10
Schizophrenia (%)	57.5	13	37	17
Major affective disorder (%)	0.0	3	0	37
Neuroses (%)	12.5	15	0	5
Personality disorders (%)	5.0	0	0	0
Psychophysiological disorder (%)	0.0	5	0	0
Transient situational disorder (%)	10.0	0	0	0
Organic brain syndrome (%)	2.5	11	29	1
Sociopathic (%)	2.5	31	0	12
Substance abuse disorder (%)	0.0	0	0	3
Behavior disorders (%)	0.0	0	44	0
Improved at discharge (%)	50.0	0	0	0
Improved at follow-up (%)	37.0	46	0	23

A casual review of Table 9–5 indicates that schizophrenia was a fairly common diagnosis and accounted for a large proportion of the hospitalized population of adolescents. Similarly, behavior disorders and psychopathic personality disorders were quite common in some hospital units. Surprisingly, the diagnostic category of affective disorders was minimally used in most studies and was absent in other studies. This diagnosis, however, has increased in recent studies.

Several follow-up studies have noted that psychiatric diagnoses made during hospitalization are fairly stable in the majority of the cases at the time of follow-up. King and Pittman (1969) reviewed the diagnoses of 55 adolescent patients 6 years after discharge. They found that the diagnoses were stable in 68% of the cases. The diagnoses of 8 patients were changed to affective disorders at follow-up. Similarly, Welner et al. (1979) reported that most of the discharge diagnoses were stable 10 years later. However, 1 patient with the diagnosis of hysteria and 7 undiagnosed patients were considered schizophrenic at follow-up. Also, 4 patients with subsequent bipolar illness with schizophrenia were misdiagnosed initially as having unipolar illness and hysteria.

Overall improvement and adaptation have usually been measured in terms of psychosocial adjustment and educational achievement (in broad categories such as good, fair, and poor) on the basis of the results of questionnaires, interviews, and adjustment scales (for example, the Witmer Social Adjustment Scale) administered at the time of follow-up. Most studies indicate that two thirds to three fourths of the population at the time of discharge show significant symptomatic improvement. These figures usually decrease with the length of follow-up to about 30% at 5 to 10 years after discharge.

Most studies have attempted to determine the outcome for various diagnostic categories. In general, the prognosis for psychoneurosis, affective disorders, and behavior disorders (conduct disorders) have been reported to be good to excellent. Eighty percent to 85% of these patients made good improvement at follow-up 3 to 5 years after discharge from the hospital. However, the outcome for schizophrenia has been poor in most studies. Masterson (1956, 1958) noted that 32 out of 34 patients with the diagnosis of psychoneuroses and 11 out of 20 patients with psychopathic personality disorders made good adjustment at follow-up. However, only 15 out of 83 schizophrenics had shown significant improvement. Seventy-five percent of the schizophrenics required more than 3 years of additional hospitalization. Annesley (1961) reported the following profile of improvement at follow-up (Table 9–7):

TABLE 9–7
Outcome of Hospitalization for Schizophrenia and Behavior Disorders

Diagnosis	% Recovered	% Improved	%No Change/Worse
Schizophrenia	19	23	58
Behavior disorders	38	22	40

Pollack et al. (1968) compared the outcome of hospital treatment among three age groups of schizophrenics: adolescent (n = 28), young adults (n = 32), and older adults (n = 31) in a 3-year follow-up study. They found that the prognosis was worse in childhood-onset schizophrenia. The prognosis also varied somewhat with the subtypes of schizophrenia, with schizoaffective subtypes showing a better prognosis than other subtypes.

Welner et al. (1979) found a poor prognosis with adolescent-onset bipolar affective disorder. In an 8- to 10-year follow-up of 12 adolescent-onset bipolar patients, 3 committed suicide, and the remaining 9 were chronically symptomatic and severely disabled. Ten of the 12 who were treated with lithium did not seem to benefit from this treatment.

A number of factors appeared to influence the outcome of follow-up studies. These factors include the following:

1. Age.
2. Sex.
3. Intellectual functioning.
4. Length of hospital stay.
5. Premorbid psychosocial adjustment.
6. Strength of family system.
7. Nature of psychopathology.
8. Severity of psychopathology.
9. Type of onset of psychopathology.
10. Utilization of treatment resources in the community.

Masterson (1958) noted that in the psychopathic group an age below 16 years was related to a good outcome. However, schizophrenic patients below 14 years of age were likely to have poor outcomes. A younger age did not seem to influence the outcome of psychoneurotic disorders. Gender differences in outcome seemed to be related to other factors such as type of psychopathology and its severity. Adolescents with a below-average intellectual potential seemed to have an unusually difficult task in overcoming their problems. The length of hospitalization is based on multiple considerations of a clinical and socioeconomic nature. Hospital stay may be terminated by staff because a patient is unmanageable within a treatment program. The patient and family, on the other hand, may leave the program with the perception that it is unhelpful. However, a few studies indicate that patients staying longer in the treatment program are not more severely ill than are the patients discharged earlier (Beavers and Blumberg, 1968). Frank (1980) compared two groups of hospitalized adolescents—those who stayed in the hospital less than 61 days and those who stayed longer than 61 days. Those who stayed longer than 61 days showed a better outcome. A good premorbid psychosocial adjustment appears to be associated with a better outcome in most follow-up studies. The severity of family dysfunction is frequently related to the outcome. This is particularly true in cases of younger adolescents who are more dependent on their families than older adolescents are and who need appropriate guiding and nuturing from their families. Schizophrenia presents the worse prognosis, while psychoneurosis and affective disorders show the best prognosis in outcome studies. The prognosis of conduct disorders falls between these two groups.

Gossett and associates (1983) emphasized the distinction between a process vs. a reactive onset of psychopathology. A reactive onset of psychopathology carries a better prognosis than does a slow and progressive onset. A schizophrenic adolescent with process schizophrenia had additional problems such as poor academic achievement, isolation from peers, extreme passivity, an early gradual and bland onset of symptoms, and a slow symptomatic response. Reif (1980) followed 45 formerly hospitalized adolescents through personal interviews and questionnaires. The inquiry covered various areas of psychosocial adjustment. The current level of psychological functioning was estimated as good, fair, or poor. The results indicated significant relationships between current levels of functioning with the type of onset of symptomatology (process vs. reactive). In other words, the type of onset of symptomatology and the severity of psychopathology were the most useful predictors of the patient's longer-term outcome. The study also indicated that those adolescents with a less severe diagnosis and better treatment outcome tended to discontinue psychotherapy.

The disposition of patients at discharge varies greatly with the type of psychopathology, degree of family dysfunction, and availability of appropriate community resources. Also, such factors as court-mandated evaluations or hospitalizations, state custody of the adolescent, and socioeconomic status influence disposition at discharge. Seventy percent to 80% of adolescent patients return to their homes at discharge. Similarly, most of the adolescents coming from foster homes return to foster homes. However, in about 20% of the cases further treatment or substitutive care is required. Frank (1980) reported that 48% of discharges from Mt. Sinai Hospital went home whereas 52% were placed away from the home, including state hospitals (30%), private hospitals (7.5%), and supervised residential placement (7.5%). Frank, however, noted that one third of the cases may have been placed in more restrictive settings because less restrictive choices were not available in the community. Adams (1977) reported the following pattern of disposition of adolescent patients discharged from short-term psychiatric hospitals located in an impoverished area of Pennsylvania:

1. Referred back to court—26%.
2. Group or foster homes—24%.
3. Long-term hospitalization—7%.
4. Went home with treatment referral to a mental health center—43%.

Kling et al. (1986) noted that 74% of their discharged adolescents went home whereas 26% required further treatment in hospitals or in substitutive care.

Criticism of Follow-up Studies

All studies have tried to determine the effects of hospitalization on the subsequent psychosocial adjustment of patients over variable periods after discharge. Healing or modification of behavior is attributed to the hospital treatment. The hospital treatment generally includes group therapy, individual therapy, family counseling, recreation, and formal education. All of these therapies are offered in outpatient clinics and are not specific to inpatient treatment. In fact, many of the patients and their families had received these therapies in outpatient clinics without successfully averting hospitalization. Whether these therapies have a more intensive effect when offered in the confined situation of the hospital is not known. It is possible that the removal of an adolescent to a hospital helps the adolescent become more responsive to these therapies. In addition, the hospital milieu may exert an important effect in modifying behavior and attitudes through the expectation that the patient must abide by certain rules through contact with sympathetic and understanding staff. None of the follow-up studies have been able to identify the specific healing factors in hospital treatment. In fact, it may not be possible to specify those aspects of hospital treatment that are different from other treatment programs such as day-care or partial hospitalization. However, the placement of an adolescent patient in the protective environment of a hospital is necessary when an adolescent is suicidal, homicidal, severely depressed, or psychotic. Perhaps it is the very act of hospitalization and the meaning of confinement that exert an important influence on the patient and make the patient more responsive to traditional therapies.

Whatever the specific therapeutic factors involved in inpatient treatment their effects have been measured in follow-up studies. Most medium- and long-term follow-up studies show that the beneficial effects are maximum shortly after discharge and tend to decrease with time, especially in certain types of psychopathology such as schizophrenia, conduct disorder, and bipolar mood disorder. The beneficial effects are especially remarkable in patients with adjustment disorder; they may recover completely without reoccurrence.

The results of follow-up studies may be diluted by a large number of factors that oppose recovery and decrease the gains made by hospital treatment. Such factors include the severity of family dysfunction, the influence of peers, the unavailability of community mental health resources, and educational and vocational difficulties.

Such factors can rarely be controlled in follow-up studies.

It appears that, in the absence of being able to identify the specific healing factors in inpatient treatment and the inability to control important influential factors after discharge, the result of most long-term follow-up studies may only indicate the course of various psychiatric disorders over a period of time. It is extremely important to define the unique therapeutic aspects of hospital treatment and to measure the expected beneficial effects from such treatment. Long-term follow-up studies have to take into consideration various postdischarge influences such as the family and the community to predict the progress or deterioration of initial psychopathology. Acute models of short-term hospitalization (discussed in Chapter 8) appear to be better suited to follow-up studies. These models define the objectives and ingredients of hospital treatment. Accomplishment of these objectives reflects the degree of success in hospital treatment.

REFERENCES

Adams M: Reflections on short-term psychiatric hospitalization for children and adolescents. *J Natl Med Assoc* 1977; 69:721–724.

Annesley P: Psychiatric illness in adolescence: Presentation and prognosis. *J Ment Sci* 1961; 107:268–278.

Avison WR, Speechley K: The discharged psychiatric patients: A review of social, social-psychological and psychiatric correlates of outcome. *Am J Psychiatry* 1987; 144:10–18.

Beavers WR, Blumberg S: A follow-up study of adolescents treated in an inpatient setting. *Dis Nerv Syst* 1968; 29:606–612.

Canfield M, Muller J, Clarkin J, et al: Issues in research design in psychiatric hospitals. *Psychiatr Hosp* 1988; 19:11–26.

Durkin RP, Durkin A: Evaluating residential treatment programs for disturbed children, in Guttentag M, Struening E (eds): *Handbook of Evaluation Research,* vol 2. Beverly Hills, Calif, Sage Publications, 1975.

Garber B: *Follow-up Study of Hospitalized Adolescents.* New York, Brunner/Mazel, 1972, p 156.

Hartmann E, et al: *Adolescents in a Mental Hospital.* New York, Grune & Stratton, 1968.

King L, Pittman G: A six-year follow-up study of sixty-five adolescent patients: Predictive value of presenting clinical picture. *Br J Psychiatry* 1969; 115:1441.

Korowitz J, et al: A follow-up study of hospitalized adolescents. *Compr Psychiatry* 1974; 15:41.

Kling V, Piggott L, Knitter E, et al: A follow-up study of psychiatrically hospitalized adolescents. *Adolescence* 1986; 21:697–701.

Masterson J: Prognosis in adolescent disorders. *Am J Psychiatry* 1958; 114:1097–1103.

Masterson J: Prognosis in adolescent disorders—Schizophrenia. *J Nerv Ment Dis* 1956; 124:219.

Pollack M, Lovenstein S, Klein D: A three-year post-hospital follow-up of adolescents and adult schizophrenics. *Am J Orthopsychiatry* 1968; 38:106–107.

Pfeiffer SI: Follow-up of children and adolescents treated in psychiatric facilities: A methodology review. *Psychiatr Hosp* 1989; 20:15–20.

Reif BA: A follow-up study of selected adolescents treated in a short-term, all-adolescent psychiatric hospital unit (Dissertation). Abstract International 41: 1980.

Welner A, Welner Z, Fishman R: Psychiatric adolescent inpatients: Eight- to ten-year follow-up. *Arch Gen Psychiatry* 1979; 36:698–700.

10 | Training and Research in Inpatient Units

The inpatient adolescent service provides an excellent opportunity for training medical students, general psychiatry residents, child psychiatry residents, pediatric residents, and trainees from social work and psychology. The inpatient environment is particularly suited for new trainees who need a great deal of supervision to learn basic psychiatry skills. There are a large number of professionals working with each patient who can provide supervision and feedback to new trainees. The fear on the part of new trainees that they might do some harm to their patients is easily dispelled by immediate positive feedback from patients and staff.

There are several areas of the psychiatric curriculum that can be taught best in the inpatient adolescent service. The curriculum may be organized into cognitive objectives and skill objectives.

Although the primary emphasis is on learning basic psychiatric skills, it should be accompanied by some discussion of the knowledge in those areas. The necessary cognitive objectives may be achieved by acquiring some knowledge in the following areas:

1. Normal adolescent development.
2. Adolescent development with a chronic illness.
3. Substance abuse by adolescents.
4. Acute and chronic models of psychiatric care.
5. Goal-oriented brief psychotherapy with the adolescent.
6. Goal-oriented brief family therapy.
7. Psychopharmacology.
8. Group therapy in an adolescent inpatient unit.
9. Management of common psychopathology in hospitalized adolescents.
10. Administrative tasks in inpatient psychiatry.
11. Legal issues in inpatient psychiatry.

It is important to explain the expectations that an inpatient service has for its trainees. Many trainees are likely to feel overwhelmed in the hospital unit because of the large number of staff involved in the care of patients. Their primary difficulty lies in trying to assess the hierarchy of various administrative and therapy staff members and their influence on patient care. The role of the trainees should be explained clearly with regard to their work, participation in various seminars and meetings, frequency of sessions with patients, and frequency of progress notes in the chart. The above curriculum may be presented in once-a-week hour-long seminars, which should be attended by all psychiatric trainees.

The following descriptions are examples of material in each of the cognitive skill areas. Certainly, more lengthy modules for each area can be organized and delivered if time permits.

NORMAL ADOLESCENT DEVELOPMENT

Adolescence is a developmental stage of intense turmoil in Western societies. The onset of adolescence is usually associated with puberty, which is a biological event characterized by increased activity of the hypothalamic-pituitary-gonadal axis and by rapid and progressive changes in the musculoskeletal system and secondary sexual characteristics. As biological development progresses, there are associated changes in intellectual functions, emotional adjustments, and social relationships. However, emotional adjustment frequently lags behind, and many adolescents find it hard to give up their childhood dependency needs and take on the responsibilities consistent with their physical and cognitive development. Sexual fantasies and scenarios involving interaction with the opposite sex become the major preoccupation of adolescent thought. Cognitive changes are as dramatic as the physical changes and include increased comprehension and abstract reasoning. These cognitive changes allow adolescents to question the values of their parents and those of the society. Slowly, they begin to blend various values into something that is unique to them or their generation of adolescents. Establishing emotional independence and self-identity are two major tasks of the adolescent years. Many adolescents are not able to establish their self-identity by the end of the teenage years. Some may suffer an identity crisis, with no clear sense of self and no plan for achieving a place in the world.

The learning objectives for trainees include the following:

1. Tanner's classification of sexual maturity in girls and boys.
2. Cognitive development of formal operations during adolescence.
3. Identity formation during adolescence.
4. Phases of adolescence.
5. The second individuation process of adolescence.
6. Adolescent turmoil.

Adolescent Development With a Chronic Illness

The presence of a chronic illness or a developmental disability puts an additional burden on the adolescent and requires extra emotional and physical efforts to cope with them. Most chronic illnesses such as asthma, diabetes, and epilepsy seem to get worse with the onset of adolescence. Emotional turmoil and difficulties in coping with the illness appear to be the major contributory factors in the worsening of the illness. All aspects of adolescent life are affected by the presence of a chronic illness or developmental disability. There is decreased interest and motivation for academic achievement, and interest in sports activities and hobbies may also diminish. The adolescent may withdraw from social contact with his peers. He may deny his illness and participate in activities that aggravate his illness. Depression and substance abuse may become the primary manifestations of an underlying difficulty in coping with a chronic illness or developmental disability.

Learning objectives for residents include the following:

1. Understanding the influences of chronic illnesses and developmental disabilities on adolescent development.
2. Learning techniques to help these adolescents to cope better with their handicaps.

Substance Abuse by Adolescents

Almost all adolescents experiment with smoking, drinking, and other psychoactive substances. Although the majority do not progress beyond the experimental stage, some become frequent and regular abusers of drugs. The learning objectives of this section are to help trainees understand the following:

1. The factors contributing to more frequent and regular abuse of drugs.
2. The effects of drug abuse on the relationships of adolescents with peers and family.
3. Changes in the level of interest in achievement and other extracurricular activities.
4. Different philosophies of treatment for substance abuse.
5. Who should be treated as an outpatient and who should be hospitalized.
6. Long-term outcome of counseling for substance abuse in inpatient and outpatient settings.

For further discussion see Chapter 2 and the works in "Suggested Reading."

ACUTE AND CHRONIC MODELS OF PSYCHIATRIC CARE

Currently psychiatric care of disturbed adolescents is provided in different types of facilities that may be grouped into three categories:

1. Short-term psychiatric care is usually provided in general hospital settings for adolescents who are hospitalized for an acute psychiatric emergency. The duration of treatment is about 4 to 6 weeks.

2. Medium-term psychiatric care is usually provided in state-funded institutions or private hospitals that can treat adolescents for much longer periods of time, usually 4 to 6 months. These adolescents are not able to derive enough benefits from short-term treatment to return to the community and need more extended psychiatric care than the short-term facilities can provide.

3. Long-term psychiatric care is provided in residential treatment centers and long-term psychiatric hospitals. The treatment may last from a few months to several years.

The learning objectives for trainees include the following:

1. Understanding of various models of short- and long-term psychiatric care.
2. Learn various indications for different types of psychiatric care.
3. Treatment outcome of short- and long-term psychiatric care.

For further discussion see "Suggested Reading" and Chapters 8 and 9.

GOAL-ORIENTED BRIEF PSYCHOTHERAPY WITH ADOLESCENTS

Most hospitalized adolescents need to sort out the factors contributing to their hospitalization. They should be helped to focus on issues that must be resolved before discharge. Adolescent patients are frequently confused about their problems and tend to blame their environment including family, peers, and school. Some therapists overly empathize with the adolescent and focus all their energies on finding fault with the environment. Obviously, this is a mistake involving transference issues. Although therapists should carefully explore all environmental factors, adolescent patients should be helped to assess the extent of their own contribution to the problem and focus on bringing about changes in those areas.

Learning objectives should include the following:

1. Understanding the adolescent's perspective on his problems.
2. Therapeutic issues related to goal-oriented brief psychotherapy.
3. Outcome studies of goal-oriented brief psychotherapy.

Further discussion can be found in Chapter 3 and "Suggested Reading."

GOAL-ORIENTED BRIEF FAMILY THERAPY

The hospitalization of an adolescent is frequently preceded by a family crisis. Although hospitalization may end the crisis, it usually leads to the emergence of guilt and self-blaming on the part of parents and other family members. Sometimes these feelings of guilt are intensified by the manipulation of the adolescent patient who may call his family and complain of being miserable in the hospital. The patient may describe the hospital staff and the program in a most negative manner. The guilt-ridden parents are frequently overcome by the unhappy plight of their adolescent and may take him out of the hospital against medical advice.

Counseling for the family of a hospitalized adolescent frequently requires an initial assessment of the role of the adolescent patient in the family, the parental capacity to set appropriate limits to adolescent behavior, and the presence of other conflicts and turmoil in the family. The family therapy sessions during the hospitalization of the adolescent are generally used to improve communication between the patient and his family and to begin an open dialogue on major issues in the family.

The learning objectives of this section (see also Chapter 3) for the trainees include the following:

1. Become familiar with the developmental process in the family system.
2. Learn about the adolescent phase of the family life cycle.
3. Learn the general systems theory of family dynamics.
4. Become familiar with the parameters of a brief family therapy.

PSYCHOPHARMACOLOGY

Most trainees in psychiatry receive lectures in psychopharmacology before rotating through adolescent inpatient psychiatry. They are generally knowledgeable about various psychotropic drugs and their therapeutic effects and side effects. Many of them have been giving these medications to their adult psychiatric patients. The learning objectives in psychopharmacology in the adolescent unit should emphasize the following:

1. Specific indications of psychotropic medications in adolescent disorders.
2. Differences in doses and side effects of psychotropic drugs between adults and adolescents.
3. Explanation of the medication's effects and side effects to both the parents and the adolescents to obtain their cooperation before prescribing medication to the adolescents.
4. Outcome studies of psychopharmacological treatment of various adolescent disorders.

For a discussion of the psychopharmacological treatment of various adolescent psychiatric disorders see Chapter 5 and "Suggested Reading."

GROUP THERAPY IN THE ADOLESCENT INPATIENT UNIT

A great deal of therapeutic work in the inpatient adolescent unit is carried out in the form of group therapy (see also Chapter 3). Adolescents, in general, seem to respond better to a group therapy format of treatment. They are more comfortable in the company of their peers and can participate in group discussions more easily. Our inpatient unit has two types of groups: general group therapy and special focused groups. Participation in general therapy groups is required of all patients. However, special focused groups (i.e., groups for adopted children, groups for adolescents of divorced parents, and groups for sexually abused girls) are voluntary for adolescents with specific problems. All therapy groups are time limited to the duration of hospitalization (4 to 6 weeks). Although most therapeutic skills are learned through apprenticeship with experienced group leaders, it is necessary for trainees to have a basic knowledge of the dynamics of short-term goal-oriented group therapy in an inpatient adolescent unit.

The learning objectives for trainees include the following:

1. Major issues in adolescent therapy groups such as limit setting, control, and rebellion against authority.
2. The role of the group therapist.
3. Setting goals in group therapy.
4. Therapeutic processes in group therapy.
5. Focused groups.

MANAGEMENT OF COMMON PSYCHOPATHOLOGY IN HOSPITALIZED ADOLESCENTS

The most common types of disorder seen in adolescent inpatient units include conduct disorders, substance abuse disorders, depression, adjustment disorders, and parent-child conflict (see Chapter 5 for the specific management of various disorders). A careful evaluation of each patient should result in a dynamic formulation of the problem that is based on a biopsychosocial model of psychopathology. It is important for trainees to understand that the treatment of most psychiatric disorders in adolescents, in addition to pharmacotherapy, includes intervention in the psychosocial factors related to the family and the community contributing to the etiology of the problems. The trainees should also plan treatment with a clear understanding of all the biopsychosocial factors related to a particular case. Since the duration of hospitalization is short and it is usually impossible to work on all the factors contributing to the psychopathology, it is necessary to select the areas of intervention that are likely to produce maximum results during hospitalization. Other factors may be left for the community mental health agencies to resolve in an outpatient therapeutic setting.

The management of acute symptoms such as aggression, anxiety, agitation, depression, and intoxication is based on the combined principles of behavioral management and pharmacological treatment. Some institutions prefer a trial of behavior management before considering drug treatment. However, in most acute cases, a combined treatment is generally more helpful.

Learning objectives for this section include the following:

1. Knowledge of the diagnosis, treatment, and prognosis of the common psychiatric disorders treated in inpatient adolescent units.

2. Treatment outcome studies of the disorders.
3. Management of acute agitation, aggression, anxiety, suicidal behavior, and intoxication in hospitalized adolescents.

ADMINISTRATIVE PSYCHIATRY

Psychiatric trainees need to communicate with various members of the psychiatric team and provide leadership. It is the ability to verbalize a thoughtful and comprehensive treatment plan that creates leadership, not the administrative authority bestowed upon the psychiatrist. Different members of the therapy team have different amounts of training and experience, and the views expressed by them may not be consistent with those of the psychiatrist. However, the role of the psychiatrist is to integrate all these varying thoughts and suggestions into a comprehensive treatment plan. Even an ideal treatment plan will fail if the members of the treatment team are unable to comprehend it and, consequently, unwilling to carry it out. New psychiatric trainees are frequently frustrated with other members of the therapy team who are viewed as obstructing their ideal treatment plan. Agreeing with the team may imply to some trainees that they have to sacrifice their desire for the best possible care for their patient and settle for a second-rate treatment. Each member of the team may feel the same way and has the same basic goal of providing the best care for his patient.

Management of the therapy team requires a special type of leadership on the part of the psychiatrist. The psychiatrist should develop the skills to integrate the different views expressed by the team members into a comprehensive treatment plan.

Learning objectives for trainees for this section include the following:

1. Understanding of the workings of a milieu.
2. Learning to work as a member as well as a leader of the therapy team.
3. Understanding the concept of sapiential authority (authority acquired through knowledge).
4. Fulfilling additional objectives including administrative theories and practices relative to leadership of a clinical psychiatric unit (i.e., unit director).

LEGAL ISSUES IN INPATIENT PSYCHIATRY

Laws relating to voluntary psychiatric hospitalization and commitment of adolescents vary somewhat from state to state, especially with regard to the input required by the department of justice in the process of commitment. However, psychiatrists themselves should be cognizant of the civil rights of each patient and should not recommend commitment unless the necessity for extended treatment cannot be worked out with the patient through therapeutic dialogue. The trainees should become aware of the state mental health code for minors, especially the sections relating to hospitalization, commitment, conditions for discharge, isolation, seclusion, restraints, and the use of medication and electroshock treatment.

In addition, knowledge of the laws relating to child abuse, sexual abuse, neglect, and the custody rights of parents are frequently necessary in dealing with the problems of hospitalized adolescents. Other laws relating to mental health, competency to stand trial, rights to treatment and rights to refuse treatment, confidentiality, and informed consent are similar to those for adult psychiatric patients.

Teaching Methods

Once-a-week teaching seminars in the inpatient adolescent unit may be sufficient to achieve most of the cognitive objectives described in the above sections. The material, however, is best integrated by the application of the knowledge to actual clinical cases seen in the inpatient unit. Teachers may ask the trainees to present relevant cases during the discussion of various topics.

SPECIFIC SKILL OBJECTIVES FOR THE INPATIENT SERVICE

1. To conduct a complete psychiatric diagnostic evaluation including a comprehensive physical and neurological examination and to record the findings in the medical record.
2. To make use of appropriate laboratory examinations, psychological testing, and other consultations as indicated in the work-up of psychiatric problems.
3. To conduct family interviews, both diagnostic and therapeutic.
4. To make accurate psychiatric diagnoses and thorough appraisals of the presenting problems, both emotional and physical.
5. To formulate a comprehensive treatment plan, mobilize resources to implement the plan, and evaluate the effectiveness of such a plan and make changes based on such evaluation.
6. To use psychopharmacological agents and other medications well while being especially aware of pharmacological effects, psychological effects, and effects on the comprehensive treatment plan.
7. To provide thorough medical evaluations on all appropriate patients through complete physical examinations, judicious use of laboratory tests, and appropriate consultation requests.
8. To conduct some inpatient group therapy meetings.
9. To work effectively within a multidisciplinary team structure in terms of patient evaluation, treatment planning, and comprehensive inpatient treatment.
10. To learn the essential elements of an effective treatment milieu.
11. To use short-term individual psychotherapy to achieve specific therapeutic goals.

12. To become aware of countertransference problems and personal idiosyncrasies as they influence interactions with patients and their families and begin to learn to deal with them constructively.
13. To carry out appropriate and comprehensive discharge planning while taking into account all available community resources and making appropriate referrals for aftercare.
14. To select appropriate patients and families for continued longer-term outpatient treatment.

Teaching Methods

The number of teaching methods used and the amount of time spent in teaching activities on the inpatient unit depend upon the availability of faculty time. Ideally, each trainee should be provided with a supervisor with whom the trainee may model himself in doing diagnostic and therapeutic work with patients and families. It is important that the primary model be provided by the teacher or supervisor of the same discipline. However, various therapeutic techniques may be taught by individuals involved in carrying out those therapies such as a group therapist or a family therapist. Unfortunately, most inpatient adolescent units have a small number of faculty with a limited amount of time. In such situations, a modified apprenticeship method may be used to provide skill training. The aforementioned skills are best learned by active participation in various diagnostic and therapeutic activities. Teachers are in the best position to demonstrate their techniques of individual therapy, group therapy, and family counseling. We find that interviewing patients of trainees with them on a periodic basis keeps the supervisor abreast of the progress of each case as well as provides new directions for the trainees for further treatment of their patients. A similar apprenticeship method is used for family therapy and group therapy. A 15- to 20-minute period must be set aside for discussion with trainees after each session.

In addition to these daily teaching activities, presentation of selected cases at a once-a-week case conference is helpful, as is a literature review relating to the cases. Similarly, brief daily morning rounds with trainees are helpful in reviewing the current treatment of each case and for planning further treatment.

ROLE OF PSYCHIATRY RESIDENTS IN THE INPATIENT UNIT

It is important to orient the new psychiatry residents in regard to their role in the unit. Most residents tend to behave quite inappropriately with regard to their role in the milieu. Some of them take over the role of an attending psychiatrist and direct the treatment of their patients without fully knowing the rules of the milieu and without consulting other members of the treatment team. These residents generally have an unpleasant experience in the unit because they quickly lose the cooperation of the milieu staff. We advise our new trainees not to make any major decision without consulting the attending psychiatrist and/or other members of the team during the first 2 weeks of their rotation. It is better for them to overcommunicate with the unit staff than undercommunicate with regard to their understanding of the treatment plan. Most adolescent units have developed set policies with regard to various privileges such as telephone times, outings, visiting with family and friends, and smoking. Residents must familiarize themselves with these policies before granting any privileges to the patients. It is essential that residents participate in the meetings of the therapy team and learn the process of making decisions regarding the treatment and discharge plan of each patient. It is also important for trainees to understand the philosophy underlying the concept of the psychiatric team in the management of the hospitalized adolescent.

Residents play a major role in teaching medical students and other trainees. They need to present themselves as models for their students. Initially, all interviews with patients should be carried out jointly by the resident and students, at least for the first week of student rotation. The students can then be allowed to spend time with patients by themselves.

RESEARCH ACTIVITIES ON THE INPATIENT UNIT

Research in an inpatient unit is essential not only to train the psychiatric residents in research methodology but also to improve the clinical care of patients. It is surprising that clinicians of various disciplines continue to hold strong beliefs with regard to the effectiveness of their interventions without any supporting scientific evidence. A lot of practices continue to exist because they seem to have public appeal and sound good when described. The idea of scientifically testing their well-established clinical practices rarely occurs to most clinicians. In order to establish an environment of investigation and research, one must create an atmosphere of willingness on the part of all clinicians to test their set routines and practices with the aim of improving their effectiveness. This is an ideal goal but is rarely accomplished, even in the best circumstances. There are those professionals who oppose research verbally and in attitude because they believe most clinical research to be a waste of time. Some are simply jealous of other people's efforts that they are unable to carry out themselves.

Mark Riddle (1989) has emphasized creation of a shared value system among the staff—a belief that increased knowledge through research will provide better care for patients. Such beliefs can be maximized by holding regular research conferences in the unit that describe new findings and their application to patient care. These conferences may also be used to describe new research studies planned for the unit. In fact, most new studies may be discussed in these conferences, even before they are submitted to the research committee for approval. The staff can be quite helpful in planning the study by pointing out various problems that may be encountered in carrying out a particular study.

Research activities on an inpatient unit should be kept within a reasonable limit in order not to overwhelm the staff or the patients. The inpatient units are generally very busy and require a great deal of time and effort on the part of each staff member. Filling out a new questionnaire or doing an extra assessment or collection of 24-hour urine may be quite taxing and should not be introduced without a great deal of planning. A medical school–affiliated service is likely to have multiple requests for carrying out new research. It is difficult for the staff to decide which research study should be given top priority over others and thus begun first. The medical director of the unit or an associate research director should have the job of assigning priority to the research studies. Although there is no easy system, the director must not sacrifice patient therapy time to the god of research.

It has become apparent in recent years that trainees not exposed to research rarely become involved in doing research themselves. Child psychiatry has lagged behind in the production of research. Several training programs are now requiring child psychiatry residents to carry out a study or at least write a paper describing a research project. This is a healthy trend and should be promoted in all child psychiatry training programs. Child psychiatry residents should be told about designing a research study or writing a paper at the beginning of their training program so that they may have ample time to think about it and discuss it with their peers and the staff. However, primary research activities should be part of the second-year curriculum. Inpatient adolescent services provide an excellent opportunity for residents to participate in ongoing research. Residents should be involved in evaluation and data collection from research patients. This participation provides the residents with a good opportunity to learn various structured interview schedules such as the KIDDIE Schedule for Affective Disorders and Schizophrenia (K-SADS), Hamilton's Depression and Anxiety scales, and structured interview for DSM III. Periodic conferences in which residents present their research proposals or papers would certainly raise the level of interest in research projects among all residents.

SUGGESTED READING

Normal Adolescent Development

Blos P: Phases of adolescence, in *On Adolescence: A Psychoanalytic Interpretation.* New York, Free Press, 1962, pp 52–157.
Blos P: Second individuation process of adolescence. *Psychoanal Study Child* 1967; 22:162–187.
Erikson E: *Identity: Youth and Crisis.* New York, WW Norton, 1968.
Keniston K: *The Uncommitted.* New York, Harcourt, Brace & World, 1965.
Piaget J: The Intellectual Development of the Adolescent, in Kaplan G, Lebovici S (eds): *Adolescence: Psychosocial Perspectives.* New York, Basic Books Inc Publishers, 1969, pp 22–26.
Tanner GM: *Growth of Adolescence,* ed 2. Oxford, Blackwell Scientific Publications, 1962.

Adolescent Development With a Chronic Illness

Gode RO, Smith MS: Effects of chronic disorders on adolescent development: Self, family, friends and school, in Smith MS (ed): *Chronic Disorders in Adolescents.* Boston, John Wright PSP Inc, 1983, pp 31–44.
Hodgman CH, McAnarney ER, Myers G, et al: Emotional complications of adolescent grand mal epilepsy. *J Pediatr* 1979; 95:309–312.
Zeltzer L, Ellenberg L, Rigler D, et al: Psychological effects of illness, II. Impact of illness in adolescents, crucial issues and coping style. *J Pediatr* 1980; 97:132–138.

Substance Abuse by Adolescents

Bailey GW: Current perspectives on substance abuse in youths. *J Am Child Adolesc Psychiatry* 1989; 28:151–162.

Friedman AS, Beschner GN: *Treatment Services for Adolescent Substance Abusers.* Rockville, Md, National Institute on Drug Abuse, 1985.

Kandel DB: Epidemiological and psycho-social perspectives on adolescent drug use. *J Am Acad Child Psychiatry* 1982; 21:328–347.

MacDonald RI: *Drugs, Drinking and Adolescence.* Chicago, Year Book Medical Publishers Inc, 1984.

Acute and Chronic Models of Psychiatric Care

Harper G: Focal-inpatient treatment planning. *J Am Acad Child Adolesc Psychiatry* 1989; 28:31–36.

Nurcombe B: Goal-directed treatment planning and the principles of brief hospitalization. *J Am Acad Child Adolesc Psychiatry* 1989; 28:26–30.

Stone LA: Residential treatment, in Noshpitz JD (ed): *Basic Handbook of Child Psychiatry,* vol 3. New York, Basic Books Inc Publishers, 1979, pp 231–262.

Goal-Oriented Brief Psychotherapy With Adolescents

Barrow JC: Coping-skill training: A brief therapy approach for students with evaluative anxieties. *Gen Am College Health* 1982; 30:269–274.

Bolten MP: Short-term residential psychotherapy: Psychotherapy in a nutshell. *Psychother Psychosom* 1984; 41:109–115.

Budman SH, et al: Advances in brief psychotherapy: A review of the recent literature. *Hosp Community Psychiatry* 1983; 34:939–946.

Haley J: *Problem-Solving Therapy.* New York, Harper & Row Publishers Inc (Colophon Books), 1976.

Moultrie MB, et al: Short-term inpatient treatment of children and adolescents. *J Sci Med Assoc* 1983; 79:30–32.

Reich J, et al: Principles common to different short-term psychotherapies. *Am J Psychother* 1984; 40:62–69.

Sifneos PE: The current status of individual short-term dynamic psychotherapy and its failure: An overview. *Am J Psychother* 1984; 38:472–483.

Goal-Oriented Brief Family Therapy

Ackerman NJ: The family with adolescents, in Carter EA, McGoldrick M (eds): *The Family Lifecycle: A Framework for Family Therapy.* New York, Gardner Press Inc, 1980.

DeShazer S, et al: Brief psychotherapy: Focused solution development. *Fam Process* 1986; 25:207–221.

Fisher SG: Time limited brief therapy with families: A one-year follow-up study. *Fam Process* 1984; 23:101–106.

Kaufmann L: The rationale for the family approach with adolescents. *Adolesc Psychiatry* 1986; 13:493–509.

O'Shea MD, et al: Multiple family therapy: Current status and critical appraisal. *Fam Process* 1985; 24:555–582.

Wellner JS: Matchmaking: Choosing the appropriate therapy for families at various levels of pathology, in Mirkin MP, Koman SL (eds): *Handbook of Adolescence and Family Therapy.* New York, Gardner Press Inc, 1985, pp 39–53.

Whitley NJ, et al: Family therapy in a hospital setting: A model for time limited treatment. *Gen Psychoactive Drugs* 1986; 18:61–64.

Psychopharmacology

Ambrosini PJ: Pharmacotherapy in child and adolescent major depressive disorders, in Meltzer HY (ed): *Psychopharmacology. The Third Generation of Progress.* New York, Raven Press, 1987, pp 1247–1254.

Campbell N, Green W, Deutsch S: *Child and Adolescent Psychopharmacology.* Beverly Hills, Calif, Sage Publications, 1985.

Campbell N, Spencer N: Psychopharmacology in child and adolescent psychiatry. *J Am Acad Child Adolesc Psychiatry* 1988; 27:269–279.

Group Therapy in the Adolescent Inpatient Unit

Butcher JN, Koss MP: Research on brief and crisis-oriented therapies, in Bergin AE, Garfield SL (eds): *Handbook of Psychotherapy and Behavior Change.* New York, John Wiley & Sons Inc, 1978, pp 725–767.

Klein RH: Some principles of short-term group therapy. *Int J Group Psychother* 1985; 35:309–328.

Pekala RJ, Siegel IM, Farrar DM: Problem-solving support group: Structural group therapy with psychiatric inpatients. *Int J Group Psychother* 1985; 35:391–409.

Poey K: Guidelines for the practice of brief dynamic group therapy. *Int J Group Psychother* 1985; 35:331–354.

Yolom ID: *The Theory and Practice of Group Psychotherapy,* ed 2. New York, Basic Books Inc Publishers, 1975.

Zabusky G, Kymissis P: Identity group therapy: A transitional group for hospitalized adolescents. *Int J Group Psychother* 1983; 33:99–109.

Management of Common Psychopathology in Hospitalized Adolescents

Shaffer D, Ehrardt A, Greenhill L (eds): *The Clinical Guide to Child Psychiatry.* New York, Free Press, 1985.

Administrative Psychiatry

Abrams RC, Sweeney JA: A critique of the process-oriented approach to ward staff meetings. *Am J Psychiatry* 1982; 139:769–773.

Borus JF: Teaching residents the administrative aspect of psychiatric practice. *Am J Psychiatry* 1983; 140:444–448.

Geraty R: Administrative issues in inpatient child and adolescent psychiatry. *J Am Acad Child Adolesc Psychiatry* 1989; 28:21–25.

Talbott J, Kaplan S: *Psychiatric Administration.* New York, Grune & Stratton, 1983.

Legal Issues in Inpatient Psychiatry

Burlingame, Amaya: Psychiatric commitment of children and adolescents, in
Schetky, Benedek (eds): *Issues, Current Practice and Clinical Impact in
Emerging Issues in Child Psychiatry and the Law,* 1985.
State mental health code relating to minors.

Research Activities on the Inpatient Unit

Riddle M: Research on a children's psychiatric inpatient service. *J Am Acad Child
Adolesc Psychiatry* 1989; 28:42–46.

11 | Mental Health Education for Patients and Families

It is generally assumed that knowledge about a disease improves the patient's cooperation with his treatment. It also reduces anxiety and improves coping skills. This hypothesis has been proved to be correct in a number of studies related to chronic illnesses (Anderson et al., 1986) such as asthma, cystic fibrosis, muscular dystrophy, and congenital heart disease. In fact, many agencies providing health care, hospitals, and drug companies utilize educational approaches to acquaint their consumers with their services and products. Regularly published newsletters by health organizations frequently include new information about diet, exercise, physical fitness, and common diseases to attract consumer attention. Similarly, book publishers and writers have seized upon the public's concern with youth and longevity so that hundreds of monographs and books are published each year on subjects such as diet, physical fitness, exercise, and cholesterol.

The educational approach in mental health has become increasingly acceptable. Most of the popular literature in this field, however, relates to child development, parenting skills, coping with stress, and assertiveness. With the exception of schizophrenia and mood disorders, other mental health problems are rarely addressed by the mass media. One of the major difficulties of communicating information about mental disorders is related to the existence of multiple explanations and theories of mental illness. Most books written for the layperson tend to emphasize one point of view such as the social, the psychological, or the biological causes of mental illness. The public, in general, tends to subscribe to social and psychological causes and is least aware of the biological mechanisms of mental disorders.

Wide dissemination of mental health information through books and the news media appears to have helped the public to become less ashamed of and less secretive about their mental problems and more willing to seek psychiatric help. Similarly, knowledgeable patients show more compliance with psychiatric treatment. Mental health education in a hospital setting is designed to help the hospitalized adolescent and his family to understand the factors contributing to their problems and to cope with them in a manner that maximizes the benefits of treatment to the patient and his family.

PLANNING A CURRICULUM

It is difficult to plan one curriculum for all psychiatric patients because of the differences in the nature and intensity of their problems. Also, the presence of emotional problems diminishes the amount of energy and interest available to invest in learning new material. The mental health curriculum should include basic ideas about mental problems. The information should be applicable to the current problems of the patients. The inpatient staff should chose a dozen topics and clearly outline the objectives to be achieved with each topic. The topics have to be fairly general so that each patient may relate to the subject matter. The nursing staff should be able to present the information and lead group discussions.

These topics should include some of the following:

1. Coping with stress.
2. Managing anger.
3. Communication with the family.
4. Communication with peers.
5. Assertiveness.
6. Self-esteem.
7. Peer pressure.
8. Methods of relaxation.
9. Problem solving.
10. Love and rejection.
11. Love and sex.
12. Legal rights of adolescents.
13. Experimentation with drugs.
14. Drug treatment.
15. Contraception.
16. Sexually transmitted diseases.
17. Problems of adopted children.
18. Dealing with separation and divorce of parents.
19. Facing a stepparent.
20. Problems and joys of teenage pregnancy.

Parents are frequently concerned about the causes of emotional problems. Commonly asked questions by parents include: "Did we cause his problems?" "What could we have done differently?" "How do we handle it now?" Answers to these questions require some knowledge of the adolescent phase of development, communication problems with adolescents, peer pressures, techniques of limit setting, and some knowledge of psychopathology.

PRESENTATION AND PROCESSING OF INFORMATION

Enticing a group of emotionally disturbed adolescents to hear a lecture may present a challenge to even the most experienced teachers. It is generally helpful to begin with a question and provide information in the form of answers. For example: "How do you feel when you feel stressed?" "What types of situations cause stress?" "What do I do when I feel stressed?" Answers are provided by the patients as well as by the teachers. Sufficient time should be provided so that each patient can express his views about a question and the information can be processed through group discussion. Teachers should also design short questionnaires and self-learning modules that can be filled out by patients as either a warm-up before the presentation of information or afterward as a test of the acquisition of knowledge.

Mental health information for parents is frequently presented to groups of multiple families. These groups prefer short lectures followed by questions from the audience period and group discussions. The psychoeducational approach is sometimes contrasted with multiple family therapy groups in which information is processed through discussion by the members of the group. The families provide support for each other. They also share their own experiences of success and failure in coping with the patient's illness. Better communication and understanding are frequently emphasized as a primary goal of multiple family therapy. Laqueur et al. (1964) emphasized that the two main objectives to be achieved in multiple family therapy are (1) improving communication within the family and (2) gaining a better understanding of the reasons for family conflicts. Multiple-family therapy groups present a special problem in the adolescent inpatient unit because they are open groups with frequent changes in the composition of members. The goals of therapy are limited and short-term, with active participation on the part of the therapist. Some particularly aggressive parents may manipulate the group enough to minimize the full participation of the other families. It usually takes a long time before a group of families develops supportive relationships with each other. Anderson et al. (1986) found no significant difference between the satisfaction level of two multiple-family groups. One of the groups received brief group therapy and the other psychoeducation.

SOME EXAMPLES OF THE PATIENT CURRICULUM

Coping With Stress

This module may be presented with an example of stress. The teacher may ask one of the patients in advance to present his situation of stress. Help the patient organize his material so that it can answer the following questions: What factors caused the stress? How does stress feel? What did they do to reduce the stress?

The information to be presented should include the following. Stress is a feeling. Different people experience this feeling differently. Some have an uneasy feeling, some become "nervous," and others become irritable and angry. Most people develop bodily symptoms such as headaches, stomachaches, general weakness, and sweating. Few people recognize that their feelings and physical symptoms are the result of stress.

Stress is caused by circumstances that are difficult to deal with. Some people are better able to deal with difficult circumstances than others are, but everybody has a breakdown point or exhaustion stage.

Different people cope with stress in different manners:

1. By avoiding stress-producing situations.
2. By dealing with the causes of stress.
3. By using substances such as alcohol or drugs that numb their senses.

Appropriate steps in dealing with stress include the following:

1. Recognize that certain feelings and bodily symptoms are stress related.
2. Find the causes that are producing the stress.
3. Think how you could handle the stress-producing factors better.
4. If the circumstances are too overwhelming, seek help from friends, relatives, and parents, or mental health professionals who are more understanding and can provide better advice.
5. Remember that stress is experienced less if a person is in good physical health and is well rested.

This information should be broken down into small sections, each represented by a question such as the following:

1. What is stress?
2. What causes stress?
3. How do different people cope with stressful situations?
4. What are some of the better ways of handling stress?

The teacher should pose one question at a time to the group and ask the group to respond (spontaneously or by directly asking different patients). The presenter should utilize a chalkboard on which to write the questions and responses. Patients should be supplied with paper and pencil to take notes if they desire.

Managing Anger

Information on this topic may include the following:

1. Anger is a normal emotion that, like fear, is an instrument for dealing with a threatening environment. In anger, a person takes action against the threat. In fear he retreats from it.
2. Sources of anger vary at different ages. Young children become angry if their physical needs and activities are interferred with. Older children and adults become angry when their possessions are taken away, someone thwarts their plans or expectations, they perceive that their rights are violated or treated unjustly, somebody takes advantage of them, or they are abused or threatened with harm.
3. Susceptibility to anger increases when a person is tired, exhausted, hungry, irritated, recovering from an illness, or living in an overcrowded quarters.

Anger may be expressed in various ways:

1. Directly to the source of anger.
2. In displacement (finding a scapegoat).
3. In a passive/aggressive manner (slow, quiet protest).
4. Losing touch with anger (repression).
5. Directing the anger against themselves (hurting oneself, verbalizations such as "I hate myself," "I am a clutz," or "I am stupid").

There are many individual differences in the expression of anger. For example, some people become very physical—hit, kick, or throw punches—while others are very verbal and use obscenities and call names. There are some who become very quiet and withdrawn and do not speak to the person with whom they are angry.

Most expressions of anger are excessive, more than the situation warrants.

Handling angry feelings is very difficult for most people. These feelings can be blocked by reasoning and affection. In order to assess the situation correctly, the angry person must calm down enough to evaluate the situation. Understanding the point of view of the other person involved in the angry exchange is important to evaluate the situation correctly. A temporary reduction in anger may be achieved by various relaxation techniques and/or punching one's own pillow. Anger may be blocked by excusing the offender, "He did not mean it." The angry person may recognize his increased susceptibility as a result of being overtired. Some people may take the responsibility for angry situations by saying "I had it coming."

The following questions should be raised in discussion to cover the aforementioned information:

1. What is anger?
2. How does it compare with other emotions such as fear and sadness?
3. Why do we get angry? (Sources of anger.)
4. How do we know when somebody is angry? (Verbal, physical, and facial gestures.)
5. How do different people express their anger?
6. What are the different ways of managing anger?

Self-Esteem

Awareness of self occurs very early during childhood. Young children focus mostly on their physical attributes to recognize themselves as unique individuals. Cognitive advances during the adolescent years allow the adolescent to think more abstractly about himself and the world around him. The adolescent becomes more capable of evaluating his behavior, feelings, emotions, and motivations.

Self-concept and self-acceptance are fairly stable in late childhood. These are based primarily on the physical attributes of the child and the type of feedback that the child receives from his parents, teachers, and peers. However, with the onset of adolescence, the self-concept becomes very unstable, with an increasing tendency toward self-criticism and the search for the real truth.

Self-esteem is the worth or value that a person ascribes to himself. This evaluation of self is based on various concrete and abstract attributes such as physical appearance, likability, acceptance by parents and peers, certain special skills, academic achievement, sports abilities, and musical talents. Different adolescents include different items in their self-evaluation. A distinction is also made between actual and ideal self-evaluations. The ideal self refers to what a person really would like to be.

The purpose of this module for adolescent patients is to enhance self-acceptance and self-respect by highlighting the positive and likable attributes of each patient. This goal may be achieved by asking each patient to list his positive attributes. Many adolescent patients are so preoccupied with negative thoughts and feelings about themselves that they do not recognize their positive attributes or are unable to focus on them. This can be helped by providing feedback from peers about their positive attributes. Some authors feel that obsessive preoccupation with negative self-feelings is intensified by the inability of most adolescents to accept positive feedback from others.

The following questions should be raised to cover the aforementioned information:

1. What is self-esteem?
2. How does it develop?
3. On what do different individuals base their self-esteem?
4. How can self-evaluation be improved?

There are several self-esteem inventories that can be utilized to help adolescent patients focus on various aspects of self-esteem. These inventories include Rosenberg's Self-Esteem Scale (1965) and the Piers-Harris Self-Concept Scale (1969).

Positive-Feedback Exercise

This exercise may be carried out in a small group of eight to ten patients. Each patient is provided with the same number of pieces of paper as there are patients in the group. Each patient writes one positive thing on each paper about every other patient. At the end every patient has ten different positive things written by ten different members of the group. The same attributes may be mentioned by different patients. The teacher should utilize a large sheet of paper secured on the wall with plastic tape, with the names of each member of the group written on the top. Each patient is then asked to read the names and the positive attributes that they have written down on their slips of paper. The teacher writes these positive attributes under each name in column format. These sheets of paper should be displayed in the unit for several days before they are put away. Each patient may want to collect all the positive slips of papers for their own keeping.

Communication Skills

Communication problems between an adolescent and his parents are fairly common. Both parties, the adolescent as well as his parents, feel that they are misunderstood by each other. The causes of communication problems lie in the very nature of the developmental stage of adolescence. Adolescents begin to develop intimate relationships with peers and experiment with drinking, smoking, and drugs. They find it difficult to share these activities and the feelings associated with them with their parents for fear of reprisal and imposition of stricter control over their activities. Parents have become sensitized by the increased number of teenage pregnancies and excessive substance abuse in teenage groups. Even a trusting relationship during the preadolescent years turns into distrust and constant suspicion during the adolescent years. Meaningful communication between the parents and the adolescent may cease because of mutual distrust and suspicion. Yelling and screaming may be the only type of communication that is left between the parents and the adolescent. Such episodes are frequently precipitated by parental refusal to allow the adolescent to engage in some activity for lack of a trusting relationship.

Basic communication skills include the following:

1. Effective listening.
2. Exploring.
3. Responding.

Active listening requires paying attention to the speaker, making eye contact, and letting the speaker know that you are listening through body posture, head nodding, or verbal sounds. Certain responses on the part of the listener such as jumping to a conclusion and preparing a reply before the speaker finishes his point interfere with effective listening.

Exploration may be carried out by asking for clarification or elaboration of the speaker's remarks. The responder may respond to the content of the remarks or the affect of the speaker. Similarly, a response can be made to the verbal as well as the nonverbal communication of the speaker. A response to the affect of the speaker usually requires greater involvement and intimacy with the speaker.

The issues to be discussed with the patient group include the following:

1. Good communication skills.
2. Problems in communication with peers.
3. Problems in communication with parents.

Practical exercises to promote communication skills should be organized in small groups of patients in which each patient has the opportunity to communicate on a given topic. The group should discuss problems in communication at the end of each exercise. It is important to practice communication skills in the peer group before the adolescent patient can apply these skills to improve his communication with his parents.

Problem Solving

An infant solves his physical problems of hunger, thirst, cold, and wetness by crying, which attracts the attention of adults who satisfy the needs of the infant. An older child may throw a tantrum in order to have adults provide some of his social and psychological needs. As children grow older, their needs become more complex and require more complex solutions. Teenagers, by virtue of their abstract reasoning, are expected to solve their problems through the use of logic. Young teenagers, however, do not quickly give up their old methods of solving their problems such as temper tantrums, angry outbursts, or crying spells. Problem solving through the use of logic is a gradually acquired process that is developed through experience and practice.

Many individuals become overwhelmed with frustration and anxiety when confronted with a problem. Excessive anxiety and frustration reduce their capacity to solve a problem. The first step in solving a problem is to cool down, relax, and overcome excessive emotions. Then do the following:

1. Identify the problem.
2. Narrow down the problem to a definite source.
3. Think of various solutions and their consequences.
4. Pick out one solution and formulate a plan.
5. Carry out the plan.
6. Evaluate the results.

Different individuals tend to use different methods to resolve their problems. There are those who jump in with both feet and let the sequence of subsequent events take care of the problem. They thus often put themselves at the mercy of uncontrollable events. Some people feel that they have to be in the midst of a problem situation in order to find the right solution. Others take the opposite view and will not face a problem situation unless they have worked out a perfect solution in their mind. However, most people take a middle approach in which they have thought through some solutions but have not come up with a definite plan before facing a problem situation.

The issues to be discussed with patient groups include the following:

1. Developmental aspects of problem solving at different ages.
2. Emotional factors reducing problem-solving capacity.
3. Steps in problem solving.
4. Individual differences in problem solving.

Practical exercises on this topic should be carried out in small groups in which each patient identifies a problem, writes various solutions and the consequences of each solution, and formulates a plan to resolve the problem. At the end of this written exercise, each patient should verbally share his problem, the solution, and the plan to resolve the problem with the group. The group can provide feedback with regard to his solutions and the plan to solve the problems.

Assertiveness

Assertiveness training is frequently confused with being aggressive. This term however, has acquired special meaning in human relations. Assertiveness is considered to be an attitude or expression that lies between passivity and aggressiveness. Although overaggressiveness has always been disliked, passivity has only recently become an undesirable attitude. In fact, human relations experts now belive that assertiveness is a normal human attitude while passivity and aggressiveness are considered abnormal.

Passive individuals hide their feelings of resentment, anxiety, and disappointment with passivity. They are afraid to express their true feelings. They allow other people to make decisions for them. Consequently, their rights may be ignored and infringed upon.

Aggressive individuals are overly preoccupied with their needs, feelings, and rights. They express their feelings at the expense of others. They do not hesitate to dominate and humiliate others to express their frustrations and anger.

Assertive individuals are not afraid to express their feelings and ideas, but they accomplish this without violating the rights of others or dominating them. They stand up for their rights without infringing on the rights of others.

The basic tenet of the assertiveness philosophy is the assumption that honest and open expression of one's feelings and ideas promotes self-respect, builds up free and honest relationships with others, and gives other people an opportunity to change their behavior and attitude.

Assertiveness training was designed initially for individuals who were shy and were unable to express their views. Current training workshops in assertiveness are viewed as helpful for all individuals in promoting personal growth and development. Aggressive individuals are as likely to benefit from such training as passive individuals.

Developmental studies indicate that passivity and aggressiveness are personality traits that develop over a long period of time during childhood and adolescence. No amount of training is likely to overcome these traits completely. However, the goal of such training is to bring the individual from the extreme ends of passivity and aggressiveness toward the middle (assertiveness). When a passive adolescent is trained to be assertive, he is usually awkward in the beginning and frequently appears aggressive in his early attempts to become assertive. Such behavior should not be discouraged, but appropriate feedback should be given to help the adolescent modify his behavior. This concept may be explained to adolescent patients with the example of how an infant learns to walk. They are awkward and fall down frequently and get hurt before they are able to walk with confidence.

The questions to be raised for a discussion of assertiveness training include the following:

1. What is a passive individual like in his behavior, feelings, and relationships?
2. What is an aggressive person like in his behavior, feelings, and relationships?
3. How is assertiveness different from passivity and aggressiveness?
4. What kinds of problems are faced by a passive or an aggressive person when he tries to be assertive?

Training in assertiveness for adolescent patients should be carried out over several sessions. Several self-inventories have been designed to assess one's degree of assertiveness. They may be utilized initially to help adolescents to think about this topic. Further training should include the following self-evaluations:

1. Evaluate yourself on a scale of 1 to 10, 1 being very passive and 10 being very aggressive.
2. List those qualities in yourself that you consider to be passive or aggressive.
3. How do you feel about your being passive or aggressive, with choices being (a) I am comfortable with it, (b) I am not comfortable with it, or (c) I hate it.

These self-evaluations will provide sufficient material for discussion in a small group setting.

MENTAL HEALTH EDUCATION TOPICS FOR FAMILY GROUPS

Some of the examples for mental health education include the following:

1. Effects of adolescent hospitalization on the family.
2. Hospital treatment and beyond.
3. Substance abuse in teenagers.
4. Family recreation patterns.
5. Setting limits for teenage children.
6. Communication problems in the family.
7. How do medications work in psychiatric problems.

PRESENTATION OF INFORMATION TO FAMILIES

Presentation of didactic material to family groups is generally easy and productive. The type of information to be presented should be planned in advance. It can be presented in a brief lecture format for 15 to 20 minutes. The points to be emphasized in the lecture should be written on a chalkboard. At least two thirds of the time should be spent in answering questions and group discussion.

Effects of Hospitalization on the Family

Hospitalization of an adolescent is frequently preceded by a family crisis. The problems of the adolescent escalate to the point where they affect the whole family, and the family is unable to control these events. Sometimes the problems appear acute without an apparent past history such as a suicidal attempt, discovery of substance abuse, and severe aggressive episodes. The family crisis generally subsides with hospitalization of the problem adolescent. However, it affects the family in several ways:

1. Parents may begin to argue about the nature of the adolescent's problem.

2. They may blame each other for contributing to the adolescent's problem.
3. Some divorced parents and members of the extended family may use this occasion to criticize the caretaker parent.
4. They may feel guilty about putting the adolescent in the hospital.
5. The remaining siblings at home may feel threatened or neglected and abandoned.
6. Some parents may become more cautious and tougher with the remaining siblings at home in the hope of avoiding similar problems.

Most of the aforementioned influences on the family are fairly universal and can be observed in most families. During discussion, the families should be asked to describe their experiences before and after the hospitalization and to describe how they handled the aftereffects, especially blaming others and feeling guilty.

Hospital Treatment and Beyond

This lecture-discussion should cover the following points:

1. Help the parents understand the nature of hospital treatment.
2. The role of parents in the recovery of the patient.
3. What can be expected from hospital treatment.
4. Importance of the aftercare plan.

The lecturer may start with a description of a typical day for the adolescent patient in the hospital and discuss each component of the therapeutic program in detail such as group therapy, individual therapy, and specialized groups. The aims of these therapies are to help each adolescent focus on his problem, find the contributing factors to his problems, and take steps to correct them. Of course, very few adolescents are able to identify the causes of their problems.

At least some of the factors contributing to adolescent problems lie in the family situation. The family may promote adolescent problems in various ways such as the presence of constant turmoil in the family system, not providing adequate supervision to the adolescent, or ignoring his problems until they become unmanageable. Family therapy sessions are extremely important to focus discussion on these issues in order to rectify them.

In most cases, hospital treatment only serves to highlight the problems rather than cure them. Hospital treatment also directs the adolescent and his family to choose a modified path of behavior and interaction in order to resolve the existing problems and avoid recurrences. A great deal of therapy has to be carried out in the community to resolve these problems. Thus, an aftercare plan becomes extremely important for the resolution of problems.

Substance Abuse in Teenagers

Most parents want to know how can they recognize whether their teenager is abusing drugs. Many parents go to great lengths such as checking the room and possessions of the adolescent, talking to his friends, and following the activities of the adolescent around town. Unfortunately, most parents cannot catch their adolescent abusing drugs. Many adolescents caught with drugs or drug paraphernalia are able to convince their parents that these belong to their friends. Most drug abuse occurs at parties, at unsupervised houses, and at school. It is almost impossible for parents to catch their teenagers in the act of drinking or smoking marijuana. We know of adolescents who got intoxicated almost every weekend without their parents ever knowing about it. They usually call home to tell their parents that they are staying overnight at a friend's house.

Initially, there are usually no changes in behavior, but as the use of drugs becomes regular, the lifestyle of the adolescent changes. Drug abuse affects the relationship with peers and adults. The adolescent begins to associate with peers who are drug abusers and decreases his association with other friends. He becomes more secretive about his activities and communicates less with adults. Lying and stealing money from his family may become a common occurrence. Academic achievement and grades drop. Skipping school and defiant behavior in the classroom may become frequent. After a while the adolescent becomes careless about hiding his drugs and drug paraphernalia, and this is usually the time when parents become aware of their adolescent's substance abuse. By the time most parents find out about the drug abuse, the adolescent has been a regular substance abuser and needs professional help. Drug use can only be confirmed by urine tests and blood tests for certain drugs.

Preventive measures are very important in decreasing substance abuse. Every family should have a conversation with their children in junior high school, irrespective of whether they are abusing drugs or not. The conversation should be carried out in a calm and friendly way. The family (including the adolescents) should spend several evenings educating themselves about different drugs of abuse and their common effects on the body and mind. There are several monographs that are written for the public and can be utilized in family self-education.

REFERENCES

Anderson CM, et al: A comparative study of the impact of education vs. process groups for families of patients with affective disorders. *Fam Process* 1986; 25:185–205.

Laqueur H, LaBurt H, Morong E: Multiple-family therapy, in Masserman JH (ed): *Current Psychiatric Therapies*. New York, Grune & Stratton, 1964.

Piers EV: *The Piers-Harris Children's Self-Concept Scale.* Nashville, Tenn, Counselor Recordings and Tests, 1969.

Rosenberg M: *Society and the Adolescent Self-Image.* Princeton, NJ, Princeton University Press, 1965.

12 | Trends in Inpatient Psychiatric Care

The psychiatric care of children and adolescents has shifted from long-term residential care to short-term hospital care. General hospitals with psychiatric units have become much more acceptable settings for children to receive short-term psychiatric care. Easy accessibility of general hospital units has increased their utilization for children who would otherwise have received outpatient or day treatment. The increased utilization of psychiatric hospitals does not necessarily imply a misuse. In fact, brief psychiatric hospitalization has helped many children and adolescents receive early treatment to avoid long-term residential treatment. The reduction in many state and county mental hospital facilities during the 1970s left a big gap in the psychiatric care of children. Short-term hospitalization in general hospitals has been able to fill this gap only partially. Unfortunately, the development of many general hospital psychiatric units was not accompanied by communitywide planning of aftercare facilities. The lack of appropriate aftercare facilities in many communities has led to ineffective and inefficient use of general hospital psychiatric services. Hospital treatment in these communities is frequently used to deal with acute mental health crises resulting from suicidal attempts, severe depression, acute psychosis, etc. Hospital treatment stabilizes most of these patients and returns them to their community for further treatment. Most communities, however, are fairly unorganized and uncoordinated in providing the appropriate mental health services to maintain the discharged patient in the community. In the absence of the appropriate services, crises recur and lead to rehospitalization. The communities that have developed an extensive network of outpatient, day treatment, and crisis centers have made the most efficient use of short-term psychiatric hospitalization.

A reduction in median and long-term psychiatric facilities has also contributed to frequent rehospitalization in general hospitals. At least half of the readmitted patients are those who require medium- or long-term psychiatric care. These readmitted patients utilize general hospital psychiatric units as a stop-gap measure when they are in a severe crisis. Only after repeated admissions in general hospitals are some of these adolescents finally accepted by state or county hospitals for long-term care.

It is the economic pressure rather than the realistic appraisal of the psychiatric needs of children that has led the way to the changing patterns of psychiatric care.

The development of psychiatric units for children and adolescents in general hospitals seems to be financially advantageous to both hospitals and insurance companies. The hospitals have been able to fill their empty beds as well as provide a necessary service to the community. Insurance companies expect to reduce the cost by having a better control over treatment in general hospitals and avoid the cost of long-term hospitalization in private psychiatric hospitals. Unfortunately, these expectations have not come true. The cost of hospital care has escalated at a much higher rate since 1979 than in the 10-year period before that. Total expenditures in current dollars for all mental health organizations increased from $3.29 billion in 1969 to $14.43 billion in 1983 (an increase of 339%). The increase has been contributed to at a much higher rate by the general hospital psychiatric units and private psychiatric hospitals than by the state and county mental hospitals. In fact, the expenditure of most county and state mental hospitals has decreased in constant dollars. There appears to be a much greater rise in cost since 1979 that has continued into the late 1980s. Most third-party payers are beginning to demand stricter criteria for hospitalization and discharge. The term "medical necessity" is frequently utilized to justify hospitalization. However, the meaning of "medical necessity" in psychiatry remains ambiguous. It is even more confusing in the psychiatric hospitalization of children and adolescents as compared with adults. For example, does the hospitalization of a child who is constantly running away from home meet the criteria of medical necessity for his own protection and for an evaluation of the cause of running away? Some insurance companies may deny such admissions. Certainly, community facilities such as crisis centers may be able to handle such situations and possibly avoid hospitalization. However, many communities lack such facilities, and hospitalization appears to be the only immediate intervention available in most communities, with the exception of juvenile detention homes and jails. Most clinicians involved in the care of hospitalized children frequently feel harrassed and pressured for early discharge by agents of the third-party payers. Even many mental health professionals working for insurance companies are unaware of the complexities of psychiatric care of children and make similar demands on their peers. New ways of conceptualization of hospital psychiatric care for children (see Chapter 8) may reduce to some degree the current frustrations as experienced by most inpatient staff who want to provide the best psychiatric care for their patients but are handicapped by time constraints. However, it appears that the financial pressure will continue to rise with the escalating cost of hospitalization, and professionals will be under greater pressure to develop less expensive methods of treating the emotionally and behaviorally disturbed children and adolescents.

In addition to the cost many other factors are likely to determine the future trends in the psychiatric care of children and adolescents, for example, the portion of children and adolescents in the general population; the availability of trained child mental health professionals; the involvement of private businesses in providing psychiatric care; and the allocation of local, state, and federal dollars for developing the appropriate community mental health resources.

TABLE 12–1.
Population Trends Under 18 Years Old*

Year	Under 18 Years Old		5–17 Years Old		14–17 Years Old	
	Population (× 1,000)	Distribution (%)	Population (× 1,000)	Distribution (%)	Population (× 1,000)	Distribution (%)
1970	69,689	34.2	52,526	25.8	15,851	7.7
1975	67,186	31.1	51,065	23.7	17,125	7.2
1980	63,724	28.0	47,265	20.8	16,139	7.0
1982	62,948	27.1	45,669	19.7	15,020	6.4
1984	62,660	25.5	44,844	19.0	14,707	6.2
1985	63,992	26.7	45,975	19.2	14,865	6.2
1986	63,271	26.1	45,143	18.6	14,797	6.1
1988†	63,613	25.8	45,348	18.4		
1990†	64,038	25.5	45,630	18.2		
1995†	66,173	25.4	48,374	18.5		
2000†	65,713	24.4	48,815	18.1		

* Data from the U.S. Bureau of Census.
† Population projections.

POPULATION TRENDS

Table 12–1 shows the actual and projected population trends for persons under 18 years of age. The population of persons under 18 years has progressively decreased between 1970 and 1984. A slight increase occurred in 1985. However, this increase was not sustained for the next 3 years. The population projection estimates indicate a small increase in this age group during the next decade. Similar trends are present in subgroups of children between the ages of 5 and 17 and 14 and 17 years. These trends indicate a continuing need for more mental health services for children and adolescents during the next decade.

TRENDS IN MENTAL HEALTH FACILITIES

There are indications that the utilization of mental health services by children and adolescents has greatly increased but the mental health services have not kept pace with this trend. The inpatient psychiatric services include primarily state and county mental hospitals, private psychiatric hospitals, and inpatient psychiatric services of general hospitals.

Table 12–2 shows the trends in development of various hospitals since 1970. There has been an overall increase in the number of mental health organizations from 3,005 in the 1970s to 4,579 in 1986 (an increase of 52%). The number of mental health organizations providing inpatient psychiatric care increased from 1,633 in 1970 to 2,305 in 1984. The increase in general hospitals with separate psychiatric services was from 797 in 1970 to 1,531 in 1982 before slightly increasing to 1,347 in 1984. The major increase shown in Table 12–2 in 1982 in general hospital psychiatric units was the result of a shift in the funding of the community mental health center (CMHC) program from categorical to block grants. The organizations that had been classified as federally funded (CMHCs) in previous years were reclassified as multiservice mental health organizations, free-standing psychiatric outpatient clinics, or psychiatric units

TABLE 12–2.
Trends in Mental Health Facilities*

Year	Total†	State & County Mental Hospitals	Private Psychiatric Hospitals	Veterans Administration Hospitals	General Hospital Psychiatric Units
1970	3,005	310	411	115	797
1976	3,480	303	513	126	870
1978	3,738	297	563	136	923
1980	3,727	280	552	136	923
1982	4,302	277	550	129	1,531
1984	4,438	277	542	139	1,347
1986	4,579	286	596	139	1,347

* Data from the U.S. National Institute of Mental Health.
† Total number includes other facilities not listed here.

TABLE 12–3.
Trends in Inpatient Psychiatric Beds*

Year	Total[†]	State & County Mental Hospitals	Private Psychiatric Hospitals	Veteran's Administration Hospitals	General Hospital Psychiatric Units
1970	524.9[‡]	413.1	29.4	50.7	22.4
1976	339.0	222.2	34.1	35.9	28.7
1978	301.0	184.1	36.7	33.8	29.4
1980	274.7	156.5	37.4	33.8	29.4
1982	247.3	140.1	37.5	24.6	36.5
1984	252.5	128.6	37.1	23.5	46.0
1986	257.0	124.8	44.8	23.5	46.0

* Data from the US National Institute of Mental Health.
† Total number includes other facilities not listed here.
‡ Values are in thousands.

of nonfederal general hospitals, depending upon the type of services they provided. The number of private psychiatric hospitals rose consistently from 411 in 1970 to 596 in 1984. The number of state and county mental health hospitals actually decreased from 310 in 1970 to 286 in 1986.

In spite of an increase in the number of psychiatric services, the number of total inpatient beds has actually dropped to less than half, from 524,000 in 1970 to 257,000 in 1986 (51% change) (Table 12–3). This decrease resulted primarily from a reduction in the bed capacity in the large state and county hospitals from 413,000 in 1970 to 124,000 in 1986 (a decrease of 70%). Although the psychiatric services of private and nonfederal hospitals have added about 37,000 new beds since 1970, these additions have not filled the gap left open in the long-term care of psychiatric patients by the reduction of state and county hospitals.

The large decreases in the number of inpatient episodes in the state and county mental hospitals are compensated only slightly by small increases in private and general psychiatric hospital services. The inpatient care episodes are defined as the number of inpatients receiving services at the beginning of the year plus the number of additions during that year. The inpatient care episodes in state and county mental hospitals dropped from 767,115 in 1969 to 459,374 in 1983 (a decrease of 40%). Inpatient care episodes increased in private psychiatric hospitals from 102,510 in 1969 to 180,822 in 1983 (an increase of 76%). A somewhat lesser increase was noticed in the patient care episodes in nonfederal general hospital psychiatric units: from 535,493 in 1969 to 820,030 in 1983 (an increase of 53%).

Another later change in the delivery of mental health care has resulted from drastic reductions in the length of hospitalization for all types of psychiatric hospitals. The median number of days of stay in inpatient service in 1980 was 22 days for state and county mental hospitals, 19 days for private psychiatric hospitals, and approximately 11 for nonfederal general hospital psychiatric units. The number of days, however, varied according to the primary diagnosis, being higher for schizophrenia and other psychosis.

MENTAL HEALTH FACILITIES FOR PERSONS UNDER 18 YEARS OF AGE

About 81,532 persons under the age of 18 years were admitted to inpatient psychiatric services of all types of mental hospitals in 1980. Table 12–4 shows that there was a decrease in the number of admissions to state and county hospitals by about 37% between 1970 and 1980.

There was a major increase in the number of admissions to private psychiatric hospitals (159%) and a smaller increase in the nonfederal general hospital psychiatric service by about 9%. The general hospital census included about 4,900 patients under 18 years of age admitted to multiservice centers. In 1980 the admissions were distributed across the hospitals as follows: 20% in the state and county mental hospitals, 21% in private psychiatric hospitals, and 59% in general hospital psychiatric services. The individuals under 18 years composed about 7.5% of the total population in all three types of hospitals in 1970. This percentage increased slightly in 1980 to 8.03%.

Table 12–5 shows that the rate of admissions of persons under the age of 18 years per 100,000 population admitted to selected hospitals decreased in state and county hospitals and increased in private and general hospitals.

The median number of days that individuals under 18 years of age stayed decreased for county and state hospitals, remained the same for private hospitals, and slightly decreased for general hospital psychiatric units since 1975 (Table 12–6).

Further analysis of the population under the age of 18 years indicated that groups between 15 and 17 years of age accounted for the major portion of the hospital admissions (Table 12–7).

TRENDS IN SUBSTANCE ABUSE

Adolescents between the ages of 12 and 17 years appear to have increased their consumption of alcohol, marijuana, and other psychoactive drugs. Table 12–8 shows the data collected by the U.S. National Institute on Drug Abuse through a national

TABLE 12–4.
Number of Admissions of Persons Under 18 Years of Age to Selected Inpatient Psychiatric Hospitals*

Hospital Type	1970	1975	1980	Change (%)
State and county mental hospitals	26,352	25,252	16,612	36.9
Private psychiatric hospitals	6,452	15,426	16,735	159.3
Nonfederal general hospitals (psychiatric units)	44,135	42,690	48,185	9.1

* Data from the US Department of Health and Human Services.

TABLE 12–5.
Rate of Admissions of Persons Under 18 Years of Age Per 100,000 Population in Selected Psychiatric Hospitals*

Hospital Type	1970	1975	1980	Change (%)
State and county mental hospitals	37.8	38.1	26.1	30.9
Private psychiatric hospitals	9.3	23.3	26.3	182.7
Nonfederal general hospitals (psychiatric units)	63.3	64.4	68.5	8.2

* Data from the US Department of Health and Human Services.

TABLE 12–6.
Median Days of Stay for Admissions of Persons Under 18 Years of Age to Selected Psychiatric Hospitals*

Hospital Type	1970	1975	1980	Change (%)
State and county mental hospitals	74	66	54	27.0
Private psychiatric hospitals	36	36	36	0.0
Nonfederal general hospitals (psychiatric units)	9	17	14	55.5

* Data from the US Department of Health and Human Services.

TABLE 12–7.
Percent Distribution of Admissions of Persons Under 18 Years of Age to Selected Psychiatric Hospitals*

Hospital Type	Age Groups (%)		
	Under 10 Years	10–14 Years	15–17 Years
State and county mental hospitals	5	29.8	65.2
Private psychiatric hospitals	4.3	29.2	66.5
Nonfederal general hospitals (psychiatric units)	4.8	27.1	68.1

* Data from the US Department of Health and Human Services.

TABLE 12–8.
Trends in Drug Abuse by Youths 12 to 17 Years of Age*

Types of Drugs	Percentage Ever Used			Percentage Current User		
	1974	1982	1985	1974	1982	1985
Marijuana	23.0	26.7	23.7	12.0	11.5	12.3
Inhalants	8.5	NA†	9.1	0.7	NA	3.6
Hallucinogens	6.0	5.2	3.2	1.3	1.4	1.1
Cocaine	3.6	6.5	5.2	1.0	1.6	1.8
Heroin	1.0	0.5	0.5	0.5	0.5	0.5
Analgesics	NA	4.2	5.9	NA	0.7	1.9
Stimulants	5.0	6.7	5.5	1.0	2.6	1.8
Sedatives	5.0	5.8	4.0	1.0	1.3	1.1
Tranquilizers	3.0	4.9	4.8	1.0	0.9	0.6
Alcohol	54.0	65.2	55.9	34.0	26.9	31.5
Cigarettes	52.0	49.5	45.3	25.0	14.7	15.6

* Data from the US Department of Health and Human Services.
† NA = not available.

TABLE 12–9.
Trends in the Current Use of Marijuana and Alcohol by Youth: Percentage of the 12- to 17-Year-Old Population*

Type of Drug and Gender	1972	1976	1979	1982	1985
Marijuana	7	12	17	12	12.3
Current users (total)					
Male	9	14	19	13	13.2
Female	6	11	14	10	11.2
Alcohol	24	32	37	27	31.5
Current users (total					
Male	27.	36	39	27	33.7
Female	21	29	36	27	29.0

* Data from the US Department of Health and Human Services.
† NA = not available.

household survey on drug abuse in 1985. This table shows that the use of tranquilizers, sedatives, stimulants, and analgesics has decreased since 1974 and the use of alcohol has increased during the past several years. The use of heroin has remained confined to a small group of hard drug abusers. Also, the percentage of individuals who have ever used any drugs has increased in the past 10 years.

Table 12–9 shows a further analysis of the data on commonly abused drugs such as marijuana and alcohol by sex distribution and indicates that the use of alcohol and marijuana may be on the rise during the past few years, both by male and female teenagers.

TRENDS IN THE QUALITY OF MENTAL HEALTH CARE

A great deal of concern has been expressed over the quality of psychiatric care provided in the short-term inpatient hospitals. Some clinicians feel that short-term hospitalization does not give sufficient time to the staff to do any in-depth psychotherapy. Primary therapeutic efforts are focused on supportive measures for the patient and his family. This type of therapy seems to promote denial on the part of the patient. The patient begins to think that talking about feelings and conflicts is not necessary because none of the staff encourages the expression of those feelings. Jemerin and Philips (1988) believe that short-term psychiatric hospitalization of children has fragmented the psychiatric care of children and has decreased the focus on understanding children. They believe that in short-term hospitalization so much time is spent in collecting basic data and coordinating the care with community agencies that little time is left for understanding the child. The inpatient staff develops a "triage mentality" rather than one of spontaneously helping the disturbed child (Philips, 1986). Hospital staff members spend a great proportion of their time in aftercare planning, which blurs the boundary between hospital and social service system.

A work group on consumer issues of the American Academy of Child and Adolescent Psychiatry (Chaired by David Pruitt, 1988) expressed concern over the increasing short-term hospitalization of children. The group believed that "public perceptions regarding the increasing role of hospitalization in child and adolescent psychiatric treatment can damage the profession as successfully thoroughly as any reality."

The group suggested a fact sheet containing 11 questions for the families to understand the nature of hospital treatment and avoid any misunderstanding of the hospital treatment. These concerns are justified in the present state of hospital care. Most of the hospitals provide a package of services that include milieu therapy, group therapy, recreation, and education. These services are designed to take care of all the adolescent patients and are rarely individualized. Group therapy sessions, for example, focus on general issues of adolescents such as strained relationships with families, problems with peer relationships, and substance abuse. So-called "comprehensive treatment plans" written by the staff for each patient read alike and focus on general categories of problems as mentioned above. Very little effort is spent in understanding each child and his specific conflict. These services perform a very important function— to take care of hospitalized adolescents—but depend upon the psychiatrist to provide direction for the hospital staff to take care of their patients. These services can be improved by individualizing the care of each patient. Psychiatrists should take the lead in understanding their patients and sharing the information with the inpatient staff and guiding them in working on specific conflicts and issues with each patient.

REFERENCES

Admission Rate to State and County Psychiatric Hospitals by Age, Sex and Marital Status, United States, 1975. Rockville, Md, National Institute of Mental Health, Statistical Note 142, Nov 1977.

Admission Rate to State and County Psychiatric Hospitals by Age, Sex and Race, United States, 1975. Rockville, Md, National Institute of Mental Health, Statistical Note 140, Nov 1977.

Diagnostic Distribution of Admissions to Inpatient Services of State and County Hospitals, United States, 1975. Rockville, Md, National Institute of Mental Health, Statistical Note 138, Aug 1977.

Jemerin J, Philips I: Changes in inpatient child psychiatry: Consequences and recommendations. *J Am Acad Child Adolesc Psychiatry* 1988; 27:397–403.

Length of Stay of Discharge From Non-federal General Hospital Psychiatric Inpatient Units, United States, 1975. Rockville, Md, National Institute of Mental Health, Statistical Note 133, May 1977.

Mourderscheid RW, Barrett S: *Mental Health, United States, 1987.* Rockville, Md, US Department of Health and Human Services, 1987.

Philips I: The decay of optimism: The opportunity for change. *J Am Acad Child Adolesc Psychiatry* 1986; 25:151–157.

Provisional Data on Patient Care Episodes in Mental Health Facilities, 1975. Rockville, Md, National Institute of Mental Health, Statistical Note 139, Aug 1977.

Provisional Patient Movement and Administrative Data of State and County Psychiatric Inpatient Services, July 1, 1974–June 30, 1975. National Institute of Mental Health, Statistical Note 132, 1976.

Pruitt DB (chairperson): Eleven questions to ask before psychiatric hospital treatment of children and adolescents, in *Facts for Families,* no. 32. *Am Acad Child Adolesc Psychiatry* 1988.

Tauhe C, Barrett S: *Mental Health, United States, 1985.* Rockville, Md, US Department of Health and Human Services, 1985.

A | Assessment in Group Setting

Name: _____ Age: _____

Date of Admission: _____ Date of Assessment: _____

Type of Group: _____

1. OPENNESS-SECRETIVENESS
   (a) Shares his problems with the group rather too openly in an inappropriate manner (quality of naiveté).
   (b) Shares his problems with group openly in an appropriate manner.
   (c) Takes time to warm up to others but then shares his problems openly and spontaneously.
   (d) Has to be asked to share problems but then is fairly open.
   (e) Does not respond to questions from peers or adults but seems to be attentive to others' problems.
   (f) Withdrawn, nonparticipating, but no other inappropriate behavior.
   (g) Withdrawn, nonparticipating, manifests inappropriate behavior.
   (h) May whisper to a peer but is very reluctant to share his thoughts openly.
   (i) Communicates mostly with gestures.

2. OUTGOING-SUBMISSIVE
   (a) Overly outgoing, bossy, argumentative.
   (b) Appropriately assertive in making his point.
   (c) Gives his position up easily when challenged by peers.
   (d) Quite submissive and will go along with everybody's suggestion.

3. HELPFUL-DISRUPTIVE
   (a) Participates in the discussion about other adolescents and makes helpful comments.
   (b) Participates in the discussion about other adolescents but usually puts them down or makes negative comments.
   (c) Tries to dominate group discussion with irrelevant details.
   (d) Only interested in himself and does not want to be helpful to others.

B | Self-Assessment on Substance Use

1. Do you smoke cigarettes? (Circle)   Yes   No

2. How long ago did you start smoking cigarettes?

   _____ Months _____ Years

3. How many cigarettes *a day* did you smoke in the past 6 months?

   number of cigarettes _____ or packs _____

4. Have you tried smoking marijuana (pot, grass)? _____ Yes _____ No

5. How often did you smoke marijuana in the past 6 months? (Circle one)

   Daily   Once or twice weekly   Once or twice monthly   Less often   Never

6. Circle all the other drugs with their frequency that you have tried in the *past 6* months:

		Frequency		
Drugs	Daily	Once or Twice a Week	Once or Twice a Month	Less Often
Alcohol	_____	_____	_____	_____
LSD (acid)	_____	_____	_____	_____
Hashish	_____	_____	_____	_____
Mushrooms	_____	_____	_____	_____
PCP	_____	_____	_____	_____

		Frequency		
Drugs	Daily	Once or Twice a Week	Once or Twice a Month	Less Often
Cocaine	_____	_____	_____	_____
Stimulants (uppers)	_____	_____	_____	_____
Barbituates (downers)	_____	_____	_____	_____
Others:				
_____	_____	_____	_____	_____
_____	_____	_____	_____	_____
_____	_____	_____	_____	_____
_____	_____	_____	_____	_____

7. Have you been using drugs more often than a year ago:
   Yes   No (Circle one):

   Same as before   Twice as much   Several times more
   Less than before

8. Where do you use drugs (including alcohol)? (Circle one)

   At parties   At home   With friends   Alone

9. Why do you use drugs (including alcohol)? Check *all* that apply to you:

   _____ To join the company of friends   _____ Relaxes me

   _____ Just to be social in parties   _____ Makes me feel more social

   _____ Makes me feel good   _____ Makes me forget my troubles
   _____ Makes me feel excited

   List any other reasons below:

   _____

   _____

10. How has your school attendance been in the *past 6 months*? (Circle one)

    Frequently tardy   Skip school often   Good attendance

11. What were your school grades *a year ago*? (Circle one)

    Mostly F's   Some F's   C's & D's   Mostly B's   Mostly A's

12. What were your grades *last semester*? (Circle one)

    Mostly F's   Some F's   C's & D's   Mostly B's   Mostly A's

13. Do most of your close friends use drugs?   Yes   No

15. Do you have frequent arguments with your parents?   Yes   No

16. How did you get along with your parents *1 or 2 years ago*? (Circle one)

    Same as now   Better than now   Worse than now

17. Do you play a sport now?   Yes   No   Occasionally

18. Did you play a sport *a year ago*?   Yes   No   Occasionally

19. Do you have a lot of free time?   Yes   No

20. Are you bored a lot of the time (nothing to do?)   Yes   No

21. Have you stolen money or things to buy drugs (including alcohol)?
    Yes   No

22. Do you lie frequently to avoid punishments?   Yes   No

23. Have you been in trouble with the law?   Yes   No

For what reason: _____

_____

_____

When: _____

_____

_____

C | Recreational Interest Survey

This survey may ask adolescents to describe the following:

1. A typical weekday.

2. Number of hours left after school, homework, and house chores.

3. How are those hours spent during the weekdays?

4. Describe a typical weekend.

5. Interest in physical activities such as

_____ Swimming   _____ Playing team sports

_____ Exercise   _____ Others

_____ Biking   _____ Bowling

6. Interest in artistic activities

_____ Painting   _____ Photography

_____ Drama   _____ Crafts

_____ Carpentry   _____ Sewing

_____ Ceramics   _____ Others

7. Interest in various hobbies.

8. Extent of knowledge of leisure activities available in the community.

9. Satisfaction with current leisure activities.

10. Desire to try new activities.

D | Topics of Nursing Evaluation and Observation

This evaluation may include the following:

1. General appearance
2. Hygiene
3. Sleeping habits
4. Eating habits
5. Interaction with peers
6. Interaction with adults
7. Religious interest
8. Overall mood
9. Energy level
10. Acceptance of treatment program
11. Willingness to work on personal problems

Index